The Longevity Matrix

THE
LONGEVITY
MATRIX

HOW TO LIVE BETTER, STRONGER, AND LONGER

MICHAEL T. MURRAY, N.D.

NEW YORK

LONDON • NASHVILLE • MELBOURNE • VANCOUVER

The Longevity Matrix

How to Live Better, Stronger, and Longer

Published in New York, New York, by Morgan James Publishing. Morgan James is a trademark of Morgan James, LLC. www.MorganJamesPublishing.com

ISBN 9781631951374 paperback
ISBN 9781631951381 eBook
Library of Congress Control Number: 2020936312

Cover Design by:
Megan Dillon
megan@creativeninjadesigns.com

Interior Design by:
Chris Treccani
www.3dogcreative.net

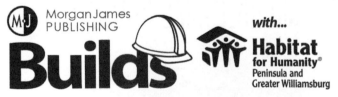

Morgan James is a proud partner of Habitat for Humanity Peninsula and Greater Williamsburg. Partners in building since 2006.

Get involved today! Visit
MorganJamesPublishing.com/giving-back

TABLE OF CONTENTS

PREFACE:

A New Approach to Anti-aging and Longevity

My purpose in writing this book is to share a strategy to help you achieve an extreme level of wellness and vitality. You see, it is not enough to live longer. The desire should be to live better and stronger with a tremendous amount of health, energy, fulfillment, and joy. If you focus on accomplishing these goals, living longer will naturally take care of itself.

In naming this book, I chose a descriptive title. To understand the meaning of a Longevity Matrix, let me give the formal definition of a matrix in biology. It refers to a set of conditions that provides a system in which something grows or develops. In this context, the "Longevity Matrix" refers to creating the best set of conditions to develop longevity. If that happens, not only will it lead to a longer life, but it also allows the systems within body and mind to function at the highest possible capacity.

The systems within us are composed of very complex interconnectedness. Everyone knows the answer to "What determines the strength of a chain?" is the weakest link. The same concept applies with a systems approach to our body and health, they are just much more complex than a simple chain. Every system in the body affects the other. So, the strength of our health is ultimately determined by the weakest body system. What I offer in this book is a step-by-step approach to improve the function of each body system and if there is a weak link, I am going to help you make it as strong as possible.

You might be thinking, who is Dr. Michael Murray and why should I allow him to guide me? Well, I am someone who has created a life full of incredible health, vitality, and meaning. I am someone who has walked his talk and sowed the benefits from applying what I detail in this book. I want to share what I have learned in a way that will allow you to feel a higher degree of wellness in your life no matter what circumstances you currently find yourself. And, why do I want to share and help YOU? Because I love the feeling of making a difference in a person's life and I want to make difference in yours. As for my credentials, I am a Doctor of Naturopathic Medicine—a N.D. licensed as a primary care physician in the States of Arizona and Washington, I graduated from Bastyr University in Seattle, WA, in 1985. What is naturopathic medicine? It is a system of medicine that is all about the art and science of harnessing the power of nature to prevent and treat illness in order to achieve the highest level of health possible. My particular areas of focus are the use of diet and natural products such as dietary supplements and herbal extracts to promote health and healing. I also take advantage of the discoveries in the new field of positive psychology and my lifestyle is impeccable in its focus on health and personal growth.

When people refer to me as an expert in "alternative" medicine, I really don't like that label. What is so alternative about using food as medicine? Hippocrates, the father of Western medicine said, "Let your food be your medicine and your medicine be your food." And, how is a helping people develop a positive attitude and live a health promoting lifestyle considered alternative as well? What is considered "mainstream" or "alternative" today may trade places in the future or be entirely displaced by advances in our understanding of what really impacts health. One thing that I want to make clear here is that I am very pragmatic in my approach, it supersedes any philosophical dogma. I am a proponent of what I like to refer to as *rational* medicine.

I am certainly not against *rational* aspects of modern medicine. It can make a true life-or-death difference when it is needed. As far as improving our general level of health, however, I believe that modern medicine is often completely *irrational.* There is simply no drug or pill that can take the place of diet, lifestyle, and attitude. Modern medicine is clearing failing us in moving patients to a higher level of wellness. It is obvious if we look at the general health of the population as a whole in the United States and most other "developed" countries. Do the current medical treatments of such things as depression, digestive disturbances, poor sleep quality really help in the long run? And, what about the treatments of most chronic degenerative diseases such as heart disease, high blood pressure, arthritis, and diabetes? Often, in the long run, current drug treatments in these conditions and others end up causing more side effects and harm than benefits. Here is what I believe with 100% congruency: Rather than relying on drugs as biological band-aids to suppress symptoms, it makes more sense to use diet, lifestyle, attitude, and natural products to address the underlying core issues—the root causes of our illnesses. To me that is a *rational* approach and simply just good medicine.

My interest in, and commitment to, natural medicine is the result of deep personal experience. Years ago, when I was a freshman at the University of Oregon, I underwent a four-hour knee operation to repair damage from a long-standing injury. The orthopedic surgeon told me that I'd be lucky if I walked without a limp. When the cast was removed three months later, I did everything I could to rehabilitate my knee. I wanted to have a full and physically active life, and that meant taking part in basketball games, racquet sports, and jogging. But after a year and a half I was still unable to put any significant stress on my knee. At the suggestion of my father, I went to see Ralph Weiss, N.D., a doctor of natural medicine.

I was skeptical. I knew that Dr. Weiss had helped a lot of people, including members of my family, but I had been treated by one of the top knee specialists in the world. What could Dr. Weiss do that conventional medicine couldn't? I soon learned.

In our first meeting, Dr. Weiss expressed concern not just about my knee but also about my diet and lifestyle. He explained things in terms I could understand. He spoke with confidence and wonder about the body's tremendous ability to heal itself. All we had to do, he said, was remove the obstacles that were preventing my knee from healing properly. His technique was to use electro-acupuncture and some unique physical therapy machines. As soon as the treatment began, I could literally feel my leg come alive again. Within minutes it was almost as strong as my healthy leg. That evening, I played basketball again—without pain—for the first time in years.

It was a life-changing experience—a miracle actually for me. As a result, I changed my major from history (I had planned to go on to law school) to pre-med and soon fulfilled the entrance requirements to attend what is now Bastyr University to pursue a degree in naturopathic medicine. What inspired me was the deep inner desire to learn as much as I could about how to make ME healthy so I could then help others. It is the classic example of reaching for your own oxygen mask in an emergency situation on an airplane before assisting others. I have walked the talk of health and wellness my entire adult life and it shows in the way that I feel and look. I am not bragging; I am simply stressing the points because I want to have confidence in my words to you.

There is so much that I want to share in this book, but it is a process. So, let me first stress that there are several themes, or threads, running through this book. Here are some of the main ideas you will encounter in the chapters ahead.

- *The health of the body depends on the health of each individual cell.* These very complex living factories connect to form tissues and organs. In order for a cell to function at its peak, it requires oxygen and a steady stream of compounds. The cell will use these as energy; building blocks to build cell structures, agents to assist in assembling other cell molecules, or in order for the cell to protect itself from damage. Some of these compounds are nutrients like fats, amino acids (the building blocks of proteins), vitamins, and minerals; some are plant-derived chemicals; and some are compounds supplied by other cells of the body. In addition to basic cell function, cells use the steady stream of compounds to support their constant remodeling, healing, and the ability for the cell to reproduce itself.

- *The body strives to be healthy.* Health is our natural state. Your body tells you when something is wrong and takes steps to correct the problem. To give a simple example, if you are dehydrated, your body causes you to feel thirsty. By listening to the body, we can sense when we have fallen out of balance. We can also pay attention to the alarms our body sends us that something is out of balance. We call these alarms symptoms! It is important to understand what the symptom is telling us. We don't get a headache because we lack aspirin. A deficiency of Prozac or Wellbutrin is not what causes us to be depressed. And, joint pain is not the result of our body screaming to feed us ibuprofen. One of my primary goals in this book is to provide you with information and guidance to get you on to a program that will get to the root cause of your symptoms instead of using drugs.

- *Each human being is biologically unique.* We all share the same basic structure. But our genes and how they are expressed make us unlike anyone else who has ever lived. We each have our own biological needs and our own responses to the world around us. What works for one person may not work for another. That is exactly why this book has so many questionnaires that can help you pinpoint your personal needs and take the personalized steps to living better, stronger, and longer.

CAUTION

Although this book discusses numerous health conditions and offers ideas for preventing or managing them, it is not intended as a substitute for appropriate medical care. Please keep the following in mind as you read:

- Do not self-diagnose. Proper medical care is critical to good health. If you have symptoms that suggest an illness described in this book, please consult a physician, preferably a naturopathic doctor (N.D.), holistic medical doctor (M.D.) or doctor of osteopathy (D.O.), chiropractor, or other natural health care specialist.

- If you are currently taking a prescription medication, you absolutely must work with your doctor before discontinuing any drug or altering any drug regimen. Make your physician aware of all the nutritional supplements or herbal products you are currently taking.

- If you wish to try a nutritional supplement or herbal product as a therapeutic measure, discuss it with your physician first especially if you are taking any prescription medication. Doing so can help avoid potential side effects and adverse interactions.

- Many nutritional supplements and herbal products are effective on their own, but they work best when they are used as part of a comprehensive natural approach to health that incorporates diet and lifestyle factors.

It is my sincere hope that you—or someone you care about—will use the information provided in the following pages to achieve greater health and happiness.

Live Better, Stronger, and Longer!
Michael T. Murray, N.D.

CHAPTER 1:

Priming for Success

"Nature is doing her best each moment to make us well. She exists for no other end. Do not resist. With the least inclination to be well, we should not be sick."
Henry David Thoreau

Of all nature's miracles, the human experience is the most amazing. As Thoreau realized, nature works constantly to ensure that your body functions well. Health is our natural state. We just need to remove obstacles and support the nature within us to do its job of making and keeping us well.

Our being—the matrix of body, mind, and emotions—is complex and intricate. It is a collection of interweaving systems, each dependent on the other. At each moment, every cell in the body tries to maintain the ideal conditions it needs to carry out its tasks. The technical term for this the process of maintaining balance is *homeostasis*. It is the basic function of any living cell. And, each cell is constantly striving to maintain the optimal state. Mechanisms in our cells, tissues, and organs to promote homeostasis are a lot like a thermostat in your house. If the temperature rises too high, the thermostat kicks in the air conditioner to cool things back down to normal. If homeostatic mechanisms cannot overcome the forces that threaten it, like stress, then the system falls out of balance. The result is *dis-ease*—a disruption in the ability of a body system or part to carry out its normal function. By keeping our systems in fine tune, we can protect ourselves against disease and enjoy the benefits of health.

No matter how old you are or what your current state of health is, you can take steps to help your body function better. You can work better, feel better, look better—all by taking measures to help your body maintain its optimal homeostasis. For starters, read through the following set of questions. The more "yes" answers you give, the greater your need to prime yourself to become a better, healthier version of YOU!

- Do you feel that you are not as healthy and vibrant as other people your age?
- Do you want to have more energy?
- Do you want greater mental clarity?
- Do you often feel blue or depressed?
- Do you get more than one or two colds a year?
- Do you struggle with your weight?
- Do you suffer from lack of libido or impotence?
- Do you have digestive disturbances?
- Do you have weak, brittle, or cracked nails?
- Is your hair dry and lifeless?
- Do you have dark circles under your eyes?
- Are you constantly hungry?
- Do you have trouble getting to sleep or do you want to sleep all of the time?
- Do you have high cholesterol levels or blood pressure?
- Do you feel anxious or stressed out most of the time?
- Do you suffer from premenstrual syndrome, fibrocystic breast disease, or uterine fibroids?
- Do you crave sweets?
- Do you suffer from allergies?
- Do you lose your temper easily?

- Do you have bad breath or body odor?
- Do you suffer from chronic post-nasal drip or hay fever-like symptoms?

These symptoms are often nothing more than a squeaky wheel in need of maintenance. What I am offering in the Longevity Matrix is a tune up to take care of underlying issues. With the right strategy and action not only will these symptoms improve or disappear, you will experience some general benefits such as these:

Increased energy
The quality of a person's life is often directly related to their energy levels. The greatest improvement most people notice with a tune-up is a higher energy level. The Longevity Matrix gives them the power to live with more passion and joy.

Improved protection against disease
All of us want to be well and stay well. Your body does its best to fight illness. But you must provide the nutrients your body needs to build strong tissues and vigorous immune cells. You must also consistently have the right mental and emotional state as well as health promoting lifestyle. The Longevity Matrix provides the framework for optimal health.

Better moods and mental function
When we feel better physically, we feel better emotionally too. The body and mind are interconnected. When one is affected so is the other. The Longevity Matrix will help you by elevating your mood and help you think and feel clearer, with greater focus and clarity.

Better appearance
It's not vain to want to look your best. It's a sign of self-respect. The same strategies for keeping your internal systems humming

also work on the external ones—skin, hair, nails. The Longevity Matrix builds good health from within that radiates to our exterior.

Greater ability to deal with stress

In today's society, pressure comes from all directions. The demands of work, family, and society all take their toll. Constant stress wears you down both mentally and physically, putting you at risk of serious illness. Some of the most ground-breaking research over the last forty years has documented how stress causes or contributes to a wide range of health problems, from infections to infertility. The Longevity Matrix will show you how to reduce your stress as well as strengthen your ability to deal with stress.

Better sex

It's natural and normal to enjoy an active sex life for as long as we choose. But if our body isn't functioning right, both our interest in sex and our ability to engage in it can plummet. The Longevity Matrix will help you replenish energy reserves and increase muscle strength and improve circulation. When the hormonal and electrical systems in our body and mind are working at their peak, and when our emotions are in healthy balance, we are more responsive to sexual stimulation and better able to express our most intimate feelings with our partners.

Weight control

If you have unsuccessfully tried to lose weight, you are not alone. Diet and exercise alone are often not enough. The Longevity Matrix can help you bring your weight under control—and keep it there—by focusing on improving appetite control and resetting your metabolism.

A happier attitude

Your attitude is like your physical body, it needs to be conditioned. It is easy for people to fall into the trap of a "negative" attitude if they are too tired, stressed, or unhappy. Your tune-up can help you see the world differently. Your attitude is like a lens through which you filter your life's experiences. Your tune-up will adjust the lens properly and help you see life as a rainbow of miracles and possibilities. Such awareness will naturally make you want to live as well and as long as possible—if for no other reason than just to see what happens next!

Slower aging and living longer

When your body is functioning better and stronger, it kicks in anti-aging mechanisms. Key factors responsible for aging will be highlighted throughout the book. Just be assured that by focusing on becoming healthier and stronger, you will be slowing down the aging process.

The First Step

O.K., one thing you are going to find out in reading this book is that I am going to ask you to do some work. To start things off, I want to give you something that is going to change your life immediately. It costs absolutely nothing, and it is the most basic key to living better, stronger, and longer. In fact, I can tell you with 100% confidence that based upon detailed scientific analysis it is the most important first step you can take to a better, longer life. It isn't a particular diet, exercise program, or supplement plan and it certainly isn't a drug. It is something that is woven into every major religion and expressed by many great philosophers and thinkers throughout history. The key I am referring to is cultivating a spirit of gratitude into your life.

One of Plato's greatest observations was that "*a grateful mind is a great mind which eventually attracts to itself great things.*" I want great things for you! So, I want to help you cultivate a grateful mind. There is a large growing body of scientific work showing that people who are more grateful and kind have higher levels of well-being and are happier, less depressed, less stressed, more satisfied with their lives and social relationships, and live longer. Wow!

Recent research also shows exactly what Plato observed as detailed studies have shown that expressing gratitude leads to other kinds of positive emotions, such as enthusiasm and inspiration, because it promotes the savoring of positive experiences. The end result is that gratitude helps people optimize feelings of enjoyment, no matter what their circumstances are in life.

Several studies have now shown that gratitude appears to be the strongest link to health (and happiness) of any character trait. But, perhaps the best evidence that feelings of gratitude (and kindness) promote health are with studies in which gratitude exercises are used as an intervention.

One of the leading experts in the importance of gratitude as a therapy is Martin Seligman, PhD, former president of the American Psychology Association and one of the major thought leaders in the discipline of positive psychology. Back in 2005 I read a review article published in the journal *American Psychology* by Dr. Seligman that made a huge impact on me. Seligman described a study in which participants were randomly assigned to one of six therapeutic interventions designed to improve their overall quality of life. Of these six interventions, it was found that the biggest short-term effects came from a "gratitude visit" in which participants wrote and delivered a letter of appreciation to someone in their life. This simple gesture caused a significant rise in happiness scores and a significant fall in depression scores. This positive effect lasted up to one month after the visit. In other studies, the act of keeping "gratitude journals," in which participants wrote down three things they were grateful for every day, had even longer-lasting effects on happiness scores. The greatest benefits usually occurred around six months after journal keeping began. Similar practices have shown comparable benefits.

Two studies from Utrecht University in the Netherlands were designed to test the potential of positive psychological interventions to enhance the quality of life in university students. The interventions focused on "thoughts of gratitude" and "acts of kindness," respectively, in two separate randomized controlled trials.

In the first study, participants were asked to think of people that they were grateful for and instructed to focus their gratitude each day on a different passage in their lives. For example, on the first day they were instructed to think back on their years in elementary school and remember a person there were close to and of whom they were grateful to in reference to a specific event, e.g., a friend or family member who helped them with an accomplishment or task. They were also asked to write down a short note whom they wanted to express gratitude towards and why.

In the kindness study, participants of the kindness condition were instructed to pay close attention to their behavior toward the people around them at university and perform at least five acts of kindness per day and report on them in the evening, including the responses of others they received. Examples of acts of kindness included holding a door for someone, greeting strangers in the hallway, helping other students in preparing for an exam, etc. In both studies, subjects in the control group were given random tasks such as recalling their activities of the day.

Using very sophisticated questionnaires, results revealed that the gratitude intervention had a significant positive effect on daily positive emotions and that it may have a cumulative effect on increasing positive emotions. However, results from this study did not show the same impact as previous studies. The difference is that in previous studies there was a much deeper expression of gratitude. For example, in Seligman's study participants not only had to write a gratitude letter, but actually deliver and read the letter to the person they were grateful of as well. It is likely that by doing so, positive feedback from the recipient was provoked, which might have boosted positive emotions among the participants

The kindness intervention had a positive influence on both positive emotions and academic engagement. Based upon the researcher's analysis, the acts of kindness intervention were much stronger than the effects of thoughts of gratitude. One explanation is that the kindness intervention was more intensive than the gratitude intervention (i.e., five acts of kindness per day versus one thought of gratitude per day). Another possibility is that the acts of kindness evoked immediate positive feedback. Positive reactions of people towards the participants were likely to strengthen the effects of the acts of kindness.

The takeaway message is the stronger the act of appreciation or kindness, the bigger the impact on positive emotions and social engagement

Your Assignment

While many may argue that the need to feel loved is the greatest emotional need we have, I believe there may be no greater emotional need than appreciation. The funny thing is that the things we really want in life are usually best obtained when we give the exact same thing. In other words, if you want to feel more appreciation in your life, begin with expressing more appreciation.

To help you feel the power of gratitude, I would like you to challenge you with the following assignments:

- Assignment A: Create a gratitude visit or call in your life. We all have had people touch our lives in profound ways. Pick a worthy recipient and preferably someone whom you have not had much recent contact with. Then figure out a way to make a special acknowledgment, and watch the magic unfold. The more special you make it for the recipient, the more special it will be for you.
- Assignment B: I want you to be more aware in your daily life of opportunities to acknowledge people and seize chances to say thank you. Be bold! Put an effort into making at least three people smile today.
- Assignment C: When you are putting yourself to sleep, make the last conscious thoughts those of giving thanks in your mind and

heart for at least three wonderful things you have in your life. Think of the love, joy, peace, and happiness those things give you and feel the gratitude in your heart.

If you make these three assignments a daily habit, the impact on your life, your relationships and your health can be absolutely incredible. Gratitude is the most powerful magic bullet for a better life that I know. It's simple, safe, has no side effects and it is still very powerful medicine.

Priming for What You Want!

Next, I have another daily habit I want to share with you that I have found critically important to my life. I call it "priming" and it is a breathing, prayer, and meditation practice that I have found really works for me. One of my skills is asking great questions. And, one of the most powerful questions that I ask often in my life is "How can I make this _____ better?" That is exactly what I asked as I was learning various meditation techniques over the years. Eventually it led to a priming exercise that I love.

The problem for me with some forms of meditation and prayer was I found it impossible to quiet my mind. That whole concept of trying to shut down my mind just didn't ring authentic for a Type A person like myself. I thought "What if instead of quieting my mind, I used my mind like a radio antenna to call out into the Universe what I wanted to attract into my being and into my life?" That question led me to developing a form of priming that changed my life in a powerful way.

What I want you to do first is think of four things that you absolutely desire to have more of in your life. Things that you want at the very core of your being. Now, you may have a challenge right now thinking of four things you really want. So, let me help you by sharing mine.

I realized that what my soul really wanted more of was four states: Love, Joy, Peace, and Happiness. I found these were powerful feelings that I could associate to and feel in my priming. The more we can associate to positive feelings, the more they can ignite a charge within us that can spread throughout our entire being. In fact, the literal definition of priming is something that is used to ignite a charge. Another way to look at what happens when we create the vibrations of these positive states within us is that our soul acts as a tuning fork and starts sending out a vibration of these very same frequencies. It all sound great, right?

Here is how I do my priming. I like to do it on my bed, but you can also do it in a chair. I sit up straight. I breathe in and out through my nose. As I take in a big breath, I raise my hands as far into the Universe as I can reaching up and grabbing as much Love as I possibly can and then exhale through my nose as I pull that Love into my being. Then I quickly take in another breath as I again reach into the Universe to pull down as much Joy as I possibly can as I exhale, then I do the same for Peace and Happiness. I do this process seven times. I do it fairly quickly on most occasions, but you can experiment to find the pace that works for you. Sometimes I do it rapid fire, sometimes I do it much slower.

After going through the progression seven times, I then lie back on the bed, put my hands on my heart and perform a different breathing exercise. As I take in a slow breath, I repeat to myself "I AM LOVE, I AM LOVE, I AM LOVE, I AM LOVE" then as I exhale, I associate as much as I possibly can to the feeling of Love. Then I do it for Joy, then Peace, and finally Happiness and then I repeat it once more.

Then I pop up and once again do the first progression and reach high into the Universe and pull down all the Love, Joy, Peace, and Happiness as I possibly can seven times. Then I lie back and perform the "I AM Love, Joy, Peace, and Happiness" statements on the inhale and the association to the feeling on the exhale. Then I repeat both progressions so that I have done each three times. How long does it take me? Less than 7 minutes.

If you can start your day with priming as well as possibly do variations of it at other times during the day, it will change your life. For example, I perform the "I AM _____" breathing as I put myself to sleep, during a massage, on an airplane, and as much as I possibly can. Why? Because I can feel these states growing inside me to higher and deeper levels every single day. We are limitless in our abilities to create these feelings that will fuel us to WANT to live longer, better, and stronger.

One caution regarding "I AM" statements. They are powerful. What you put after these two words you become. Too many times people use "I AM" to reinforce what they don't want in their life (e.g., I am fat, I am bored, I am stupid, etc.). Be careful what you reinforce with I am statements. Also, because I am statements make strong impressions on our subconscious mind, it is important that the subconscious mind buys into what you are saying. If you are obese, in my opinion, saying "I AM THIN" is not going to produce a positive result because the subconscious mind is going to resist or flat out reject it. During my priming what I like about my "I AM" statements is that I genuinely feel Love, Joy, Peace, and Happiness during the exercise. I am literally filling my mind, heart, soul, and entire being with these powerfully positive feelings. My subconscious mind is occupied because it is flooded with conscious focus and the physiology that is produced by each "I AM" statement.

The Importance of Leverage: The Power of Why

I was interviewed recently on the subject of longevity for an online summit, the host Brian Vaszily, asked me what the most important step was in living a longer life, and I responded, "Creating a Powerful Why." I went on to explain that if someone is struggling through life, in pain, suffering, with low energy, depression, etc., the idea of living longer may feel like a tortuous burden. One of the pitfalls with most of us is that we have a tendency to think that everyone of us has the same values and thoughts on life as we do. For me (and hopefully you as well), life is about purpose, mission, growth, and being as healthy as possible so that we can have the full spectrum of the human experience. I could not imagine not wanting to live life to its full potential because that is how I am wired. I have hundreds of reasons "why" I want to be healthy and live longer. Do you?

One of the most popular TED Talks of all time is Simon Sinek's " The Power of Why: How Great Leaders Inspire Action. Here is the link if you have not seen it, https://www.ted.com/talks/simon_sinek_how_great_

leaders_inspire_action. Sinek applied this concept to business, but I think it is beyond that. We need to use the Power of Why to guide our own lives. Sinek draws what he refers to as the "Golden Circle." At the center of the Golden Circle is WHY. The next concentric circle is HOW. And finally, the outermost circle is WHAT.

Let me transpose this framework into the Longevity Matrix. I would like you to start a personal journal. The first entry I want you to make is to create a list. The Top Ten Reasons I Want to Live Longer, Better, and Stronger. Here are mine in no particular order:

- To better fulfill my mission and purpose in life.
- To be an inspiration to my children.
- To express gratitude for the experience I have been given in this life.
- Because I enjoy life and the wonder that it brings.
- I want to experience as much of life as I can.
- It has become part of my personal identity. It is who I am.
- To share more fully love and connection with those close to me.
- Because I love my children and want to delay the pain of my loss of health or life until it is later in their lives.
- I want to see how the story of humankind evolves in my ultimate lifetime.
- I am passionate about self-actualization and my legacy.

Once you know you reasons WHY, the next step is HOW. This step involves creating the values, beliefs, and practices that will guide your actions and decisions on a day-to-day basis. The HOW will be woven throughout this book. In regard to WHAT, that simply reflects actually taking action. I can lead you, but you have to actually do the work.

Longevity Matrix Lifestyle Tune-Up #1–Cultivate a Positive Attitude

At the end of each chapter, I will introduce an important general Longevity Lifestyle Key. I start with attitude because it another critical factor not only for optimal health, but for an optimal quality of life as well. As I have seen over and over in my patient's lives (and my own), it is not what happens in our lives that determines our direction; it is our *response* to those challenges that shapes the quality of our life and determines our destiny. Surprisingly, it is often true that hardship, heartbreak, disappointment, and failure serve as the spark for joy, ecstasy, compassion, and success. If you can condition your attitude to be positive, I can promise that you will be happier, more successful, and healthier.

- *Become an optimist* - We humans, by nature, are optimists. The term comes from the Latin word *optimum*, meaning "the greatest good." Optimism is the philosophy that looks for the best possible outcome and that focuses on the most hopeful aspects of a situation. Some studies have found that people who adopt a positive outlook live longer and suffer from fewer and less severe diseases.

- *Improve the way you talk to yourself* - We all conduct a constant running dialogue in our heads. In time the things we say to ourselves percolate down into our subconscious mind. Those inner thoughts, in turn, affect the way we think and feel. Naturally, if you feed yourself a steady stream of negative thoughts—"I am not good enough, I am not lovable, I am helpless"—your subconscious will respond in kind. Become aware of your self-talk, and then consciously work to feed positive self-talk messages to your subconscious mind.

- *Ask better questions* - The quality of your life is equal to the quality of the questions you habitually ask yourself. For example, if you experience a setback, do you think, "Why am I so stupid? Why do bad things always happen to me?" Or do you think, "Okay, what can I learn from this so that it never happens again? What can I do to make the situation better?" Clearly, the latter response is healthier. Regardless of the specific situation, asking better questions is bound to improve your attitude. Here are some questions to start you off that you may want to answer in your personal journal:
  - What am I most happy about in my life right now?

- What am I most excited about in my life right now?
- What am I most grateful about in my life right now?
- What am I enjoying most in my life right now?
- What am I committed to in my life right now?
- Who do I love? Who loves me?
- What must I do today to achieve my long-term goal?

- *Set positive goals* - Learning to set achievable goals is a powerful method for building a positive attitude and raising self-esteem. Achieving goals creates a success cycle: you feel better about yourself, and the better you feel about yourself, the more likely you are to succeed. Here are some guidelines for setting health goals:
  - State the goal in positive terms and in the present tense; avoid negative words. It's better to say, "I enjoy eating healthy, low-calorie, nutritious foods" than to say, "I will not eat sugar, candy, ice cream, and other fattening foods."
  - Make your goal attainable and realistic. Start out with goals that are easily attainable, like drinking six glasses of water a day and switching from white bread to whole wheat. By initially choosing easily attainable goals, you create a success cycle that helps build a positive self-image. Little things add up to make a major difference in the way you feel about yourself.
  - Be specific. The more clearly you define your goal, the more likely you are to reach it. For example, if you want to lose weight, what is the weight you desire? What body fat percentage or measurements do you want to achieve?
  - Write it down. Enter your goals in your personal journal. Writing them down provides clarity, focus, and makes you feel accountable to fulfill them.

CHAPTER 2:

Keys to Anti-Aging and a Longer Life

mmortality is an interesting concept, but I am not sure it is a natural or desired part of the human experience. There are seasons in our lives and perhaps a finite mortal life creates a greater sense of value, meaning, and purpose. That said, I also believe that our soul is eternal. It is housed in this vessel we call the body and mind allowing us to experience those things that we can only do in the human form. Hence, my goal in making sure that my vessel serves me long and well.

Slowing down the aging process and extending life has been a goal of humans since long before Ponce DeLeon's search for the mythical fountain of youth. Since the early 1980's, a number of books advocating the use of vitamins, minerals, hormones, drugs, and other compounds to extend life have made the best-seller lists. That trend continues. Many—though not all!—of the recommendations to slow down the aging process do make sense and appear to be scientifically sound. This chapter will focus on such recommendations.

First, some definitions: *life expectancy* refers to the average number of years of life a person is expected to live in a given population while *life span* refers to the maximal obtainable age by a member of a species. *Health span* refers to the number of years of healthy life—our true goal. After all, why live longer if you are debilitated, living in a nursing home and don't recognize your children…

On the surface it appears that in the United States, impressive gains in extending life from birth have been made since the beginning of the 20th century. In 1900 the average life expectancy was 45 years. Now it is 75.6 years for men and 80.8 years for women. However, if we really examine what was responsible for this increase in life expectancy, it is almost entirely due to decreased infant mortality. If infant mortality is taken out of the equation, life expectancy really only improved at a maximum of 6 years during this time. In adults reaching 50 years of age, life expectancy has increased a few years at best.

A rational strategy for increasing life expectancy involves reducing causes of premature death. Obesity, smoking, and alcohol abuse contribute greatly to premature death and in many cases are the underlying contributors to the majority of the top ten causes of death. As detrimental as smoking is due to the large number of Americans who are now obese, obesity has become the most important risk factor for premature death as well as shortened health span.

Table 2.1 - Top Ten Causes of Death for 2017

Condition	Number of Deaths
1. Heart disease	647,457
2. Cancer	599,108
3. Accidents (unintentional injuries)	169,936
4. Chronic lower respiratory diseases	160,201
5. Stroke (cerebrovascular diseases)	146,383
6. Alzheimer's disease	121,404
7. Diabetes	83,564

8. Influenza and Pneumonia	55,672
9. Chronic kidney disease	50,633
10. Intentional self-harm (suicide)	47,173

Longevity Myths and Reality

Myths still circulate about certain groups of people (the Hunzas of Pakistan, Georgian Russians, and Andean villages in Ecuador for example) who are reported to live to an extremely old age, between 125 and 150 years. However, detailed scientific reports have refuted these claims.

For example, one group of investigators studying the people of Vilcabamba, Ecuador, to determine whether the degree of bone loss that occurred during aging was different in that population compared to the U.S. population made a revealing discovery. They did an initial survey and 5 years later went back for a follow-up. After this 5-year interval a number of individuals reported being 10 years older than they had been during the first survey. From studying existing birth records, it became obvious that there was considerable exaggeration of age. In this society as well as in the other societies associated with longevity, social standing increases with increasing age.

In the Georgia region of Russia, it has been demonstrated that the majority of reported centenarians (people older than 100 years) are actually in their seventies and eighties, they just look like they are 140 years old as a result of their tough lives.

The current official world record of longevity is 122 years reached by a French woman, Jeanne Louise Calment. However, some researchers believe that she died much earlier and that her daughter Yvonne assumed her identity to avoid estate taxes in 1934.

Table 2.2 - The 10 Oldest Living People Based on Confirmed Records

Rank	Name	Birth date	Death date	Age	Country of death or residence
1	Jeanne Calment	2/21/1875	8/4/1997	122 years, 164 days	France
2	Sarah Knauss	9/24/1880	12/30/1999	119 years, 97 days	United States
3	Nabi Tajima	8/4/1900	4/21/2018	117 years, 260 days	Japan
4	Lucy Hannah	7/16/1875	3/21/1993	117 years, 248 days	United States
5	Marie-Louise Meilleur	8/29/1880	4/16/1998	117 years, 230 days	Canada
6	Violet Brown	3/10/1900	9/15/ 2017	117 years, 189 days	Jamaica
7	Emma Morano	11/29/1899	4/15/2017	117 years, 137 days	Italy
8	Chiyo Miyako	5/2/1901	7/22/2018	117 years, 81 days	Japan
9	Misao Okawa	3/5/1898	4/1/2015	117 years, 27 days	Japan
10	María Capovilla	9/14/1889	8/27/2006	116 years, 347 days	Ecuador

What Causes Aging?

Answers to the question "What causes aging?" are coming rapidly as a result of research in gerontology, the science of aging. There are many interesting theories of aging, however, only the most significant will be briefly discussed below. There are basically two types of aging theories: programmed theories and damage theories. Programmed theories believe there is some sort of a genetic clock ticking away which determines when old age sets in, while damage theories believe aging is a result of cumulative damage to cells and genetic materials. My opinion is that both are valid. Arguments like this seem to repeat themselves in science—case in point is the nature of light. It functions as both a particle and a wave. Well, human aging is the result of both programmed cell life and cellular damage.

The Hayflick Limit

In 1912 in a laboratory at the Rockefeller Institute, Dr. Alexis Carrel, one of the foremost biologists of his time, began an experiment that would last over 34 years. Dr. Carrel set out to find out how long he could keep chicken fibroblasts dividing. Fibroblasts are connective tissue cells which manufacture collagen. Fed with a special broth containing an extract of chick embryo, the chicken fibroblasts grew quite well in flasks. They would divide and form new cell with the excess cells being periodically discarded. The "tissue culture" system kept dividing for 34 years, until two years after the death of Dr. Carrel when his co-workers discarded the culture. Dr. Carrel's work prompted the idea that cells are inherently immortal if given an ideal environment.

This idea was not discarded until the early 1960s when Dr. Leonard Hayflick observed that human fibroblasts in tissue culture wouldn't divide more than about fifty times. Why the discrepancy? It appears Dr. Carrel had inadvertently added new "fresh" fibroblasts contained in his embryo broth used as nutrition for the tissue culture. New cells had repeatedly been added to the tissue cultures.

Hayflick found that if he froze cells in culture after 20 divisions, they would "remember" that they had thirty doublings left when they were thawed and refed. Fifty cell divisions or doublings is called "the Hayflick limit." As fibroblasts approach fifty divisions, they begin looking old. They become larger and accumulate an increased amount of lipofuscin, the yellow-brown pigment responsible for "age-spots"—those brownish spots that appear on the skin as the result of cellular debris and lipofuscin clumping together. *age spots cellular debris + lipofuscin*

The Telomere Shortening Theory

Based on the Hayflick limit, experts on aging theorized there is a genetic clock ticking away within each cell that determines when old age sets in. The latest, and most likely, program theory of aging is the telomere shortening theory. Telomeres are the end-cap segments of DNA (our genetic material).

Each time a cell replicates, a small piece of DNA is taken off the telomere and gets shorter. The shorter the telomere gets, the more it effects gene expression. The result is cellular aging.

In addition to serving as a clock for aging, the telomere is also involved in protecting the end of the chromosome from damage; controlling gene expression and aiding in the organization of the chromosome. In short, the telomere not only determines the aging of the cell, but our risk for cancer, Alzheimer's disease, and other degenerative diseases associated with aging.

The Free Radical Theory

The best damage theory is the free radical theory of aging. This theory contends that damage caused by free radicals contributes to aging and age-associated disease. Free radicals are defined as highly reactive molecules which can bind to and destroy cellular compounds. Free radicals may be derived from our environment (sunlight, X-rays, radiation, chemicals), ingested foods or drinks, or produced within our bodies during chemical reactions. The majority of free radicals present within the body are actually produced within the body. However, exposure to environmental and dietary free radicals greatly increases the free radical load of the body. In addition to aging, free radicals have been linked to virtually every disease associated with aging including atherosclerosis, cancer, Alzheimer's disease, cataracts, osteoarthritis, and immune deficiency.

Telomeres appear to be especially susceptible to oxidative damage, so telomere shortening may actually fit very nicely as the underlying result of cumulative free radical damage. The energy producing compartments of the cells, the mitochondria, are also very susceptible to free radical damage and decreased mitochondrial function is one of the hallmark features of an aging cell.

Cigarette smoking is a good example of what happens to our health when there is an increased free radical load. Much of the deleterious health effects of smoking are related to extremely high levels of free radicals being inhaled. Other external sources of free radicals include radiation; air pollutants; pesticides; anesthetics; aromatic hydrocarbons (petroleum-based products); fried, barbecued and char-broiled foods; solvents; alcohol; coffee; and solvents like formaldehyde, toluene, and benzene found in cleaning fluids, paints, gasoline and furniture polish. Obviously, reduced exposure to these sources of free radicals is recommended in a life extension program.

Most free radicals in the body are toxic oxygen molecules. It is ironic that the oxygen molecule is the major source of free radical damage in our bodies. Oxygen sustains our lives in one sense, yet in another it is responsible for much of the destruction and aging of the cells of our bodies. Similar to the formation of rust (oxidized iron), oxygen, in its toxic state, is able to oxidize molecules in our bodies. As you probably already know, compounds that prevent this type of damage are referred to as antioxidants.

In addition to damaging cell membranes and proteins, free radical damage extends to our DNA. The genetic material is responsible for transmitting the characteristics of one generation of species or cells to another. Damage to the DNA structure results in mutations (expression of different genetic material) or the cells simply die or are destroyed. DNA is constantly bombarded by free radicals and other compounds that can cause damage. Fortunately, the body has enzymes which (mostly) repair damaged DNA. The differences in life spans among mammals is largely a result of an animal or human's ability to repair damaged DNA. For example, human maximal life span (about 120 years) is more than twice as long as a chimpanzee (about 50 years) because our DNA repair is much more effective.

Research has shown that old cells are not able to repair DNA as rapidly as young cells. It appears that nature has set the rate of DNA repair at less than the rate of damage, so that animals can accumulate mutations and evolve. If repair were perfect, there would be no evolutionary processes.

Glycosylation and Aging

Another damage theory that deserves mentioning is the glycosylation theory. In a nutshell, this theory involves the continued attachment of blood sugar (glucose) molecules to cellular proteins until finally the protein ceases to function properly. For example, cholesterol-carrying proteins that have been glycosylated do not bind to receptors on liver cells that halt the manufacture of cholesterol. As a result, too much cholesterol is manufactured. Excessive glycosylation and the formation of what are referred to as advanced glycation end-products (AGEs) has many adverse effects: inactivation of enzymes, damaging structural and regulatory proteins, impaired immune function, and increased likelihood for autoimmune diseases. Like free radical damage, AGEs are associated with many chronic degenerative diseases. Diets that promote glycosylation and poor glucose control are also linked to telomere shortening.

Obviously, we want to avoid excessive glycosylation. How is this done? By keeping blood sugar levels under control by consuming a low glycemic diet (and if needed using special nutritional factors like alpha-lipoic acid and others).

Inflammaging, Garb-aging, and Mitochondrial Decline

Accelerated human aging is characterized by a state of chronic, low-grade, inflammation. This process is referred to as inflammaging. There are a few triggers of inflammaging. A big one is poor blood sugar control. Another is the continuous stimulation of macrophages, a type of white blood cell that is responsible for digesting cellular debris, infectious organisms, and other molecular "garbage." The aging process is associated with not only macrophage stimulation leading to inflammation, but also a decreased ability of macrophages to dispose of molecular garbage. The term "garb-aging" is used to describe this link. The inability of macrophages to clear cellular debris and inflammatory molecules further worsens the inflammatory state.

Another key factor that is part of the inflammaging equation is reduced mitochondrial function. Typically, as people age there is a decline in mitochondrial numbers and function. With the decreased energy that is the result of this process, it leads to the leakage of inflammatory compounds from mitochondria as well as just a greater formation of cellular garbage within the cell itself. Within an individual cell, it is not the macrophage that is responsible for clearing this debris, it is the process of autophagy. The term literally means the "eating of one's self." Decreased autophagy is another hallmark feature of aging and is closely tied to mitochondrial function. The end result is that what happens when the mitochondria become damage or are not functioning properly is that the cellular debris that is created is not cleared through autophagy and as a result is another big trigger of chronic inflammation.

What is the point that I am trying to make here? To slow down aging we must protect and improve mitochondrial function; preserve autophagy; and support the function of macrophages to be able to properly process and dispose of cellular garbage. Fortunately, actions can be taken to accomplish these goals through following the Longevity Matrix. For example, I believe that exercise, body movement, and diaphragmatic breathing are the key factors that keep macrophages functioning properly in clearing cellular debris and fighting inflammaging. Hence, a key reason I will be stressing the importance of these activities throughout this book. The same is true for fighting against cellular and mitochondrial damage.

Extending Life Span

Can life span be increased, and the aging process slowed? The answer is definitely yes. It is happening and many people are living proof (humbly, myself included). There is no single "magic bullet" to halt the aging process. Instead I want you to realize that the best steps that can be taken to slow down the aging process and reduce the risk for the major causes of premature death is to adopt the strategies that will unfold here in subsequent chapters.

One life extending strategy that I want you to embrace and celebrate is exercise. Researchers have estimated that for every hour of exercise, there is a two hour increase in longevity. That is quite a return on an investment. The bottom line is that the better physical shape that you are in, the greater your odds of enjoying a healthier and longer life. Much of the benefit is reducing the risk for heart disease. Most studies have showed that the risk of having a heart attack or stroke in a physically unfit individual carries with it an 8-fold greater risk than a physically fit individual.

The Importance of Preserving Muscle Mass and Preventing Sarcopenia

Maintaining muscle mass must be a major goal in any life extension plan. Muscle mass increases in childhood and peaks during the late teens through the mid-to late 20s. After that there starts a decline in muscle mass that is rather slow, but unfortunately very consistent. From the age of 25 to 50 the decline in muscle mass is roughly 10%. In our 50's the rate of decline is slightly accelerated, but the real decline usually begins at 60 years. After 50 years of age, approximately 1% to 2% of muscle mass is expected to be lost per year, after 60 it accelerates to as much as 3% per year. By the time a person reaches the age of 80 their muscle mass is a little more than half of what it was in their twenties.

Sarcopenia is the degenerative loss of skeletal muscle mass and strength as we age. Sarcopenia is to our muscle mass what osteoporosis is to our bones. The degree of sarcopenia as we age is a very strong predictor of mortality and disability. In addition to a significantly shorter life expectancy, sarcopenia is linked to decreased vitality, poor balance, slower gait speed, more falls, and increased fractures. Just like in the prevention of osteoporosis where we want to build the bone while we are young to help us preserve it longer through the aging process the same is true for sarcopenia. And, just as it is important to engage in dietary, lifestyle, and exercise strategies to fight osteoporosis in our later years we must do the same to fight sarcopenia. You must build muscle to maintain your health.

Interestingly, the same dietary factors linked to accelerated aging are linked to sarcopenia while the dietary practices associated with good health are associated with protection against sarcopenia. While diet is unquestionably critical, for most people perhaps the most important step to preventing sarcopenia is to engage in a regular strength training program—that is lift weights or perform resistance exercises. The benefits of strength training are vast, particularly for women and for people over 50. In addition to helping burn more fat, a larger muscle mass is associated with a healthier heart, improved joint function, relief from arthritis pain, better antioxidant protection, better blood sugar control and a higher self-esteem. While many women do not strength train because they fear gaining weight, just the opposite occurs. Building muscle mass actually helps to more effectively burn calories.

Whey Protein for Fighting Sarcopenia

Dietary protein is also essential in supporting muscle growth and fighting sarcopenia, especially when combined with exercise. The best choice for protein supplementation is whey as it has the highest biological value of all proteins. Biological value is used to rate protein based on how much of the protein consumed is actually absorbed, retained and used in the body. One of the key reasons why the biological value of whey protein is so high is that it has the highest concentrations of glutamine and branched chain amino acids (BCAAs) found in nature. These amino acids are critical to cellular health, muscle growth, and protein synthesis. Whey protein is also high in cysteine, which promotes the synthesis of glutathione which plays a major role in helping us get rid of toxins.

Although the most popular use of whey protein is by body builders and athletes looking to increase their protein intake, whey protein is also used to support recovery from surgery, preventing the "wasting syndrome" of AIDS, and to offset some of the negative effects of radiation therapy and chemotherapy. This increased efficiency of protein use is particularly important in battling sarcopenia. Whey protein supplementation has also been demonstrated in clinical trials compared to a placebo as well as other types of protein to produce greater strength and muscle mass gains in elderly subjects involved in a weight training program.

The typical recommendation to boost protein levels is 25 to 50 grams daily; though for severe sarcopenia the dosage recommendation is one gram for every two pounds of body weight.

Table 2.3 - A Comprehensive Nutritional Approach to Prevent Sarcopenia

- Reduce the amount of saturated fat, trans fatty acids, cholesterol, and total fat in the diet by eating only lean sources of protein and more plant foods.
- Increase intake of omega-3 oils by eating flaxseed oil, walnuts, and cold-water fish such as salmon. Eat at least two, but no more than three, servings of fish per week.
- Increase the intake of monounsaturated fats and the amino acid arginine by eating regular, but moderate amounts of nuts and seeds, such as almonds, Brazil nuts, coconuts, hazelnuts, macadamia nuts, pecans, pine nuts, pistachios, and sesame and sunflower seeds; and using a monounsaturated oil, such as olive, macadamia, or avocado oil for cooking purposes.
- Eat five or more servings daily of a combination of vegetables and fruits, especially green, orange, and yellow vegetables; dark colored berries; and citrus fruits.
- Limit the intake of refined carbohydrates. Sugar and other refined carbohydrates lead to the development of insulin resistance which in turn is associated with increased silent inflammation, a key contributor to sarcopenia.
- Utilize the benefits of whey protein by taking 25 to 50 grams of whey protein daily.

Whey protein is also a rich source of the sulfur containing amino acids methionine and cysteine that are also important components of a life extension plan. Typically, as people age the content of these amino acids in the body decreases. Since supplementing the diets of mice and guinea pigs with cysteine increases life span considerably, it has been suggested that maintaining optimum levels of methionine and cysteine may promote longevity in humans.

The mechanism may be because methionine and cysteine levels are a major determinate in the concentration of sulfur-containing compounds, such as glutathione, within cells. Glutathione assumes a critical role in defense against a variety of injurious compounds and by combining directly with these toxic substances to aid in their elimination. When increased levels of toxic compounds or free radical are present in the body, the body needs higher levels of glutathione, hence methionine and cysteine. Good dietary sources are whey protein, fish, eggs, Brewer's yeast, garlic, onions, and nuts.

Dietary Antioxidants

The free radical theory of aging and its offshoots the mitochondrial theory of aging really as well as the role of inflammaging really lend themselves to nutritional and supplementation interventions. Compounds that prevent free radical damage are known as "antioxidants" or free radical "scavengers." The body has several enzymes which prevent the damage induced by specific types of free radicals. For example, superoxide dismutase (SOD) prevents the damage caused by the toxic oxygen molecule known as superoxide. Catalase and glutathione peroxidase are two other antioxidant enzymes found in the human body.

Here is an interesting factoid: the level of antioxidant enzymes as well as the level of dietary antioxidants determine the lifespan of mammals. Human beings live longer than chimpanzees, cats, dogs, and many other mammals because we have a greater quantity of antioxidants within our cells. Some strains of mice live longer than other strains because they have higher levels of antioxidant enzymes. Presumably, the reason why some people outlive others is that they have higher levels of antioxidants in their cells. This line of thinking is largely the reason that leads many nutrition experts and physicians to recommend increasing the level of antioxidants through dietary intake and supplementation.

There is little argument that diets rich in antioxidants can definitely increase life expectancy and reduce the risk for cancer, heart disease, and many other diseases linked to premature death. There is a large number of studies that have clearly demonstrated this link. Dietary antioxidants of extreme significance in life extension and fighting chronic diseases include vitamins C and E; zinc and selenium; carotenoids like beta-carotene, astaxanthin, lutein, and lycopene; flavonoids and polyphenols; and sulfur containing amino acids. Nonetheless, while dietary intakes of antioxidant nutrients consistently show benefits in fighting against aging-related diseases, studies with dietary supplements have largely been disappointing.

I have several thoughts on why the research shows dietary intake works and supplementation does not. The major shortcoming of most of these studies is that researchers often focus on the effects of just one nutrient antioxidant. In a way, this practice is like judging an entire symphony by listening to a single trombone. Such research has its value, but it's not complete and often raises more questions than it answers. It seems that many researchers become too focused on the tree instead of looking at the forest. They fail to understand the importance of the way that individual antioxidants interact within the entire antioxidant system of the human body to produce their anticancer benefits.

When it comes to mopping up free radicals, not all antioxidants are created equal. Each may have a somewhat different (and usually very narrow) range of activity. For example, beta-carotene is an effective quencher of a free radical known as singlet oxygen but is virtually powerless against the dozens of other types of free radicals. As a result, it has a very narrow range of benefit and is very susceptible to being damaged itself without additional support.

Most antioxidants require some sort of "partner" antioxidant that allows it to work more efficiently. And scientists have discovered that it is quite easy for one antioxidant nutrient like beta-carotene to become damaged if it's used alone (that is, without its partner antioxidants vitamin C, vitamin E, and selenium). Similarly, selenium functions primarily as a component of the antioxidant enzyme glutathione peroxidase. This enzyme works closely with vitamin E to prevent free radical damage to cell membranes. Studies looking only at vitamin E's ability to reduce cancer and heart disease are often faulty because they failed to factor in the critical partnership between selenium and vitamin E not to mention the interrelationship between vitamin E and coenzyme Q10.

Further adding to the shortcoming of many of the studies on antioxidant nutrients is the lack of consideration on the importance of phytochemicals and plant derived antioxidants that in addition to exerting benefit on their own are well-known to potentiate the activities of vitamin and mineral antioxidants.

There are three main points to keep in mind about antioxidants:

- The antioxidant system of the body relies on a complex interplay of many different dietary antioxidants.
- Taking any single antioxidant nutrient is not enough. Total protection requires a strategic, comprehensive supplement program.
- Although nutrient antioxidants like vitamin C and E are extremely important, they do not provide complete protection alone or in combination.
- Phytochemical antioxidants can fill in the gaps of protection left open by nutrient antioxidants.

Basic Dietary Recommendations to Fight Aging

I am going to simply introduce the seven important keys to eating a health promoting diet that will be stressed throughout the subsequent chapters:

1. *Eat to control blood sugar levels.* Refined sugars, white flour products, and other sources of simple sugars are quickly absorbed into the bloodstream, causing a rapid rise in blood

sugar leading to poor blood sugar regulation, obesity, type 2 diabetes, and an earlier death.

2. *Each day eat five or more servings of vegetables and two servings of fruit.* A diet rich in fruits and vegetables is your best bet for preventing virtually every chronic disease. This fact has been established time and again in scientific studies on large numbers of people. A serving is defined in most cases as 1 cup raw or ½ cup cooked vegetable or fruit.

3. *Focus on organic foods.* In the United States, more than 1.2 billion pounds of pesticides and herbicides are sprayed or added to food crops each year. That's roughly five pounds of pesticides for each man, woman, and child. There is a growing concern that in addition to these pesticides directly causing a significant number of cancers, exposure to these chemicals through food consumption damages your body's detoxification mechanisms, thereby increasing your risk of getting cancer and other diseases.

4. *Reduce the intake of meat and other animal products.* Many studies have shown the higher your intake of meat and other animal products, the higher your risk of heart disease and cancer, especially for the major cancers like colon, breast, prostate, and lung cancer. If you choose to eat red meat:
   - Limit your intake to no more than three or four ounces daily—about the size of a deck of playing cards. And choose the leanest cuts available, keeping in mind that the USDA allows the meat and dairy industry to label fat content by weight rather than by percent of calories.
   - Avoid consuming well-done, charbroiled, and fat-laden meats.

- Consider buying grass-fed or free-range meats, or wild game.

5. ***Eat the right type of fats.*** The goal is to *decrease* your intake of saturated fats, and omega-6 fats found in most vegetable oils, including soy, sunflower, safflower, and corn; and *increase* the intake of monounsaturated fats from nuts, seeds, avocados, and olive oil while insuring an adequate intake of the omega-3 fatty acids found in fish and flaxseed oil.

6. ***Keep salt intake low.*** Too much sodium in the diet from salt (sodium chloride) not only raises blood pressure in some people, it also increases the risk of cancer. Here are some tips for reducing your sodium intake:
   - Take the saltshaker off the table.
   - Omit added salt from recipes and food preparation.
   - Learn to enjoy the flavors of unsalted foods.
   - Use salt substitutes such as my PerfeKt Salt, or NoSalt and Nu-Salt. These products are made with potassium chloride and taste very similar to sodium chloride.
   - Try flavoring foods with herbs, spices, and lemon juice.
   - Choose low-salt (reduced sodium) products when available.
   - Read food labels and avoid high-sodium foods.

7. ***Drink sufficient amounts of water.*** Water is essential for life. The average amount of water in the human body is about 10 gallons. The recommendation to drink at least 48 ounces of water per day to replace the water that is lost through urination, sweat, and breathing is valid.

Let me stress the importance of drinking enough water more thoroughly. Even mild dehydration impairs physiologic and performance responses. Many nutrients dissolve in water so they can be absorbed more easily in the digestive tract. Similarly, many metabolic processes need to occur in water. Water is a component of blood and thus is important for transporting chemicals and nutrients to cells and tissues. Each cell is constantly bathed in a watery fluid. Water also carries waste materials from cells to the kidneys for filtering and elimination. Water absorbs and transports heat. For example, heat produced by muscle cells during exercise is carried by water in the blood to the surface, helping to maintain the right temperature balance. The skin cells also release water as perspiration, which helps maintain body temperature.

Several factors are thought to increase the likelihood of chronic mild dehydration: a faulty thirst "alarm" in the brain; dissatisfaction with the taste of water; regular exercise that increases the amount of water lost through sweat; living in a hot, dry climate; and consumption of the natural diuretics caffeine and alcohol.

There is currently a great concern over the U.S. water supply. It is becoming increasingly difficult to find pure water. Most of the water supply is full of chemicals, including not only chlorine and fluoride, which are routinely added, but also a wide range of toxic organic compounds and chemicals, such as PCBs, pesticide residues, and nitrates, and heavy metals such as lead, mercury, and cadmium. It is estimated that lead alone may contaminate the water of more than 40 million Americans. You can determine the safety of your tap or well water by contacting their local water companies; most cities have quality assurance programs that perform routine analyses. Or, you can take matters into your own hands and either invest in a water purifier or drink bottled purified water.

Basic Supplementation Program to Fight Aging

Below are my foundational supplement recommendations. In Chapter 12, I provide more advanced superfood and supplement recommendations for those wanting ultimate antiaging support. That said, these foundational supplements go a very long way in supporting antiaging mechanisms, especially fighting inflammaging.

1. ***Take a high potency multiple vitamin and mineral formula.*** Your body needs essential vitamins and minerals—each in the right amount—in order to function properly. Vitamin and minerals function as components of enzymes, which are molecules that trigger and control chemical reactions. Since most enzymes in the body have both a vitamin portion and a mineral portion, it is vitally important to ensure optimal levels of these nutrients by taking a high potency formula that provides at least 100% of the RDI of both vitamins and minerals. High potency multiple vitamin and mineral providing at least 100% of the RDI for all vitamins and minerals.

2. ***Take extra key anti-aging nutrients.*** I think it is worthwhile to take at least these two anti-aging nutrients:
   - Vitamin C: 500 to 1,000 mg daily
   - Vitamin D3: 2,000-4,000 IU daily

   Studies show that vitamin C can reduce telomere shortening by up to 62% compared to controls in cultures of human cells. Even more helpful may be vitamin D3. A 2007 study published in the *American Journal of Clinical Nutrition* scientists examined the effects of vitamin D on the length of telomeres in white blood cells of 2,160 women aged 18 to 79 years. The higher the vitamin D levels, the longer the telomere length. In terms of the effect on aging, there was a 5-year difference in telomere length in those with the highest levels of vitamin D compared to those with the lowest levels. Obesity, smoking, and lack of physical activity can shorten the telomere length, but the researchers found that increasing vitamin D levels overcame these effects. What this 5-year difference means is that a 70-year-old woman with higher vitamin D levels would have the biological age of 65 years.

3. ***Take a pharmaceutical grade, high-quality fish oil supplement.*** The health benefits of the long-chain omega-3 oils from fish oils are now well known. Using a high-quality fish oil supplement is the perfect solution to people wanting the health benefits of fish oils without the mercury, PCB's, dioxins, and other contaminants often found in fish. For optimum benefit, take a dosage of fish oil sufficient to provide a combined total of 1,000 to 2,000 mg of EPA+DHA+DPA daily. If you have one of the 60 or more health conditions shown to benefit from EPA+DHA, especially inflammatory, autoimmune, heart, or brain- related conditions like attention deficit disorder, depression, etc., then bump up the dosage to 3,000 mg EPA+DHA+DPA daily.

4. ***Take a plant-based antioxidant.*** Phytochemicals and plant derived antioxidants exert many benefits of their own, but also potentiate the activities of vitamin and mineral antioxidants. Choose one of the following:
   - Grape seed extract (>95% procyanidolic oligomers): 150 to 300 mg daily
   - Pine bark extract (>90% procyanidolic oligomers): 150 to 300 mg daily
   - A curcumin product with enhanced absorption such as Theracurmin (90 to 180 mg per day) or Meriva (1,000 to 2,000 mg per day).
   - Green tea extract (>80% polyphenol content): 300 to 500 mg daily
   - Ginkgo biloba extract (24% ginkgo flavonglycosides): 240 to 320 mg daily
   - Resveratrol: 500 mg daily.

- A "super greens formula" or other plant-based antioxidant that can provide an oxygen radical absorption capacity (ORAC) of 3,000 to 6,000 units or higher per day.

5. *Use appropriate natural products to deal with any "weak links."* Throughout the rest of the book, part of the focus will be using natural products to bolster any weak links in our physiology. For one person, it might be a weak immune system. For another, it could be poor digestive function or circulation. Used in the context of nutritional support, many dietary supplements and other natural products produce significant therapeutic effects. Chapter 12 also provides guidance on additional superfoods and supplement recommendations to maximize anti-aging effects.

Longevity Matrix Lifestyle Recommendation #2: Creating an Effective Exercise Program

Exercise is clearly one of the most powerful medicines available. Just imagine if all of the benefits of exercise could be put in a pill. Unfortunately, it is not that easy. The time you spend exercising is a valuable investment towards good health.

One of the keys to successfully starting and keeping with an exercise program is to identify your personal barriers to exercise and then find creative solutions to overcome these barriers. Rather than making excuses, find a way to overcome these obstacles and make exercise a daily commitment. To help you develop a successful exercise program, here are seven steps to follow.

Step 1. Consult your physician if necessary

If you are not currently on a regular exercise program, get medical clearance if you have health problems or if you are over 40 years of age. The main concern is the functioning of your heart. Exercise can be quite harmful (and even fatal) if your heart is not able to meet the increased demands placed on it. It is especially important to see a physician if any of the following applies to you:

- Heart disease
- Smoking
- High blood pressure
- Extreme breathlessness with physical exertion
- Pain or pressure in chest, arm, teeth, jaw or neck with exercise Dizziness or fainting
- Abnormal heart action (palpitations or irregular beat)

Step 2. Make a solid commitment to exercise

Realize the importance of physical exercise. The first step is realizing just how important it is to get regular exercise. I cannot stress enough just how vital regular exercise is to your health. But, as much as I emphasize this fact it means absolutely nothing unless it really sinks in and you accept it as well. You must make regular exercise a top priority in your life. If you have time to eat and sleep, you have time to exercise. It's really a matter of priorities. If exercise is important enough, you will find the time and expend the energy. Examine all of the things that keep you from exercising and find solutions to those barriers.

Step 3. Select an activity you can enjoy

If you are fit enough to begin with, the next thing to do is select an activity that you would enjoy. The key to getting maximum benefit from exercise is to make it enjoyable. Choose activities that you like and have fun with. If you can find enjoyment in exercise, you are much more likely to exercise regularly.

One way to make it fun is to get a workout partner or join a workout class. Another, using the list below, is to choose from one to five of the activities, or fill in a choice or two of your own. Make a commitment to do one activity a day for at least 20 minutes and preferably an hour. Make your goal to derive pleasure from the activity. The important thing is to move your body enough to raise your pulse a bit above resting.

- Bicycling
- Walking
- Swimming
- Golfing
- Tennis
- Jogging
- Jazzercise
- Dancing
- Stationary bike
- Treadmill
- Stair climbing
- Weightlifting
- Yoga
- Pilates
- Tai Chi
- Skiing
- Hiking

Step 4. Monitor exercise intensity

Exercise intensity is determined by measuring your heart rate (the number of times your heart beats per minute). The best method of monitoring is to use a heart rate monitor. A quick and easy way to determine your maximum training heart rate is to simply subtract your age from 185. For example, if you are 40 years old your maximum heart rate would be 145. To determine the bottom of the training zone, simply subtract 20 from this number. In the case of a 40-year-old this would be 125. So, the training range for a 40-year-old would be between 125 and 145 beats per minute.

For maximum health benefits you must stay in this range and never exceed it. Your heart rate monitor may allow you to set it to beep if you are above or below this zone.

If you don't have a heart rate monitor, you can use pulse measurements. This determination can be quickly done by placing your index and middle finger of one hand on the side of the neck just below the angle of the jaw or on the opposite wrist. Beginning with zero, count the number of heartbeats for 6 seconds. Simply add a zero to this number and you have your pulse. For example, if you counted 14 beats, your heart rate would be 140. Would this be a good number? It depends upon your "training zone."

Step 5. Do it often

You don't get in good physical condition by exercising once, it must be performed on a regular basis. A minimum of 15 to 20 minutes of exercising at your training heart rate at least three times a week is necessary to gain any significant cardiovascular benefits from exercise. For weight control, you should strive to exercise for an hour on most days.

Two or three weight workouts per week and three or four aerobic workouts is a good balance for most people who want to lose weight and keep it off. It is better to exercise at the lower end of your training zone for longer periods of time than it is to exercise at a higher intensity for a shorter period of time.

Step 6. Make it fun

The key to getting the maximum benefit from exercise is to make it enjoyable. Choose activities that you enjoy and have fun with. If you can find enjoyment in exercise, you are much more likely to exercise regularly. One way to make it fun is to get a workout partner. For example, if you choose walking as one of your activities there is a great way to make it fun. Find one or two people in your neighborhood who you would enjoy walking with. If you are meeting one or two people, you will certainly be more regular than if you depend solely on your own intentions. Commit to walking three to five mornings or afternoons each week for least 30 minutes.

Step 7. Stay motivated

No matter how committed a person is to regular exercise, at some point in time they are going to be faced with a loss of enthusiasm for working out. Here is a suggestion—take a break. Not a long break, just skip one or two workouts. It gives your enthusiasm and motivation a chance to recoup so that you can come back with an even stronger commitment.

Here are some other things to help you to stay motivated:

- Follow an inspiring Instagram or Facebook account, or read or thumb through fitness magazines like Self, Men's Fitness, and Muscle & Fitness. Looking at pictures of people in fantastic shape is motivating. In addition, these magazines typically feature articles on new exercise routines.
- Set exercise goals. Success breeds success, so make a lot of small goals that can easily be achieved. Write down your daily exercise goal and check it off when you have it completed.
- Appreciate your progress. Keep a record of your activities and progress. Sometimes it is hard to see the progress you are making, but if you write in a daily journal you'll have a permanent record of your progress. Keeping track of your progress will motivate you to continued improvement.

Step 8: Add variety

Variety is the spice of life. Variety is very important to help stay interested in exercise. Many people exercise for a while and then quit because it becomes too monotonous. Doing the same thing every day also puts you at risk of overuse injuries, especially if you are very heavy or you are working out a bit too long or hard for your level of conditioning. I encourage you to cross train. A typical example would be 2 strength workouts per week, 3 brisk walks, 1 swim and a day of rest. Another week might include a treadmill workout a couple of time per week rather than an outdoor walk or a bike ride when the weather is really nice.

You now have all the information to create an exercise plan that will work for you. So, write down your exercise plan in your journal for the next week. Be sure to be as detailed as possible in terms of activity, time, duration, and intensity.

CHAPTER 3:

Health Begins with the Digestive System

Hippocrates said it well, "All health begins in the gut." It is also often said "you are what you eat," but there is more to the story. While high-quality nutrition is critical to optimum health, it is really what you digest and absorb from the food you eat that nourishes your body. The gut is the central hub to all functions of the human body. Consider the following:

- 70% of the immune system is found in the gut.
- 90% of all brain chemicals (neurotransmitters) are produced within the GI tract.
- The digestive tract itself is the largest and most complex organ of the endocrine system.
- We have 10 times more microbes living in our digestive tract than human cells in our entire body.
- Functional gastrointestinal disorders such as occasional heartburn, bloating, gas, and constipation affect one in three American adults.

One of the hottest topics in medical research and among health enthusiasts these days is the microbiome. The gut *microbiome* refers to in in the genetic material within the microbes that we harbor in our body. The number of *microbiota* - bacteria, viruses and fungi - that live on or in the human body is enormous. Estimates are that approximately 100 trillion microbial cells from 1,000 different species of microorganism live within or on us in a truly symbiotic relationship. In fact, to a very large extent the human microbiome plays an integral role in our overall health.

The future of medicine and nutrition will undoubtedly include focusing on the microbiome. This complex and diverse system is composed of the genetic material from trillions of microorganisms. The microbiome is an important contributor to health and wellness. Research shows that the microbiome has a profound impact on a variety of systems and plays crucial roles in digestive, immune and mental health. An imbalance in the intestinal microbiome may lead to a wide range of issues, ranging from occasional symptoms of digestive distress like gas and bloating, to broader systemic challenges such as obesity, diabetes, Alzheimer's disease, inflammation, etc.

The truth is that while the science of how to influence the microbiome is in its infancy, there are certain undeniable facts that are well established. One of the key aspects of a healthy microbiome is a rich diversity of microorganisms. So, how do we insure microbial diversity? What is well-established in the scientific literature is that dietary diversity is the biggest determinant for diversity within the microbiome. Therefore, eat a diverse diet rich in those foods and compounds known to be associated with health, mainly an assortment of high fiber foods (especially vegetables) and the right types of fat (especially mono-unsaturated fats from nuts, seeds, olive oil, avocados, etc.; and the long-chain omega-3 fatty acids from cold-water fish and fish oil supplements).

One of the beneficial features of most healthy diets, like the Mediterranean diet, is that they are a rich source of compounds that promote the growth of beneficial organisms and microbiome diversity. Although olive oil gets a lot of credit, it is actually the synergistic effects of a multitude of different food components that are responsible for the observed health benefits of the Mediterranean diet. Many of these benefits may reflect the microbial diversity produced by the dietary variety.

But, in order for even the healthiest diet to actually promote health and feed the microbiome in a healthful way, it is essential that our digestive system be functioning properly.

The Importance of Chewing Thoroughly

Though chewing thoroughly is an important step to digestion, the process of digestion actually begins a short time before your meal even enters your body. Odors from food tickle your nose. In response, the brain sends signals to your digestive organs, telling them to get ready for the incoming food. For example, the brain tells the glands in your mouth to release saliva. The production of other digestive juices also begins. You don't actually need to smell food to begin the process. Often the mere thought of a meal is enough to literally get the juices flowing.

The act of chewing your food sends another batch of signals to your digestive organs. Chewing mixes the food with saliva. Saliva contains enzymes that immediately kick off the breakdown process. For example, the enzyme salivary amylase whittles molecules of starch into smaller sugar molecules. Chewing thoroughly is important for getting the most nutrition out of the food you eat. As part of your tune-up, make an effort to chew each bite completely before swallowing. You'll be doing your digestion a favor.

Case History: Something to Chew Over

For a year I'd been working with Trevor, a 45-year-old real estate developer, trying to find a way to relieve his feelings of bloating after meals. He was also bothered by frequent burping and belching. I suspected a deficiency of stomach acid (hydrochloric acid) or perhaps an insufficient supply of digestive enzymes. Nothing I tried worked.

Then one day I happened to go out to lunch with him. It wasn't a pretty sight. Trevor talked non-stop while eating. He took huge bites and barely chewed before swallowing. And he ate too fast. He was looking at the dessert menu while I was still finishing my salad.

Watching him eat, I immediately knew that I had missed the diagnosis. Trevor's problem was *aerophagia*—a fancy name for swallowing air while eating. When I called this to his attention, he didn't believe me. I insisted that he take it seriously, and that he should try eating more slowly and chewing each bite thoroughly—and that he NOT talk during the meal.

To make a long story short: Trevor's cured. Now that's food for thought.

The Stomach

Once food enters the stomach, digestion kicks into high gear. The food gets broken down in two ways: physically and chemically. Muscular contraction in the stomach churn the food so it mixes with digestive juices. At the same time, these motions trigger release of a hormone, gastrin, that "switches on" glands in the stomach lining. These, in turn, release the digestive juices.

The digestive juice you're probably most familiar with is stomach acid, technically known as hydrochloric acid HCL. Sitting by itself in a test tube, this stuff is pretty potent. Inside your stomach, though, it's diluted with saliva, water, and other substances.

The main function of hydrochloric acid is to provide the right environment for the real workhorse of stomach digestion, an enzyme called *pepsin*. Without enough hydrochloric acid (HCL) and pepsin, proper protein digestion will not occur. The acid environment of the stomach also fights off the undesirable overgrowth of bacteria in the stomach and small intestine, and it encourages the flow of bile and pancreatic enzymes. Hydrochloric acid also facilitates the absorption of many nutrients, including folate, vitamin B12, ascorbic acid, beta-carotene, iron, and some forms of calcium, magnesium, and zinc.

The bottom line is that without HCL and pepsin proper protein digestion and nutrient absorption will not occur. In addition, a lack of HCL and/or pepsin can adversely affect the gut's microbial flora including the promotion of an overgrowth of the bacteria *Helicobacter pylori* that is associated with ulcer formation and gastric cancer.

Stomach cells also produce a thick, sticky mucin that protects the cells of the stomach lining from damage from exposure to acid and pepsin.

Stomach cells also produce fat-digesting enzymes (gastric lipases) and a substance called intrinsic factor, which plays a vital role in helping you absorb vitamin B_{12} in the small intestine. People who don't produce enough intrinsic factor are vulnerable to vitamin B_{12} deficiency.

Once the food passes out of the stomach and into the small intestine, other nerve impulses tell the stomach to ease up until the next meal comes along. Food usually remains in the stomach until it is reduced to a semi-liquid. Depending on the types of food you eat, that process lasts between forty-five minutes and four hours. Liquids and carbohydrates are the first to move on. Generally, the more fat or fiber in the food, the longer it stays in the stomach.

The stomach phase of digestion is largely a warm-up act. Only small amounts of water, glucose, salts, alcohol, and certain drugs are absorbed in the stomach. Most digestion and absorption actually take place in the small intestine.

Low Acidity

Although much is said about hyperacidity conditions, a more common cause of indigestion is a lack of gastric acid secretion. Hypochlorhydria refers to deficient gastric acid secretion while achlorhydria refers to a complete absence of gastric acid secretion. There are many symptoms and signs that suggest impaired gastric acid secretion including heartburn, and a number of specific health conditions have been found to be associated with insufficient gastric acid output.

The stomach's optimal pH range for digestion is 1.5-2.5. The use of antacids and acid-blocker drugs will typically raise the pH above 3.5. This increase effectively inhibits the action of pepsin, an enzyme involved in protein digestion that can be irritating to the stomach. Although raising the pH can reduce symptoms, it blocks the effects of both hydrochloric acid and pepsin on digestion.

Table 3.1 - Common Signs and Symptoms of Low Gastric Acidity

- Bloating, belching, burning, and flatulence immediately after meals
- A sense of fullness nearly immediately after eating
- Indigestion, diarrhea or constipation
- Multiple food allergies
- Nausea after taking supplements
- Itching around the rectum
- Weak, peeling and cracked fingernails
- Dilated blood vessels in the cheeks and nose
- Iron deficiency
- Chronic intestinal parasites or abnormal flora
- Undigested food in stool
- Chronic candida infections
- Upper digestive tract gassiness

Table 3.2–Health Conditions Associated with Low Gastric Acidity

- Addison's disease
- Asthma
- Celiac disease
- Dermatitis herpetiformis
- Diabetes mellitus
- Eczema
- Gallbladder disease
- Grave's disease

- Chronic auto-immune disorders
- Hepatitis
- Chronic hives
- Lupus erythematosus
- Myasthenia gravis
- Osteoporosis
- Pernicious anemia
- Psoriasis
- Rheumatoid arthritis
- Rosacea
- Sjogren's syndrome
- Thyrotoxicosis
- Hyper- and hypothyroidism
- Vitiligo

The ability to secrete gastric acid tends to decrease with age. Some studies have found low output of stomach HCL in over half of those over age 60. The overgrowth of the bacteria *Helicobacter pylori* in the stomach has also been linked to lack of HCL secretion as well as gastroesophageal reflux disorder (GERD) and peptic ulcers. Low gastric output is thought to predispose to *H. pylori* colonization and *H. pylori* colonization increases gastric pH, thereby setting up a positive feedback scenario. This overgrowth chronically damages the lining of the stomach resulting in progressive thinning and loss of the cells that secret hydrochloric acid.

Digestive Assessment Part A:
Ruling out lack of stomach acid secretion (hypoacidity)

Circle the number that best describes the intensity of your symptoms on the following scale:

0 = I do not experience this symptom
1 = Mild
2 = Moderate
3 = Severe

Bloating, belching, burning, and flatulence immediately after meals	0	1	2	3
A sense of fullness after eating	0	1	2	3
Indigestion, diarrhea or constipation	0	1	2	3
Multiple food allergies	0	1	2	3
Nausea after taking supplements	0	1	2	3
Itching around the rectum	0	1	2	3
Weak, peeling, and cracked fingernails	0	1	2	3
Dilated blood vessels in the cheeks and nose	0	1	2	3
Acne	0	1	2	3
Iron deficiency	0	1	2	3
Undigested food in stool	0	1	2	3
Chronic candida infections	0	1	2	3

Add the numbers circled and enter that subtotal here: _____

Circle the number that applies to you.
Have you ever had a diagnosis of:

Asthma	No = 0	Yes = 3
Eczema	No = 0	Yes = 3
Hepatitis	No = 0	Yes = 3
Chronic hives	No = 0	Yes = 3
Osteoporosis	No = 0	Yes = 3
Psoriasis	No = 0	Yes = 3
Rheumatoid arthritis	No = 0	Yes = 3
Rosacea	No = 0	Yes = 3
Vitiligo	No = 0	Yes = 3

Add the numbers circled and enter that subtotal here: _____
Add the two subtotals and enter that total here: _____

Scoring
- 9 or more: High Priority
- 5-8: Moderate Priority
- 1-4: Low Priority

Interpreting Your Score

A score of 9 or higher indicates a possible deficiency of hydrochloric acid secretion. Low acid means food doesn't break down as quickly, so it remains in the stomach longer than is normal. Feeling full for a long time after meals is a sign of low acid. Poor appetite may indicate that hunger signals are not being generated, which normally happens after the stomach has been empty for a while. The question about fingernails may have surprised you. But people who have slow digestion may not be able to absorb certain fats at the right rate. Without these nutrients, the nails can weaken and dry out.

Dealing with Hypoacidity

The recommended adult dosage for HCL replacement therapy is one or two 500 mg capsules with meals up to three times daily. The product should contain pepsin as well. For best results I recommend the HCL challenge method:

- Begin by taking one capsule with meals. If this does not aggravate symptoms, at every meal after that of the same size take one more tablet or capsule. (One at the next meal, two at the meal after that, then three at the next meal.)
- Continue to increase the dose until reaching 7 capsules or when you feel warmth in your stomach whichever occurs first. A feeling of warmth in the stomach means that you have taken too many capsules for that meal, and you need to take one less tablet for that meal size. It is a good idea to try the larger dose again at another meal to make sure that it was the HCL that caused the warmth and not something else.

- After you have found that the largest dose that you can take at your large meals without feeling any warmth, maintain that dose at all of meals of similar size. You will need to take less at smaller meals.
- When taking a number of capsules, it is best to take them throughout the meal.
- As your stomach begins to regain the ability to produce the amount of HCL needed to properly digest your food, you will notice the warm feeling again and will have to cut down the dose level.

Safety:
Cautions: Do not take HCL on an empty stomach. Consult a health care practitioner prior to use if suffering from active peptic ulcer, during pregnancy or while breastfeeding. Keep out of reach of children.
Side Effects: May cause mild gastrointestinal side effects such as nausea and stomach upset.

Indigestion, Heartburn, and GERD

The term indigestion is often used to describe heartburn and/or upper abdominal pain as well as difficulty a feeling of gaseousness, swallowing, feelings of pressure or heaviness after eating, sensations of bloating after eating, stomach or abdominal pains and cramps, or fullness in the abdomen. The most common medical term used to describe indigestion is gastroesophageal reflux disorder (GERD), but other terms such as functional dyspepsia (FD) and non-ulcer dyspepsia (NUD) are also used.

GERD is a common condition with up to 25% of the general population experiencing symptoms at least one time per month. The incidence of reflux is increasing because of growing numbers of obesity, increased longevity, and the increased use of medications that impact esophageal function. In fact, the prevalence of GERD is 50% higher in the U.S. in studies carried out after 1995 compared to those carried out before 1995.

The degree of irritation and damage to the lining of the esophagus usually correlates to the severity of symptoms. However, this is not always the case. A multiple-site, double-blind, randomized clinical trial failed to demonstrate a correlation between the severity of self-reported heartburn symptoms and the presence of endoscopically graded esophagitis. Although there was no correlation between severity and underlying esophagitis, there was a strong correlation between the frequency of heartburn episodes and increasing severity of esophagitis.

The severity of the damage to the esophagus in GERD varies from no erosive damage to significant damage. Barrett's esophagus, erosive esophagitis, and esophageal cancer are severe complications associated with erosive forms of GERD. Fortunately, endoscopy reveals that most symptomatic patients have "non-erosive reflux disease" and "functional heartburn." These terms are often used to separate out the common forms of GERD from the more serious versions. The inability of the esophageal mucosa to withstand injury is a determining factor in the development of the more severe forms of GERD. When factors such as reflux, alcohol, heat, various drugs, etc., overwhelm the ability of the cells that line the esophagus to defend themselves that is ultimately what causes the damage.

GERD Diagnostic Summary

- Burning sensation in the esophagus, regurgitation, teeth erosion
- Symptoms chronic and periodic
- Epigastric tenderness and guarding
- Gastric analysis showing acid in all cases, with hypersecretion in about one half the patients with duodenal ulcers
- Ulcer crater or deformity usually occurring at the duodenal bulb (duodenal ulcer) or pylorus (gastric ulcer) on radiography or fiberoptic examination
- Positive test for occult blood in stool

What causes GERD?

GERD is most often the result of altered function of a circular valve that separates the esophagus from the stomach known as the lower esophageal sphincter (LES). Sometimes the dysfunction is due to mechanical factors, such as a hiatal hernia or during pregnancy or with obesity. It can also be the result of overeating or poor digestive function. With relaxation of the LES, there is a reflux of stomach contents up into the esophagus. The reflux is composed of acid, bile, pepsin, and other enzymes that leads to damage or irritation of the esophagus.

The LES is a valve that opens and shuts that acts as a physical barrier preventing gastric contents from refluxing into the esophagus. This sphincter typically opens in response to swallowing and the rhythmic contraction (peristalsis) of the esophagus and is designed to stay shut while the stomach is churning to digest a meal. Only a small minority of patients with GERD have a constantly weak, malfunctioning LES, which permits reflux every time after a meal or when there is increased pressure in the stomach. In patients with GERD, transient LES relaxations account for 48% to 73% of reflux episodes, and thus account for most gastroesophageal reflux episodes.

Other causes of GERD include cigarette smoking, chocolate, fried foods, carbonated beverages, alcohol, caffeine, and many prescription and over-the-counter drugs. The common thread among these factors is that they decrease lower LES tone. Symptoms may be particularly bad when a person is lying down. The process of esophageal acid clearance involves peristalsis as well as the swallowing of bicarbonate and is an important protective mechanism against the development of GERD. Impaired esophageal clearance can be caused by an increase in volume of the refluxate and occasionally from an underlying condition such as scleroderma. In experimentally induced or spontaneous reflux, patients with GERD have been found to present acid clearance times that are two to three times longer than those of subjects without GERD.

One of the surprising causes of GERD is low output of stomach acid or hypochlorhydria and/or lack of digestive enzymes. When food is inadequately broken down and stays in the stomach for longer periods of time it leads to an increase in gastric pressure and reflux of gastric contents into the esophagus. In many cases, supplementation with hydrochloric acid and/or digestive enzymes is very effective in relieving symptoms of GERD. The role of HCL and digestive enzymes in the treatment of GERD is discussed below.

The use of certain medications can lead to the development of GERD and can also worsen existing reflux symptoms. Mechanisms by which drugs cause or aggravate reflux include a reduction in LES pressure, delayed gastric emptying, and inducing/facilitating esophageal inflammation and damage.

Table 3.3 - Drugs and GERD

Reducing LES Pressure	Inducing/Facilitating Esophageal Inflammation	Delayed Gastric Emptying
• Beta-adrenergic agonists • Alpha-adrenergic antagonists • Anticholinergics • CCB/Nitrates • Benzodiazepines • Estrogen • Progesterone • Theophylline • SSRIs • Tricyclic antidepressants	• Bisphosphonates • Aspirin and NSAIDs • Iron salts • Ascorbic acid • Potassium chloride • Quinidine • Tetracycline • Doxycycline • Clindamycin • Chemotherapeutic agents	• Calcium channel blockers

The Folly of Acid-Blocking Drugs

Drugs used to relieve symptoms of GERD by blocking acid production are among the most popular in North America and yet several review articles have concluded in the treatment of GERD, "that the efficacy of current drugs on the market is limited at best." The at best signifies the fact that often these drugs cause more problems than they help. While there are a variety of drugs used in the treatment of GERD, as well as indigestion and the medical labels of FD, NUD, and GERD as well as the irritable bowel syndrome; but since my goal here is not to show you how ludicrous all of these drugs are in their attempt to treat these functional disorders, I want to focus on the most popular—acid-blocking drugs. These drugs work by blocking one of the most important digestive processes—the secretion of hydrochloric acid by the stomach.

Acid-blocker drugs are divided into two general drug groups. One group is the older histamine-receptor antagonist drugs like Zantac, Tagamet and Pepcid AC. The other is the newer and more potent group of drugs called proton-pump inhibitors (PPIs) that include Nexium, Prilosec, Protonix, Prevacid, and Aciphex.

These drugs are a huge business with estimates of total prescription and over-the-counter (OTC) sales of these drugs exceeding $13 billion in annual sales. The drug companies love them because they are for them perfect drugs in that they are expensive, don't produce a true cure, but do tend to suppress symptoms. In short, when people start taking these drugs, they often become dependent upon them. For good reason, these drugs interfere with the body's natural digestive processes to produce significant disturbances in the gastrointestinal tract as well as other side effects including promoting an early death (discussed below). And, while these drugs are typically quite expensive, I like what my colleague Jacob Schor, N.D. says about these drugs: "New research on their side effects says that the money spent on acid blocking drugs may be the least of the costs of using them."

Acid-blocking drugs will typically raise the gastric pH above the normal range of 3.5, effectively inhibiting the action of pepsin—an enzyme involved in protein digestion that can be irritating to the stomach. Although raising the pH can reduce symptoms, it also substantially blocks a normal body process, namely digestion. The manufacture and secretion of stomach acid and the action of pepsin are very important not only to the digestive process, but also because it is an important protective mechanism against infection. Stomach secretions can neutralize bacteria, viruses and molds before they can cause gastrointestinal infection. As far as the digestive process, stomach acid is not only important in the initiation of protein digestion it ionizes minerals and other nutrients for enhanced absorption; and without sufficient secretion of HCl in the stomach the pancreas does not get the signal to secrete its digestive enzymes. Long term use of PPIs is associated with numerous side effects and here are just a small number of examples:

- *Early death*—In a nearly six-year study of U.S. veterans it was shown that PPI use carried with it about a 20% increased risk in overall mortality.

- *Alzheimer's Disease* - PPIs get into the brain and cause an increase in the beta-amyloid deposits characteristic of Alzheimer's disease. Regular use of PPIs is associated with 44% increased risk due for dementia.

- *Heart attacks or stroke*—A review of 37 studies showed that use of PPIs was associated with a 68% increased risk of mortality (dying) and a 54% increased risk of having a heart attack or stroke. In one study, Stanford researchers examined over 16 million clinical documents on 2.9 million individuals and found regular use of PPIs was linked to a two-fold increase in dying from heart disease. It turns out that PPIs inhibit the enzyme required by the cells that line the vascular system that metabolizes a substance produced during metabolism that makes them more rigid as well as promotes inflammation and clot formation.

- *Increased fractures*—people taking high doses of acid-blocking drugs for longer than a year had a 260 percent increase in hip fracture rates compared to people not taking an acid blocker. Evidence suggests that these drugs may disrupt bone remodeling making bones weaker and more prone to fracture.

- *Vitamin B$_{12}$ insufficiency*—acid blocking drugs not only reduce the secretion of stomach acid, but also intrinsic factor (a compound that binds to and assists the absorption of vitamin B$_{12}$). Vitamin B$_{12}$ deficiency is among the most common nutritional inadequacy in older people. Studies indicate that 10 to 43 percent of the elderly are deficient in vitamin B$_{12}$ making them at risk for a number of health conditions including dementia. Many elderly put away in nursing homes for Alzheimer's disease, may simply be suffering from vitamin B$_{12}$ deficiency.

- *Pneumonia*—People using acid blockers were 4.5 times as likely to develop pneumonia as were people who never used the drugs. Apparently, without acid in the stomach, bacteria from the intestine can migrate upstream to reach the throat and then lungs to cause infection.

- *Disruption of the intestinal microbiome*—PPIs dramatically affect the intestinal environment and change the collection of microorganisms in the stomach and intestines leading to potentially serious infections as well as small intestinal bacterial overgrowth (SIBO, a condition linked to gas, bloating, and intestinal inflammation).

Natural Self-Care for GERD

Most individuals who suffer heartburn and acid reflux self-treat their symptoms. That is the reality. Unfortunately, this self-care is usually in the form variety of over-the-counter drugs such as antacid formulations, histamine H2-receptor antagonists (H$_2$RAs such as Pepcid and Tagamet), and proton-pump-inhibitors like Nexium and Prilosec. Instead of relying on this dead end of a drug approach, what I want to outline here is a more rational approach. Here are some categories of GERD with recommendations that are more fully discussed below:

- *Occasional heartburn.* The best natural approach is alginate raft therapy on an as needed basis.

- *Mechanical factors.* If you are obese, pregnant, or have a hiatal hernia the best natural approach is alginate raft therapy. If you are overweight, weight loss is often curative of GERD.

- *Irritation due to ingestion of certain foods.* Sometimes symptoms of GERD are due to the ingestion of coffee, carbonated beverages, alcohol, chocolate, fatty foods, citrus fruits, spicy foods, etc. Elimination and avoidance of these foods is recommended, but a person can also use alginate raft therapy on an as needed basis.
- *Lack of hydrochloric acid or digestive enzymes.* Insufficient output of stomach acid and digestive enzymes can result in GERD symptoms. A simple challenge protocol for HCL supplementation is given below. Sometimes a person with lack of HCL will still experience GERD symptoms with supplementation. In those situations, alginate raft therapy can also be used.
- *Nighttime heartburn.* Raising the head of the bed six inches is often helpful. Alginate raft therapy is effective and so is melatonin.

Alginate Raft Therapy

Alginate, also called alginic acid, is a dietary fiber found in the cell walls of brown algae. Alginate has a unique ability to hold upwards of 200-300 times its own weight in water, making it a naturally gelling substance. When taken with natural buffering agents like calcium carbonate, the alginate it produces a very effective raft that floats on top of the stomach contents to block reflux of gastric contents into the esophagus.

When alginate reaches the acidic environment of the stomach, it forms a pliable gel. At the same time, the calcium carbonate mixes with gastric acid to produce carbon dioxide bubbles that gets trapped in the gel causing it to float to the top of the stomach contents. It literally is like a foam raft sitting on top of the stomach contents. The raft-forming process takes less than a minute the raft can survive in the stomach for as long as four hours. As it makes its way through the intestinal tract it partially digested and behaves as other dietary fibers until it is finally passed out of the body. Alginate is a very safe and effective treatment of GERD.

Alginate formulations are a well-proven treatment for GERD based on 14 human clinical studies and detailed meta-analyses. As far as comparing alginate to a PPI, there are two basic forms of GERD, one characterized by erosion of the esophagus (ERD) and another where there is no esophageal erosion (NERD). It most people in the world, the NERD form is the most common. Comparative clinical studies show no difference in effectiveness between giving a PPI or alginate, especially in NERD.

Considering the confirmed efficacy and remarkable safety profile and lack of side-effects, alginate therapy should be considered as a first line approach to symptomatic relief. It is safe for use during pregnancy.

Digestive Assessment Part B:
Ruling out ulcers or excess stomach acid secretion (hyperacidity)

Use the same rating scale as in Part A. Some items are scored as either Yes or No. When adding your total, score 0 for each No answer and 10 for each Yes.

Stomach pains	0	1	2	3
Stomach pains just before and/or after meals	0	1	2	3
Dependency on antacids	0	1	2	3
Chronic abdominal pain	0	1	2	3
Butterfly sensations in stomach	0	1	2	3
Stomach pain when emotionally upset	0	1	2	3
Sudden, acute indigestion or heartburn	0	1	2	3
Relief of symptoms by carbonated beverages	0	1	2	3
Relief of stomach pain by drinking cream/milk	0	1	2	3
History of ulcer or gastritis	0	1	2	3
Black stool (not caused by taking iron supplements)	0	1	2	3
Current ulcer	NO=0		YES=10	
Is the pain improved with antacids?	NO=0		YES=10	

Do have a current diagnosis of peptic   NO=0   YES=10
ulcer?

TOTAL _____

Scoring
- 9 or more: High Priority
- 5-8: Moderate Priority
- 1-4: Low Priority

Interpreting Your Score:

Scores of moderate of low

A score above 9 in this section may indicate an ulcer. To be on the safe side, you must consult a physician for further evaluation if you think you have an ulcer.

WARNING - Peptic ulcers are potentially serious disorders.

Left untreated, severe complications can develop, including bleeding, perforation (a hole penetrating completely through the stomach, causing leakage of stomach contents), and obstruction. These medical emergencies require immediate hospitalization. Patients with peptic ulcer should be monitored by physicians, even if they are taking any natural remedies.

Peptic Ulcer

A peptic ulcer is a hole that develops in the lining of the stomach or first part of the small intestine. In up to ninety percent of cases of ulcers, a corkscrew-shaped bacterium known as *Helicobacter pylori*—*H. pylori* for short—appears to be a significant factor. The bacteria—one of the few that manages to survive in the acidic environment of the upper digestive tract –burrows under the mucus layer and attach itself to the underlying cells. This weakens the protective layer and exposes the cells to acid juices. *H. pylori* also produce ammonia and other toxic substances, which may further reduce mucus production and trigger inflammatory reactions in the cells and thus lead to ulcer formation.

People who secrete high amounts of stomach acid tend to develop peptic ulcers more frequently. The chronic use of aspirin or other nonsteroidal anti-inflammatory drugs (NSAIDs) can also cause ulcers. Smoking cigarettes or eating certain foods are other causes.

Some people may experience no symptoms from a peptic ulcer. Others feel pain or abdominal discomfort forty-five to sixty minutes after a meal or during the night. My patients typically tell me that the pain is gnawing, burning, cramp-like, or aching. Sometimes they describe it as "heartburn," but that's a different problem. Usually taking antacids relieves symptoms in a short time. However, antacids won't kill *H. pylori*.

To detect the presence of *H. pylori*, the levels of antibodies your body produces in response to the bacteria can be measured in the blood or saliva. There is also a test called the urea breath test that reflects *H. pylori* overgrowth.

Guidelines for Using Antacids for Occasional Gastric Irritation

Antacids are usually safe and effective when taken occasionally to treat acute heartburn. The most popular natural antacids are those that contain calcium carbonate (e.g., Tums). Although fast-acting and potent, calcium carbonate can produce what is known as acid rebound three or four hours after use. This means that the body will try to overcompensate for the neutralization of gastric acid by secreting even more acid. While this may not be a problem when treating indigestion, it may play a role in delaying ulcer healing. Be careful not to abuse antacids.

Regular use can lead to such side effects as malabsorption of nutrients, bowel irregularities, and kidney stones.

Many people take sodium bicarbonate (baking soda) for relief of acid indigestion. (Alka-Seltzer is simply ordinary baking soda in a fizzy form.) Although sodium bicarbonate can be useful in the short term, using it often or regularly can increase your sodium intake to unnecessarily high levels. Long-term administration can cause systemic alkalosis (excessively high pH levels throughout the body), leading to such complications as the formation of kidney stones, nausea, vomiting, headache, and mental confusion.

Magnesium salts such as magnesium oxide, hydroxide, or carbonate can also be used in place of calcium, just avoid all antacids that also contain aluminum. These products (such as Maalox, Rolaids, Digel, Mylanta, and Riopan) are potent and effective, but their aluminum content raises concerns about their long-term safety.

Dealing with Peptic Ulcers

The natural approach to peptic ulcers is first to identify and then eliminate or reduce any factors that may contribute to their development. These include food allergies, a low-fiber diet, cigarette smoking, stress, alcohol, coffee and drugs, especially NSAIDs (aspirin, ibuprofen, and related drugs). Try eating more slowly and chewing food thoroughly. You might see some improvement if you eat smaller meals more frequently. Once these factors have been controlled or eliminated, we then take steps to heal the ulcer and promote tissue resistance.

These steps also seem to help to eliminate H. pylori:

- *Eliminate sugar and refined carbohydrates* such as white flour from your diet.
- *Drink 16 to 24 ounces of vegetable juice per day*, including the regular consumption of cabbage juice. Back in the 1950s,

physicians at Stanford University showed that cabbage juice could be an effective treatment for peptic ulcers. The lead researcher, Garnett Cheney, believed that cabbage juice contained a substance he called "vitamin U" (for "ulcer"). Although this factor was never identified, Cheney clearly demonstrated that fresh cabbage juice relieved peptic ulcers, usually in less than seven days. Here's one of Dr. Cheney's favorite juice recipes:

1/2 head or 2 cups of green cabbage

2 tomatoes

4 ribs of celery

2 carrots

Green cabbage is best, but red cabbage is also useful. Cut the cabbage into long wedges and feed through the juicer followed by the tomatoes, then the celery and carrots. Drink up!

- *Take mastic gum.* It is effective against H. pylori and in one randomized, placebo-controlled trial, 77% of people with dyspepsia who took mastic gum at a dosage of 350 mg three times a day for 3 weeks had improvements in symptoms of indigestion, including stomach pain, upper abdominal ache, stomach pain when anxious and heartburn.

- *Use deglycyrrhizinated licorice (DGL) to promote healing of ulcers as well as fight H. pylori.* DGL is produced by removing glycyrrhetinic acid from concentrated licorice. This compound in licorice can cause elevations in blood pressure due to sodium and water retention. (Yes, eating too much licorice candy can raise blood pressure.) Because the glycyrrhetinic acid has been removed, DGL does not raise blood pressure. DGL stimulates the normal defense mechanisms that prevent ulcer formation. It improves both the quality and quantity of the protective substances that line the intestinal tract, increases the lifespan of the intestinal cell, and improves blood supply to the intestinal lining. There is also some evidence that it inhibits growth of *H. pylori*. Numerous clinical studies over the years support my experience. In several head-to-head studies, DGL has been shown to be more effective than Tagamet, Zantac, or antacids in both short term treatment and maintenance therapy of peptic ulcers. Take one or two chewable tablets of DGL 20 minutes before meals. Continue DGL for 8 to 16 weeks after symptoms abate to ensure complete healing.

The Small Intestine

Once the stomach has done its part, muscular contractions of the stomach force the digested material (now called chyme; pronounced KIME) out of the stomach and into the small intestine. This narrow muscular tube is about twenty-one feet long and has three sections, each of which plays a somewhat different role:

- The duodenum. the first ten to twelve inches is where most of the minerals in your food get absorbed.
- The jejunum, about eight feet long, is the middle section, and is responsible for absorbing water-soluble vitamins, carbohydrates, and proteins.
- The ileum is the last and longest section, measuring about twelve feet, and handles absorption of fat-soluble vitamins, fat, cholesterol, and bile salts.

The inner lining of the small intestine contains thousands of tiny fingerlike projections called villi (plural of villus). These projections, which form a velvety surface, absorb the nutrients as they flow by. If the entire absorptive area of the small intestine were laid flat, it would be the size of tennis court. Disorders of the small intestine often lead to malabsorption and various nutritional deficiencies.

The Pancreas

For intestinal digestion to proceed smoothly, your body needs to continue producing the right mix of fluids at the right time. As the chyme enters the duodenum, its presence triggers the release of secretions from the pancreas. The pancreas produces about a quart and a half of digestive juice each day. The juice flows through a duct leading directly into the duodenum. Pancreatic juice is packed with enzymes needed to digest each of the main types of nutrients: proteases for proteins; lipases for fats; and amylases for starches and sugars.

Pancreatic secretions serve other functions as well. They are responsible for keeping the small intestine free from unwanted critters including bacteria, yeast, and parasites. There are 100 trillion of microorganisms in your intestines, but the initial portion of the small intestine is supposed to stay virtually free from microbes. Low levels of pancreatic enzymes can increase the risk of intestinal infection, such as chronic yeast (candida) infections.

Insufficient pancreatic enzymes can cause a range of digestive problems, including cramps, belching and gas, and diarrhea.

Digestive Assessment Part C:
Ruling out lack of digestive enzymes

Circle the number that best describes the intensity of your symptoms on the following scale:

0 = I do not experience this symptom
1 = Mild
2 = Moderate
3 = Severe

Abdominal cramps	0	1	2	3
Indigestion or belching 13 hours after eating	0	1	2	3
Fatigue after eating	0	1	2	3
Lower bowel gas	0	1	2	3
Alternating constipation and diarrhea	0	1	2	3
Diarrhea	0	1	2	3
Large, greasy (shiny) stools	0	1	2	3
Stool poorly formed	0	1	2	3
Three or more large bowel movements daily	0	1	2	3

Foul smelling stool or flatulence	0	1	2	3
Dry, flaky skin and/or dry brittle hair	0	1	2	3
Pain in left side under rib cage	0	1	2	3
Acne	0	1	2	3
Food allergies	0	1	2	3
Abdominal cramps	0	1	2	3
Indigestion or belching 13 hours after eating	0	1	2	3

TOTAL _____

Scoring

- 9 or more: High Priority
- 5-8: Moderate Priority
- 1-4: Low Priority

Interpreting Your Score:

If you scored higher than 9 in Part C of the Digestive Assessment, consider taking digestive enzymes. In my experience, this approach is a very effective strategy for dealing with most common digestive complaints.

Digestive Enzymes 101

Enzymes are biologically active proteins found in all living cells. They are responsible for building new molecules or breaking down others by acting to build or break chemical bonds. Enzymes give us life. For simplicity, there are two types of enzymes. *Metabolic enzymes* act within the human body and are essential for cellular function and overall health. *Digestive enzymes* are secreted by the digestive system to breakdown the food to provide the necessary nutrients that are body needs for energy and various other biological processes.

Digestive enzymes are secreted along the digestive tract to break food down into nutrients and waste. Some of the enzymes are secreted by the salivary glands, the lining of the stomach and intestines, and the liver and gallbladder, but the major producer of digestive enzymes is the pancreas.

The pancreas is a gland, about six inches long, that is shaped like a flat pear and is just below and behind the stomach. It empties its digestive enzymes in the first part of the small intestine. When food enters the stomach, the pancreas starts its release of enzymes into a canal (duct) that joins with the bile duct before it empties into the small intestine. Sometimes the pancreas may not produce or secrete enough enzymes, and this can lead to gas, bloating, indigestion, irritable bowel syndrome, and malabsorption of food. Taking supplemental digestive enzymes can overcome this insufficiency much like taking supplemental thyroid hormone or insulin helps when the body is not making enough of a hormone.

Each major food group, i.e., protein, carbohydrates, and fat, have specific enzymes responsible for their breakdown. Here are some of the important enzymes to know:

- *Proteases* break down proteins into amino acids. With insufficient protease activity is insufficient undigested it can lead to a host of potentially toxic molecules being formed and a disrupted intestinal microbiome (the collection of gut microbes that play such an important role in so many body functions).

- *Lipases* breakdown of dietary fats. They also assist in the absorption of the fat-soluble vitamins A, D, E, and K. Lipase insufficiency can lead to not only gas and bloating, but also fat malabsorption and diarrhea. Lipase supplementation is an important consideration in people consuming a ketogenic (keto) or high fat diet. Lipase also plays a major role in influencing the microbiome.

- *Amylases* breakdown carbohydrates and, specifically, starches. A deficiency in amylases leads to undigested carbohydrate molecules to pass into to the colon where bacteria and yeast can break them down, literally fermenting them, to produce carbon dioxide and water, which leads to flatulence, cramping, and diarrhea. Amylases also plays a major role in influencing the microbiome.

- *Disaccharidases* are digestive enzymes that breakdown two simple sugars bound together, e.g., sucrase breaks down sugar, maltase breaks down maltose (malt sugar), and lactase breaks down the lactose found in dairy products. Of these, deficiency of lactase is the most significant. Nearly all African American, Native Americans, and Asian adults are lactose intolerant , while northern Europeans adults have a lower rate of 18% to 26% lactose intolerant. Lactose intolerance is characterized by gas, bloating, and diarrhea.

- *Cellulase* and *xylanase* breakdown plant cell walls.

So, what causes decreased production or release of digestive enzymes? Genetics certainly plays a role and there a number of specific disorders associated with enzyme insufficiency such as cystic fibrosis and diabetes. But, the biggest culprits for most people are the effects of stress and aging. Aging actually leads to actual structural changes in the pancreas as well as reduced output of digestive enzymes. It is not uncommon for people who have eaten foods they love for years without complaints to all of a sudden having symptoms every time they eat these foods. Symptoms may range from minor gas, pain, nausea, and bloating to severe cramping and diarrhea when there is an insufficiency of digestive enzymes.

Exocrine Pancreatic Insufficiency

Exocrine pancreatic insufficiency (EPI) is a medical condition that reflects an insufficient output or action of the digestive enzymes secreted by the pancreas. EPI is often silent of significant symptoms other than gas, bloating, and indigestion until output is reduced by more than 90% that results in significant malabsorption characterized by diarrhea and/or a greasy, foul smelling stool.

Many people suffer with digestive complaints for years before EPI becomes worse enough for them to seek medical help. The diagnosis of EPI is primarily made by clinical symptoms and measuring the level of two protease enzymes in the stool—elastase and chymotrypsin. However, this determination only shows the presence of these enzymes and not if they are active or not.

The dominant treatment of EPI is pancreatic enzyme replacement therapy (PERT) using hog pancreas extracts. While it is still the "gold standard," it is an outdated, inferior treatment option. Hog pancreas enzymes have been used in medicine for well over 100 years, but newer forms of digestive enzymes are producing even better results. These newer forms use enzymes derived from vegetarian sources from plants and microbial fermentation. There are certain reasons why these vegetarian enzymes exert greater benefits than those from hog pancreas. Most important is they are stronger in digesting proteins, fats, and carbohydrates and are generally more resistant to degradation within the harsh environment of the intestine. They also exert high activity across a broader pH range. Studies in humans and animals suggest that these new digestive enzyme preparations are more effective in EPI and may also be more effective in reducing digestive symptoms like bloating, gas, and abdominal pain not only in people with EPI, but also in those people who seem to secrete normal levels of enzymes into the digestive tract.

Supplementing with Digestive Enzymes vs. Probiotics to Improve Digestion

One of the greatest areas of confusion that I have often heard around natural digestive health is the difference between supplemental digestive enzymes and probiotics. Both offer incredible benefits when taken correctly, for the correct reasons. Here is the thing, most people with digestive complaints like gas and bloating may not be taking the type of product that can actually provide relief.

Most people have heard the term probiotic and know these beneficial bacteria are found in foods such as yogurt, aged cheeses, and kombucha as well as their availability through supplementation in capsules and tablets. Essentially, probiotics are live bacteria that can reside within our digestive system. While sometimes "bacteria" can cause infections, in the case of probiotics, these are beneficial organisms that play an immense role in the functions of our body. From foundational digestive health to supporting our overall immune function and even influencing our mood, probiotics can be an incredible addition to most people's supplement regime.

Unfortunately, probiotics are of limited value in helping deal with common digestive complaints like indigestion, gas, bloating, and food intolerances. The reason is simple, probiotics do NOT digest food. We need digestive enzymes to accomplish this task. While probiotics are marketed as a cure-all for almost any digestive concern, the reality is the relief that people are seeking to find is best obtained through supplementation with digestive enzymes

Unlike probiotics, enzymes make an immediate difference in your meal. That is because they actually help digest food, probiotics do not. Many people who have occasional digestive difficulties will feel a change from taking a digestive enzyme supplement in minutes. This is because the enzymes are directly working with the body to break down your meal. Many digestive symptoms are simply the result of improper breakdown of food by enzymes.

The bottom line is that many people suffering from digestive issues may not be secreting enough active digestive enzymes or may need additional help. Digestive complaints that can respond to digestive enzyme supplementation affect nearly one in three adults in the United States. Digestive enzymes supplements have been shown to:

- Help relieve bothersome symptoms. Improperly digested food is a big factor in producing digestive issues such as gas, bloating, occasional heartburn and/or indigestion, and altered bowel function.
- Soothe digestive distress. If food is not digested properly, it can irritate and potentially damage the sensitive intestinal lining. Over time, this irritation may reduce our digestive capacity and inhibit our ability to gain the benefits of the food that we eat.

- Improve the microbiome and bowel function. Promoting proper digestion encourages a healthy intestinal environment and help relieve occasional constipation and irregularity.

Vegetarian enzymes are the most popular choice of supplemental enzymes. They are grown in a laboratory setting and extracted from certain types of fungus and probiotics. The enzymes harvested from aspergillus are called vegetarian, or fungal. Of all the choices, vegetarian enzymes are the most potent. This means they can break down more fat, protein and carbohydrates than any other source.

Examples of plant-based enzymes are bromelain and papain. Bromelain is a proteolytic (breaks down protein) and milk-clotting enzyme derived from the pineapple stem. Papain is an enzyme derived from the latex of papaya.

Enzymedica is by far the leading brand of digestive enzyme supplements in the United States. They have achieved this success because of their Thera-blend™ process. This process involves blending the very best enzyme variants in a way that insures enzymatic activity at multiple pH levels. This effect is very important because the pH in the digestive track can range from very acidic to more alkaline. For example, the pH in the stomach is 1.5 (acidic) and up to 8.3 in the intestines (alkaline). Independent lab tests prove Enzymedica Thera-Blend enzymes are 3X Stronger and work more than 6X Faster than other leading enzyme supplements make it the superior choice.

Digest Gold from Enzymedica almost outsells all other leading enzyme products combined according to SPINS data that tracks retails sales of dietary supplements. For most people with common digestive issues, taking one capsule before a meal provides immediate improvements. Many people benefit from a 14-day trial with Digest Gold. In the 14-day challenge simply take one or two capsules of the Digest Gold before each meal for 14 days.

Digestive enzyme preparations are typically very well tolerated and usually have no side effects. A very small percentage of people have reported upset stomach and a soft stool (more frequent and softer bowel movements) when first beginning to take a high-potency digestive enzyme supplement. If stomach upset occurs, take the enzymes early in a meal instead of on an empty stomach. As with any adverse effect, discontinue use and consult a health care practitioner if needed.

Digestive Enzymes Are Helpful in IBS and SIBO

The irritable bowel syndrome (IBS) is referred to as a functional disorder of digestion. What this means is that there is no disease process per se or evidence of accompanying structural defect. It simply reflects that the digestive process is not functioning as it should. IBS is characterized by some combination of abdominal pain or distension; altered bowel function, constipation, or diarrhea; hypersecretion of colonic mucus; symptoms of indigestion such as flatulence, nausea, or loss of appetite; and varying degrees of anxiety or depression.

There are four main causes of IBS that have been identified over the years: stress, insufficient intake of dietary fiber, food intolerance/allergy, and meals too high in sugar. However, lack of digestive enzymes is clearly a factor for many with IBS and supplementation with digestive enzymes can be quite effective in many cases. That is particularly true if the IBS is also associated with small intestinal bacterial overgrowth (SIBO). The presence of microorganisms overgrowing in the small intestine produces a lot of gas as other digestive symptoms. SIBO includes all of the typical symptoms of IBS along with other associated symptoms including:

- Brain "fogginess"
- Fatigue
- Joint pain
- Skin issues: acne, eczema, rashes, or rosacea
- Weight loss

Taking a high potency digestive enzyme formula with each meal is an important remedy in IBS and SIBO. The enzymes act as a deterrent for bacterial and yeast overgrowth in the small intestine. In addition, digestive enzymes prevent the formation of biofilm—a collection of bacteria closely packed together that adhere to the lining of the small intestine within a slimy, gluey matrix. In general, biofilm forming yeast and bacteria are often more difficult to clear. Basically, these organisms form the biofilm when threatened. It is one of the reasons why antibiotics are rarely effective long-term for SIBO. The bacteria from the biofilm and wait till the environment is safe for them to grow again. Digestive enzymes are capable of eating away at the biofilm matrix exposing the bacteria to the natural factors that keep the small intestine relatively microbe free.

Additional Recommendations for IBS

In addition to lack of digestive enzymes, there are some dietary causes of IBS such as too much refined sugar in the diet, lack of dietary fiber, or food allergies. Simply eliminating sugar and increasing the intake of plant food in the diet is effective is many cases. Try to eat foods containing soluble fiber, such as vegetables, fruits, oat bran, and legumes (beans, peas, and so on). This kind of fiber produces a softer stool, which is easier to pass during a movement. (The fiber found in whole wheat is insoluble.) As a bonus, soluble fiber is better at lowering cholesterol levels.

Dietary fiber supplements rich in watersoluble fibers can also be quite helpful. Choose formulas that contain one or more of these fiber sources: psyllium seed husks, tapioca fiber, gum acacia, and partially hydrolyzed guar gum. For best results, take 3 to 5 grams of fiber at night, an hour or so before going to bed. The goal is to trigger an easy bowel movement in the morning.

Nearly two out of three patients with IBS have allergies to one or more foods. The most common foods causing problems in IBS are milk and dairy products, corn, wheat, eggs, peanuts, and chocolate. I recommend eliminating all of these foods for at least a week in order to determine if a food allergy is the problem. After a week, if symptoms improve, slowly add one food back every three or four days. If symptoms return, you are likely allergic to that food.

If you have followed the above steps as well as digestive enzyme supplementation, but still have symptoms of IBS, you may want to try enteric-coated peppermint oil. The typical dosage is 0.2 to 0.4 ml twice daily between meals. An entericcoated preparation prevents the oil from being released in the stomach, allowing it to reach the small and large intestines where it relaxes intestinal muscles. Without enteric coating, peppermint oil tends to produce heartburn.

Several double-blind studies have shown enteric-coated peppermint oil capsules to be a very effective treatment of irritable bowel syndrome. Roughly eight out of people gain significant relief or complete elimination of their IBS symptoms. The typical recommendation for enteric-coated peppermint oil is (0.2 ml) three to four times daily, 15-30 minutes before meals, for one month.

Enteric-coated peppermint oil is thought to work by improving the rhythmic contractions of the intestinal tract and relieving intestinal spasm. An additional benefit is its effectiveness against *Candida albicans* (an overgrowth of *C. albicans* may be an underlying factor in IBS, especially in cases that do not respond to dietary advice and for those who consume large amounts of sugar).

SIBO

As mentioned above, the upper portion of the human small intestine should be relatively free of microorganisms. That's because bacterial and yeast compete with the body's cells for nutrition. When bacteria (or yeast) get to the food first, problems can occur. For example, increased gut permeability (i.e., the "leaky gut" syndrome), abdominal pain, slower passage of food through the intestine (decreased motility), and pain.

Table 3.4 - Problems Resulting from Bacterial Overgrowth of the Small Intestine

- Leaky gut syndrome
- Vitamin deficiency
- Irritable bowel syndrome

- Inflammatory bowel disease (Crohn's disease and ulcerative colitis)
- Autoimmune conditions (for example, rheumatoid arthritis)
- Colon cancer
- Breast cancer
- Skin conditions (psoriasis, eczema, cystic acne)
- Chronic fatigue

Dealing with SIBO

As far as dealing with the bacterial overgrowth, the conventional medical treatment of SIBO relies primarily on antibiotics. However, this approach ultimately creates additional problems due to further disturbance of the microbiome. In contrast, the natural approach focuses on dealing with the bacterial overgrowth by restoring the proper functioning of the protective barriers to SIBO or supplementation strategies designed to produce similar effects. Foremost is taking a high potency digestive enzyme formula like Digest Gold with each meal along with berberine (the yellow alkaloid found in barberry bark, Oregon grape root, and goldenseal).

Digestive enzymes, especially proteases and lipases, are an important protective factor against SIBO. Insufficient output of digestive enzymes from the pancreas is associated with many symptoms associated with SIBO and may represent a key underlying factor in many cases. Digestive enzymes are also the likely host defense mechanisms within the gut that prevents the formation of biofilm—a collection of bacteria closely packed together that adhere to the lining of the small intestine within a slimy, gluey matrix. Digestive enzymes are capable of eating away at the biofilm matrix as well as acting as a deterrent for bacterial overgrowth in the small intestine.

Berberine can provide benefits in SIBO by reducing the number of organisms in the small intestine. The advantage of berberine is that it exerts selective antimicrobial action as it targets a wide range of organisms linked to SIBO as well as against Candida albicans, yet exerts no action against health promoting bacterial species such as Lactobacilli and Bifidobacteria species.

There are additional factors that indicate berberine may be effective in SIBO. In animal models, berberine improves intestinal motility. This action is another key goal in patients with SIBO. And, while berberine has not been studied in SIBO, it has been studied in irritable bowel syndrome with very good results. In a 2015 double-blind study published in Phytotherapy Research, 196 patients with diarrhea predominant IBS were randomized to receive either berberine (200 mg) or a placebo (vitamin C 200 mg) twice a day for eight weeks. The berberine group, but not the placebo group, reported significant improvement in diarrhea and less urgency and frequency in defecation. The berberine group also experienced a 64.6% reduction in abdominal pain compared with initial scores at the end of the score. Berberine significantly decreased the overall IBS symptom score, anxiety score, and depression score. Lastly, and not surprisingly, berberine was associated with an increased quality of life score in patients while no such change was seen in the placebo group.

Berberine has been extensively studied in clinical trials for supporting blood sugar and cholesterol levels as well as blood pressure. I bring this up because in these studies the dosage was typically 500 mg two to three times daily before meals. This dosage level may bring about quicker results than those found in the eight-week trial in IBS and is more likely the dosage that would show more consistent results in SIBO. Berberine is my preferred herbal recommendation for SIBO especially when diarrhea is a common feature.

A word of caution here. In many cases of SIBO, probiotics do not seem to offer much benefit and on occasion may make symptoms worsen. My feeling is that it is better to focus on the intestinal environment that lead to bacterial overgrowth than supplement with additional bacteria.

Lactose Intolerance

After childhood, much of the world's population lose the enzyme (lactase) responsible for digesting the sugar (lactose) found in dairy products. This enzyme resides on the very surface of the lining of the small intestine. A primary deficiency due to lacking the necessary genes to make the enzyme is quite rare. In almost every case a secondary deficiency - due to maturation of the intestine after infancy, infection, or irritation

- is responsible. Symptoms of lactose intolerance range from minor abdominal discomfort and bloating to severe diarrhea in response to even small amounts of lactose. Perhaps seventy to ninety percent of Asian, black, Native American, and Mediterranean adults are lactase deficient. The deficiency occurs among only ten to fifteen percent of people of northern and western European descent.

Laboratory tests can determine if you are lactose intolerant, but these tests usually just tell patients what they already know: milk gives them trouble. If you are lactose intolerant, you can buy lactose-free milk. There are also digestive enzyme supplements that provide lactase in capsule that can help. But my recommendation is to stay away from milk and dairy products. You can find soy, almond, coconut, or rice-based alternatives now that taste just like the "real thing."

Inflammation or irritation of the small intestine can cause many people to become intolerant of milk. For example, intestinal flu often strips away the lactase enzyme, making you temporarily lactose intolerant. It's a good idea to avoid milk products if you are suffering from intestinal infection, irritation, or inflammation as any irritation to the intestinal lining leads to loss of lactase.

Liver, Bile, and Gallbladder

The liver continuously manufactures bile, a thick, greenish-yellow fluid. Bile is essential for the absorption of fats and fatty acids, oils, and fat-soluble vitamins. Bile also aids the action of enzymes. Bile works by breaking up large clumps of fats into smaller droplets and mixing them with water. They also bring water into the picture. This process, called emulsification, gives enzymes a head start in digesting fat molecules more effectively.

Like the pancreatic secretions, bile helps keep the intestine free from microorganisms. Bile also makes the feces soft by promoting the binding of water into the stool. Constipation, or passage of hard dry stools, may be the result of insufficient bile.

The liver secretes some bile through ducts that lead directly into the duodenum. The rest of the bile is carried over to the gall bladder, which stores bile until it is needed. Each day the intestine receives about a quart of bile, nearly all of the bile is reabsorbed and returned to the liver when it has completed its work.

Digestive Assessment Part D:
Ruling out lack of bile output

Circle the number that best describes the intensity of your symptoms on the following scale:

0 = I do not experience this symptom
1 = Mild
2 = Moderate
3 = Severe

1. Constipation	0	1	2	3
2. Small, hard, difficult to pass stools	0	1	2	3
3. Gray, shiny, soft stools	0	1	2	3
4. Pain in right side under rib cage	0	1	2	3
5. Voluminous flatulence	0	1	2	3
6. Roughage and fiber causes constipation	0	1	2	3
7. Dry, flaky skin and/or dry brittle hair	0	1	2	3
8. Indigestion 1-2 hours after eating	0	1	2	3

TOTAL _____

Scoring
- 8 or more: High Priority
- 4-7: Moderate Priority
- 1-4: Low Priority

Dealing with Low Bile Output

A sound diet, adequate water intake, and good overall health are usually all you need to produce adequate bile. However, if you have low bile output, it is possible to increase your levels by taking nutritional supplements containing choline (1000 mg) and methionine (500 mg) or by taking the extract of artichoke leaves (discussed below). Because bile can exert a mild laxative effect, increasing the output of bile is usually quite beneficial in treating constipation.

If you have had your gallbladder removed or you do not tolerate fats, oils, or high fat foods, it may be due to a lack of fat-digesting enzymes (lipases). Enzymedica's *Lypo Gold* has been formulated with a high potency lipase blend to support proper fat breakdown and absorption. Each capsule of Lypo Gold is able to digest the fat in approximately one tablespoon of coconut or olive oil, or six slices of bacon, or a cheeseburger with a small order of fries, or ½ an avocado, or six ounces of salmon. You can find Lypo Gold at your local health food store or at iHerb.com

Artichoke Extract Improves Digestion by Increasing Bile Flow

The globe artichoke (*Cynara scolymus*) is delicious and nutritious—and it also is good for the liver and digestion. Long used as a folk remedy, the value of artichoke extract is being validated by scientific studies. The secret ingredients are plant compounds known as caffeoylquinic acids.

An extract of the leaves of artichoke was shown to increase the flow of bile by up to 150 percent. Bile attracts water, and so the more bile you produce, the better your colon is able to produce soft, easily passed stools. Bile also helps keep the small intestine free from unwanted organisms.

In one study, patients who had suffered from digestive problems for an average of three years took one to two capsules of artichoke extract three times a day. After six weeks, over seventy percent of them reported significant improvement in their constipation. The treatment also relieved other problems, including vomiting, nausea, abdominal pain, and flatulence. Look for artichoke extracts standardized to contain 15-18% caffeoylquinic acids. Take 150 to 300 mg three times daily with meals.

The Large Intestine

The large intestine, also called the colon, is only about one-fourth the length of the small intestine, about five feet, but is considerably bigger in diameter (about two and half inches, compared to about one and a half for the small intestine). By the time the chyme enters the large intestine, virtually all of the nutrients from the food have been absorbed. However, the large intestine does absorb much of the water, salts, and a few other particles.

A high-fiber diet and plenty of water are essential for maintaining the health of the large intestine. Such a diet increases the frequency and quantity of bowel movements, decreases the time it takes to move stool through the intestine, and decreases the absorption of toxins from the stool. Consuming adequate fiber helps prevent colon problems, including constipation, cancer, diverticulitis, hemorrhoids, and irritable bowel syndrome.

Typically, most people have one bowel movement a day. I think that's a reasonable goal and a good sign of healthy colon activity. But each person is different. Some people might normally have two or three movements a day, while others have one movement every other day. While you should aim for at least one movement a day, what's probably most important is that you have *regular* movements, which means that you have them with a fairly predictable pattern of frequency and at approximately the same time of day. Any change in bowel habits can be a sign of trouble somewhere along the digestive tract.

Digestive Assessment Section E:
Colon function

Circle the number that best describes the intensity of your symptoms on the following scale:

0 = I do not experience this symptom
1 = Mild
2 = Moderate
3 = Severe

1.	Alternating diarrhea/constipation	0	1	2	3
2.	Lower abdominal pain or cramps	0	1		
3.	Abdominal distention or bloating	0	1		

4.	Straining at defecation	0	1		
5.	History of use of laxatives	0	1	2	3
6.	Occasional diarrhea	0	1	2	3
7.	Frequent and recurrent infections (colds)	0	1	2	3
8.	Bladder and kidney infections	0	1	2	3
9.	Rectal itching	0	1	2	3
10.	Abdominal cramps	0	1	2	3
11.	Excessive gas	0	1	2	3

12. Have you ever had a diagnosis of:

irritable bowel syndrome	No = 0 Yes = 3
diverticulitis	No = 0 Yes = 3
colon polyps	No = 0 Yes = 3
ulcerative colitis	No = 0 Yes = 3
hemorrhoids	No = 0 Yes = 3

13. Do you have bowel movements less than once a day?   No = 0 Yes = 3

TOTAL _____

Scoring

- 9 or more: High Priority
- 5-8: Moderate Priority
- 1-4: Low Priority

Constipation

One of the most common problems associated with the large intestine is constipation, which means the infrequent or difficult passage of hard, dry stools. Constipation is a problem for more than four million Americans. It occurs when stool remains in the bowel too long. The "transit time"—the time it takes for food to complete its passage through the digestive system—depends primarily on having adequate amounts of fiber in the diet. Without enough dietary fiber, waste material accumulates, and the wrong type of bacteria overgrow. Among people who consume a very high-fiber diet (100 to 170 grams a day), transit time is about 30 hours, producing about a pound of stool. Among Americans, who usually consume only about 20 grams per day, transit time is forty-eight hours or more; typically, stools weigh only about a third of a pound. Besides low fiber, other possible causes of constipation include:

- Use of diuretics (water pills), which reduce body fluid levels
- Use of medications containing codeine, which slows down the muscle and nerve activity needed to pass stools
- Hypothyroidism
- Bowel obstruction (for example from a polyp or tumor)

To prevent constipation, I recommend a diet that provides at least 25 to 30 grams of fiber per day. Each year, people in this country consume $400 million worth of commercial laxatives and "stool softeners." A lot of that money would be better spent on high fiber foods containing bran and other fiber-rich ingredients. Simple making sure you get two servings of fresh fruit each day. Pears and apples are especially helpful as is having one or two prunes daily. Be sure to drink plenty of water and get some regular exercise. Dehydration can lead to the formation of hard, difficult to pass stools. People who are sedentary often have transit times of 72 hours or more; in the elderly the time can be even longer.

Dealing with Constipation: Bowel Retraining

There is a good reason why the labels of products containing stimulate laxatives like senna and cascara should not be used on an ongoing basis. Occasional use is totally fine but relying on these products actually "train" the bowel to become constipated. People who ignore signals to have a bowel movement can also train their bowels to become sluggish. Fortunately, it is possible to retrain your body and develop a more regular pattern of bowel movements.

- Eat a highfiber diet, particularly fruits and vegetables.
- Drink six to eight glasses of fluids per day.
- Identify known causes of constipation, such as not enough fiber in the diet or the use of drugs like diuretics.
- Do not repress an urge to defecate but visit the toilet as soon as you can.
- Sit on the toilet at the same time every day (even when the urge to defecate is not present), preferably immediately after breakfast or exercise.
- Exercise at least twenty minutes, three times per week.
- Take 35 g of a gelforming fiber supplement (e.g., Metamucil or other psyllium preparations) at night before retiring.
- Do not take enemas.
- Taper off using laxatives:
  - First week: Every night before bed, take a stimulant laxative containing either cascara or senna. Take the lowest amount necessary to reliably ensure a bowel movement every morning.
  - Weekly: Each week thereafter, decrease dosage by half. If constipation recurs, go back to the previous week's dosage. Decrease dosage if diarrhea occurs.

Quick Overview of Probiotics

I wanted to save the discussion on probiotics to the end. Probiotics is the term used to describe the beneficial bacteria that inhabit the human intestinal tract. The explosion of scientific research on the microbiome has created renewed interest in the health benefits of probiotics, but humans have been consuming fermented foods containing probiotics for many thousands of years. Many of these foods rich in probiotics are still of great importance to the diets of most of the world's people. Probiotics include not only the freeze-dried bacteria in capsules available at your health food store, but also fermented foods such as cheeses, yogurt, sauerkraut, and kefir. The specific microorganisms found in these products are usually *Lactobacilli* and *Bifidobacteria*.

Table 3.5 - Health Benefits of Probiotics Based Upon Clinical Research

Promotion of Proper Intestinal Environment

Stimulation of Gastrointestinal Tract and Systemic Immunity

Prevention and Treatment of:

    Antibiotic-induced Diarrhea

    Urinary Tract Infection

    Vaginal Yeast Infections and Bacterial Vaginosis

    Eczema

    Food Allergies

    Cancer

    Irritable Bowel Syndrome

    Inflammatory Bowel Disease

        Ulcerative Colitis

        Crohn's Disease

    Traveler's Diarrhea

    Lactose Intolerance

Probiotics exert many mechanisms to improve human health. If the probiotic is a natural inhabitant of the human gastrointestinal tract (GI tract) they actually bind to the surface of the intestinal lining to act as a barrier against damage and infecting organisms. Many pathogenic (disease causing) organisms must bind to the lining of the GI tract in order to cause an infection. Some strains of Bifidobacteria and Lactobacilli can adhere to the epithelium and act as "colonization barriers" by preventing pathogens from adhering to the lining of the GI tract.

Another mechanism of action is production of antimicrobial compounds by probiotics. Many types of Bifidobacteria and Lactobacilli produce antimicrobial compounds known as bacteriocins. The release of these compounds by probiotic organisms results in a beneficial modification of the GI tract microflora. Some of the antimicrobial activity of lactobacilli has also been shown to be due to their production of hydrogen peroxide.

Probiotics can also stimulate the immune response. For example, certain bacteria can increase the secretion of immunoglobulin (Ig) A—an antibody that lines our intestinal tract to act as a first line of defense from our immune system. Certain probiotics have also shown an ability to activate key cells of our immune system (natural killer cells and macrophages).

Probiotics may also compete for nutrients that would otherwise be utilized by pathogens. This situation occurs with Clostridium difficile, a potentially disease-causing organism that can produce a very severe form of diarrhea as a consequence of taking an antibiotic. C. difficile depends on monosaccharides for its growth. Probiotic organisms in sufficient numbers can utilize most of the available monosaccharides, resulting in the inhibition of C. difficile.

The dosage of probiotic supplements most often based on the number of live organisms present in the product referred to in colony forming units (CFUs). Successful results are most often attained by taking between 5 billion and 10 billion CFUs per day. Higher dosages are not necessarily more effective. That said, the use of specific probiotics should be based upon the effects of that particular probiotic from clinical research.

Table 3.6 - The Desirable Characteristics of Effective Probiotic Organisms

Probiotic characteristic	Functional benefit
Human origin	Human origin should translate to ability to survive conditions in the human gastrointestinal tract (GIT) as well as the possibility of species-specific health effects
Gastric acid and bile salt stability	Survival through stomach and small intestine
Adherence to intestinal mucosa	Essential for immune cell modulation and competitive inhibition of pathogens

Colonization of intestinal tract	Multiplication in the intestines suggests that daily ingestion may not be needed; immune cell modulation
Safety in food and documented clinical safety	Adverse effects absent or minimal; accurate identification (genus, species, strain)
Production of antimicrobial compounds	Normalization of GIT flora; suppressed growth of pathogens
Antagonism against pathogenic organisms	Prevention of adhesion and toxin production by pathogens
Compatibility	The organism must not impair the growth or health of other probiotics

Akkermansia muciniphila: The True Probiotic Superstar

Research on the intestinal microbiome is uncovering potential new probiotic species that could revolutionize medicine. The research is also destroying some rather long-held, but limited views on how to influence the composition of the microbiome. The focus in the marketplace has been on attempt to influence the microbiome through supplementation with lactic acid producing bacteria such as *Lactobacillus* and *Bifidobacteria* species. The truth is that while these organisms are important, they play a rather small and limited role on the microbiome.

Through newer methods of identification of bacterial species in the microbiome coupled with a growing understanding of these organisms, they are other bacterial species that are showing much greater roles in impacting health and disease. There is one bacteria in particular that is exciting as it plays a key role in the health of the gut lining as well as promotes improved insulin action to help fight obesity and diabetes. In fact, it turns out that the effects are not limited to its live probiotic effects, but rather to some of the compounds that it manufactures as it has been shown to be effective when it is either a live or heat-killed organism. It is not alone in this effect, several lactic acid producing probiotic organisms have also been shown to be effective when heat-killed. So, this commercial focus on live colony forming units maybe overstated.

Akkermansia muciniphila is the best example of an important gut bacteria that not many people have ever heard of. It is not commercially available as a probiotic, but there are ways in which a person can increase their own supply of *A. muciniphila* through diet and supplementation. First, let's take a look at *A. muciniphila* and why it is so exciting.

A. muciniphila a critical role in the health of the mucin layer that protects the intestinal lining and maintains proper structure of the intestinal lining. That is why it is given its strain name muciniphila—the Latin suffix phila means love. So, muciniphila literally translates as "love of mucin." *A. muciniphila* works with the cells that line the intestines to produce the mucin that goes a long way in protecting the gut lining from damage. Not surprisingly, higher levels of *Akkermansia muciniphila* are associated with improved intestinal barrier function, reduced intestinal permeability (leaky gut), and improved overall digestive and absorptive function.

All of the effects on the mucin layer by *A. muciniphila* are exciting, but what is really making researchers (and drug companies) excited are its effects on diabetes and obesity. As the levels of *A. muciniphila* goes down in the human microbiome, the rates of obesity, diabetes, inflammation, and metabolic disorders goes up. And, as the levels of *A. muciniphila* goes up in the human microbiome, the rates of obesity, diabetes, inflammation, and metabolic disorders goes down. The assumption is that these disorders are associated with altered gut barrier function due to reduced mucin protection, which leads to the absorption of many gut-derived toxins that trigger a cascade of different systems that promote chronic inflammation and insulin resistance.

Animal studies have shown *A. muciniphila* to prevent diet-induced weight gain and there is now human evidence to support the same effect. In the July 1, 2019 online edition of the prestigious journal Nature Medicine, a pilot randomized trial of *A muciniphila* administration among individuals with metabolic syndrome and insulin resistance showed quite convincingly that *A. muciniphila* holds much promise in perhaps tiding the now worldwide epidemic of obesity and type 2 diabetes.

Thirty-two subjects with pre-diabetes and evidence of the metabolic syndrome (abdominal obesity, elevated blood lipids, high blood pressure, etc.) were randomized to getting either a placebo, or live or heat-killed *A. muciniphila*. The active treatment groups taking *A. muciniphila* took around 10 billion bacteria (either dead or alive) daily for 3 months. The primary purpose of the study was to evaluate safety. *A muciniphila* passed that test with flying colors. It also displayed effects noted on multiple markers of metabolism and overall health. Compared with placebo, insulin sensitivity increased while total cholesterol and some markers of inflammation and liver function improved. There was also a significant decrease in the white blood cell (WBC) count in those who got the bacteria. The thought is the strengthening of the gut barrier led to a reduced absorption of gut-derived toxins that could trigger an increase in white blood cell levels.

Here is the interesting part that may be disruptive to many readers of the study, the heat-killed or dead bacteria outperformed the live bacteria. I have been stressing this effect for certain bacteria for years, but mainly to deaf ears. The marketplace is focused on more and more colony forming units (CFUs) instead of focusing on results based upon clinical data. That is a mistake in helping consumers get real results with probiotics and compounds designed to impact the gut microbiome.

One of the key features of *A. muciniphila* is that it is very "slimy" because it is covered in molecules known as exopolysaccharides that prevents white blood cells from breaking down a beneficial protein known as Amuc_1100 that is found in the membrane of *A. muciniphila*. It turns out that this protein appears to be the secret to the bacteria's beneficial effects.

When purified Amuc_1100 is given to mice it exerts the same effects as the live or heat-killed bacteria. The reason why the heat-killed produces better effects than the live form of *A. muciniphila* is that it removes the exopolysaccharides coating but leaves the leaves the Amuc_1100 intact.

Enhancing the Growth of A. muciniphila in the Human Microbiome

A. muciniphila is not expected to be commercially available as a probiotic until 2021, but I don't think that is a big deal. As I have written in the past, we are becoming obsessed with the microorganisms and not focusing enough on creating the right intestinal environment to grow our own microbiome version of the Garden of Eden. Focusing on creating the right "soil" to grow *A. muciniphila* and other beneficial probiotics is in my opinion a more rational approach to establishing the optimum microbiome.

There are a few things that have been shown to be effective in promoting the growth of *A. muciniphila*, most notably is eating a diet rich in diversity of plant foods. One of the beneficial features of most healthy diets, like the Mediterranean diet, is that they are a rich source of dietary compounds that appear to promote the growth of *A. muciniphila*. What concerns me is that popular diets like the ketogenic diet and paleo diet are often very low in foods that promote this important organism. That could be a problem for some. Here are some specific recommendations to promote the growth of *A. muciniphila*.

- **Dietary Prebiotics** - Here is a list of some common foods that are high in health promoting prebiotics:
  - Vegetables: Artichokes, asparagus, broccoli, beetroot, Brussels sprouts, cabbage, cauliflower, garlic, fennel, leaks, mushrooms, okra, onions, peas, shallots.
  - Fruit: Apples, apricots, blackberries, boysenberries, cherries, dates, figs, pears, peaches, watermelon.
  - Legumes: Beans, chickpeas, lentils, red kidney beans, baked beans, soybeans.
  - Non-gluten grains: oats, amaranth, buckwheat, rice (brown, white, wild), millet, quinoa, and sorghum
- **Prebiotic Supplements** - Prebiotic fermentable dietary fibers such as inulin, various oligosaccharides (fructo-, malto-, and xylo-), pectin, tapioca fiber, acacia gum and resistant starch are

available as dietary supplements. Take 3 to 5 grams daily of one or a combination of these fibers.

- **Fish Oils** - The omega-3 fatty acids in fish oils exert profound effects on the microbiome including an ability to increase levels of *A. muciniphila*. Fish oils providing higher levels of DHA to EPA exerts a more profound effect on the microbiome and greater anti-inflammatory effects, especially in the gut. The ideal ratio appears to be DHA 4: EPA 2: DPA 1. Interestingly, this ratio is very close to what is seen in wild salmon species. I recommend the Aqua Biome fish oils from Enzymedica. Regardless, take a minimum of 600 mg of omega-3 fatty acids from fish oil daily. Ideally the dosage should be 1,000 to 2,000 mg for optimal health.

- **Berberine**—This plant alkaloid exerts significant beneficial effects on digestive health and the microbiome including increasing the levels of *A. muciniphila*. This effects partially explains its positive results in clinical trials in improving blood sugar control in type 2 diabetes, lowering blood lipid levels better than statins, and improving liver function. Take 500 mg two to three times daily if you are dealing with any of these metabolic disorders.

Longevity Matrix Lifestyle Tune-Up #3–Keys to Help Master Stress

The stomach and intestines are often hit hard by stress because the stress reaction diverts energy away from the digestive tract and toward the muscles. Under stress, the body prepares to fight or run. Digestion will just have to wait until the danger has passed. With the digestive system on hold due to stress, essential nutrients will not be absorbed. Without those nutrients, the supply of energy stored in the cells is not being replenished. Over time, as stress persists, the energy supply gets used up. As a result, we get tired, often to the point of exhaustion. At that point, disease organisms are more likely to penetrate our defenses and make us ill. The longer stress persists, the worse the problem gets. We humans are simply not designed to live under constant high stress.

In a sense, the numerous systems of the body are like a chain made of many links. Some of these links are stronger than others. Under stress, the weakest link is always the first the break. Which link is likely to snap depends on many factors. Often the first signs of chronic stress are problems with digestion. However, for someone born with a tendency to develop heart disease, stress may be more likely to cause a heart attack or stroke. Constant high blood pressure can damage blood vessels, potentially causing them to rupture. The relentless onslaught of stress hormones can inflame tissues, leading to pain and soreness in the joints or to damage in the mucous membranes of the lungs. As a result, in some people, stress can lead to a range of debilitating conditions such as arthritis or asthma. In other cases, the immune system may be the first to collapse, leaving the person vulnerable to chronic infections.

There are two main strategies for addressing the problem of stress in our lives. The first is to identify the causes of stress and take whatever steps possible to reduce the number of stressors or their severity. The other strategy is to tune up the body and provide it with all the resources it needs to fend off the damage resulting from stress. In other words, we can work to make all of the links of the chain stronger.

Throughout our lives, each of us develops our own ways of coping with stress. Some of those strategies are healthier than others. For example, one person might relieve stress by taking long, relaxing walks or watching funny movies. Another might drink alcohol, use drugs, overeat or have an inappropriate emotional outburst. If you want to be healthy (and happy), you must develop positive methods for managing stress.

One of the most important things you can do to battle stress is to learn how to breathe properly. I learned a lot about breathing by observing my first child, Lexi, when she was just a baby. Like any doting father, I often stood over her crib and watched her as she slept. I was amazed to see how fully her chest rose and fell with each breath. At one moment I became aware of how tight my own chest felt just then. Not wanting to disturb her, I had been holding my breath. As soon as I relaxed, I felt a wave of calmness and love wash over me. A baby's body is smart—it lets breathing happen as deeply and naturally as possible. Later in life, to our detriment, we begin to control breathing more consciously. Sometimes we forget how do to it right.

Proper breathing requires the use of the diaphragm, a dome-shaped muscle that separates the chest from the abdomen. When you breathe in, the diaphragm contracts and pulls downward, enlarging the chest. This helps you draw air into the lungs. When you breathe out, the diaphragm rises, helping you expel air. Using the diaphragm when you breathe directly activates the parasympathetic nerves. This, in turn, induces the relaxation response.

To improve your ability to breathe from the diaphragm, practice the following deep breathing exercise for at least five minutes a day. Of course, you can also do it as part of your "priming" exercise.

- Find a quiet, comfortable place to sit or lie down.
- Place your feet slightly apart. Place one hand on your abdomen near your navel. Place the other hand on your chest.
- Inhale through your nose and exhale through your mouth.
- Concentrate on your breathing. Notice which hand is rising and falling with each breath.
- Gently exhale most of the air in your lungs.
- Inhale while slowly counting to four. As you inhale, slightly extend your abdomen, causing it to rise about one inch. Make sure that you are not moving your chest or shoulders.
- As you breathe in, imagine the warmed air flowing in. Imagine this warmth flowing to all parts of your body.
- Pause for one second, then slowly exhale to a count of four. As you exhale, your abdomen should move inward.
- As the air flows out, imagine all your tension and stress leaving your body.
- Repeat the process for five to ten minutes or until you achieve a sense of deep relaxation.

Of course, there is more to dealing with stress that learning how to breathe. But, engaging the diaphragm is the first step. I will give you some other tips to deal with stress in subsequent chapters.

CHAPTER 4:

Detoxifying from a Toxic World

While none of us would likely ever dream of ignoring a warning light on the dash that it is time to change the dirty oil or regular maintenance, most people ignore the telltale signs that their body is in dire need of cleanup or critical support. What are some of the body's warning signs? If you answer yes to any of the following questions, it definitely is time to tune-up your detoxification processes.

- Do you feel that you are not as healthy and vibrant as other people your age?
- Do you have low energy levels?
- Do you often have difficulty thinking with clarity?
- Do you often feel depressed?
- Do you get more than one or two colds a year?
- Do you suffer from premenstrual syndrome, fibrocystic breast disease, or uterine fibroids?
- Do you have sore achy muscles for no particular reason?

- Do you have bad breath or stinky stools?

Is improving detoxification really an effective a solution to help with all of these symptoms? In most cases, the answer is absolutely yes as these symptoms often reflect nothing more than a squeaky wheel in need of maintenance. With the growing environmental burden on toxic chemicals entering the food chain, now, more than ever, it is critical for us to support the body's detoxification systems if we desire health. Toxins can damage the body in an insidious and cumulative way. Once the detoxification system becomes overloaded, toxic metabolites accumulate, and we become progressively more sensitive to other chemicals, some of which are not normally toxic.

By reducing the toxic load on the body and giving the body proper nutritional support, in most cases these bothersome symptoms will disappear. Even more important, by addressing these warning signs now we can assure better long-term health and avoid the progression of minor problems to more serious conditions.

What are Toxins?

A toxin is defined as any compound that has a detrimental effect of cell function or structure. Obviously, some toxins cause minimal negative effects while others can be fatal. Here is just a short list of some of the thousands of toxins we are all exposed to on a daily basis.

- Toxic metals (lead, cadmium, mercury, arsenic, others)
- Phthalates (plastics)
- Acrylamides (French fries, bread)
- Dioxins, Furans, PBDE's (fire retardants) & Polychlorinated Biphenyls (PCBs)
- Organochlorine byproducts of water "purification"
- Organophosphate Pesticides
- Organochlorine Pesticides
- Carbamate Pesticides
- Herbicides
- Pest Repellents & Disinfectants
- Polycyclic Aromatic Hydrocarbons (char-broiled meats)
- Volatile organic compounds (solvents)
- Tobacco smoke byproducts (over 500 potential chemicals)

The Liver

The liver is the second-largest organ in the body (your skin is the largest). It is also the largest gland (an organ that manufactures secretes substances other tissues need). The liver performs over five hundred separate jobs. Here are some of its crucial functions:

- It produces glucose (blood sugar) from nutrients other than carbohydrates.
- It converts glucose to glycogen, the form of sugar that can be stored in your cells (including liver cells) for later use. When you are running low on energy, the liver converts glycogen back to glucose and ships it off to your cells via the bloodstream.
- Inside the liver, fatty acids, amino acids, vitamins, and minerals are converted into more usable forms.
- The liver makes important cellular structural components including cell membrane compounds (phospholipids) and cholesterol. It is also the liver's job to manufacture the carrier proteins (lipoproteins) that transport these components throughout the body.
- To keep your body's supply of protein at the right level, the liver converts amino acids into glucose, proteins, or other types of amino acids, depending on what your body needs at any given moment.
- It breaks down excess amino acids to form a waste product called urea, which is then carried in the bloodstream to the kidneys and excreted in the urine.
- The liver produces many important blood proteins including immune factors, proteins involved in blood clotting and a crucial component of hemoglobin.
- Iron and vitamins A, D, and B_{12} are stored in liver cells. Old red blood cells are broken down in the liver and their components recycled to create new cells.

How important is detoxification to your well-being? The answer is, *extremely*. Detoxification uses up over eighty percent of the amount of energy your body devotes to making new molecules. In other words, most of the molecules we synthesize every day are made for the sake of getting rid of waste molecules. You can see the connection between liver function and energy levels: If your liver is overloaded—as is the case for most Americans—you may be suffering from low energy levels, since even more of your body's energy is being devoted to detoxification. That leaves very little energy for other body processes. Supporting your liver by following the guidelines in this chapter will help your energy levels soar to new heights.

Assessing Detoxification Section A

Circle the number that best describes the intensity of your symptoms on the following scale:

0 = I do not experience this symptom

1 = Mild

2 = Moderate

3 = Severe

Some items are scored as either Yes or No. When adding your total, score 0 for each No answer and 10 for each Yes.

Section A: Liver function

Yellow in white of eyes.	0	1	2	3
Bad breath	0	1	2	3
Body odor	0	1	2	3
Fatigue	0	1	2	3
Strong smelling urine	0	1	2	3
Sensitive to chemicals	0	1	2	3
Headaches	0	1	2	3
Tingling sensations in hands and feet	0	1	2	3
Mental confusion/cloudiness	0	1	2	3

Less than one bowel movement per day	0	1	2	3
More than 20 pounds overweight	No		Yes	
History of heavy alcohol use or chemotherapy	No		Yes	
Blood test reveals elevated bilirubin or liver enzymes	No		Yes	
Have or had hepatitis	No		Yes	

TOTAL _____

Scoring
- 9 or more: High Priority
- 5-8: Moderate Priority
- 1-4: Low Priority

Interpreting Your Score:

The symptoms addressed in this questionnaire are those that commonly result from the build-up of poisons or the failure of the organs to do their job. For example, one function of the liver is to metabolize hemoglobin, the red pigment left over when old blood cells die. The pigment is changed into a water-soluble form (bilirubin) and then excreted in the bile. However, if the liver is unable to keep up with the demand, bilirubin can build up in the skin or other organs, such as the whites of the eyes. This condition is called jaundice (from the Latin word for yellow). Similarly, dark-colored or strong-smelling urine may signal that the filtration system is not working effectively. The higher your score, the greater the need to address problems related to detoxification.

Heavy Metal Toxicity

Heavy metals include lead, mercury, cadmium, arsenic, nickel, and aluminum. Once they enter the body, these substances can collect inside cells, especially those of the brain, nerves, kidneys, and immune system. Like grit that gets inside the valves of your engine, the heavy metals can disrupt the ability of the cells to carry out their function. Worse, they can cause the cells to act in abnormal ways, for example by causing the buildup of abnormal substances or making the cells reproduce in an out-of-control function, leading to cancer or other serious—potentially fatal—diseases.

Most of the heavy metals that enter the body result from environmental contamination. For example, industrial processes and fossil fuels spew thousands of tons of lead particles into the air each year. Some of the particles settle in soil, where they are absorbed by plants, or are washed into the water supply. Other sources of heavy metals include lead from pesticide sprays and the solder in tin cans; cadmium and lead from cigarette smoke; mercury from dental fillings, contaminated fish, and cosmetics; and aluminum from anti-perspirants, cooking utensils, food containers, and even some antacids.

Heavy-metal toxicity can cause a range of symptoms, depending on which cells and tissues are affected. Many of the symptoms reflect damage to the central nervous system, such as headache, fatigue, tremors, dizziness, lack of coordination, and impaired ability to think and concentrate. There is a connection between heavy-metal poisoning and childhood learning disabilities, such as attention deficit disorder. Other possible symptoms include muscle aches, indigestion, constipation, anemia, and high blood pressure.

Case History: Getting the Lead Out

Carl was a 52-year old man who works in the men's clothing department at a local store when I first saw him. He came to see me for help in getting his high blood pressure under control. He told me he was frustrated with the "medical world" and absolutely hated the drugs his doctors had prescribed. The side effects (dizziness, tingling sensations and numbness in his hands and feet—not to mention impotence) were driving him nuts. Worse, the treatment did not seem to be getting his blood pressure down. His typical reading was 150/105 (a normal reading is closer to 120/80).

Carl did not fit the mold of my usual high blood pressure patients. First of all, he was not overweight. He was an avid runner and ate a health-promoting diet. Except for his high blood pressure and some frequent headaches, he considered himself to be in excellent physical health.

The medical literature and my clinical experience have taught me that when I meet a patient like Carl, who doesn't fit the typical profile, I should suspect that the blood pressure problem may involve high body lead levels. Several studies have found that lead raises blood pressure by negatively affecting kidney function.

Because I knew that people who live in large cities or areas with "soft water" typically have higher lead levels, I asked Carl where he lived. He replied that he had "a nice old house right above a major freeway in downtown Seattle." He also told me that he ran twenty-plus miles a week, mostly on a busy road along the Seattle waterfront. His route was picturesque, but I was sure that he was sucking in too much pollution. I had the nurse collect a sample of Carl's hair so that we could send it out for a hair mineral analysis. Hair analysis is a very good screening test for heavy metal toxicity.

I was shocked by the results. Carl's lead levels were literally off the charts. Despite the high levels, Carl was unaffected by symptoms commonly seen in people with high chronic lead exposure, including depression and neurological complaints such as visual disturbances.

For some patients with high lead levels I will recommend intravenous chelation therapy. This process involves slowly infusing EDTA (ethylenediaminetetraacetic acid), an amino-acid-like molecule, into the bloodstream. EDTA chelates (binds with) minerals such as calcium, iron, copper, and lead and carries them to the kidneys, where they are excreted. EDTA chelation has been commonly used for lead poisoning, but it is also used for treating patients with atherosclerosis (hardening of the arteries).

In Carl's case, though, I thought oral (as opposed to IV) chelation might work to reduce his lead levels. I was optimistic because although Carl consumed a healthy diet, he did not take any nutritional supplements. I felt that we could "get the lead out" and lower blood pressure simply by flooding his body with the nutrients it was starving for: calcium, magnesium, and zinc, as well as vitamins such C, E, and the B vitamin. I prescribed the basic dietary recommendations given later in this chapter along with following supplements:

- A high-potency multiple vitamin and mineral formula–2 tablets 3 times daily (twice the normal dosage)
- Vitamin C–1,000 mg 3 times daily
- Garlinase 4000, a high-potency garlic preparation–1 pill twice daily (twice the normal dosage)

Garlic and onions are rich sources of sulfur-containing compounds that are helpful in escorting heavy metals out of the body. Interestingly, patients with high blood pressure typically have low levels of sulfur-containing compounds in their blood. To lower cholesterol and/or blood pressure, fresh garlic or garlic products that clearly state the "allicin potential" or "allicin yield" should be used. To lower blood cholesterol and/or pressure, the recommended dosage of fresh garlic is roughly one or two cloves of garlic. An equivalent amount for a garlic product (preferably an "odor controlled" tablet) would be an allicin potential or allicin yield of 4,000 mcg. For helping the body eliminate heavy metals it does not matter as much if the garlic is fresh. Cooked garlic (as well as onions) is still rich in sulfur compounds. The bottom line here is that for removing heavy metals is to try to include as much garlic in any form into your diet as possible.

I thought that, for the time being, Carl should continue to take his prescribed blood pressure medication (Atenolol, a beta-blocker). But I urged him to monitor his blood pressure carefully. Carl's blood pressure slowly started coming down after about a month. By the end of two months he needed only half the dosage of Atenolol, and after three months he was totally off the drug and his blood pressure had dropped to 110/70. He still runs, but I convinced him to change his route to one of Seattle's gorgeous parks overlooking Puget Sound. The view is still spectacular—but instead of lead, he's inhaling fresh sea breeze.

Toxic Chemicals

Toxic chemicals that affect the liver include:

- certain chemicals such as food additives or colorings (especially tartrazine, a yellow coloring)
- solvents such as cleaning materials or formaldehyde
- pesticides
- herbicides
- drugs (illicit, over-the-counter, and prescription)
- alcohol
- naturally occurring toxins in foods and herbs

Since all of these toxic chemicals are broken down by the liver, chronic exposure to these substances can damage liver function. Typically, symptoms of liver toxicity show up as problems involving the brain and nerves. Other parts of the body may also be affected. Most common are psychological and neurological symptoms such as depression, headaches, mental confusion, mental illness, tingling in the hands and feet, abnormal nerve reflexes, and other signs of impaired nervous system function. The nervous system is extremely sensitive to these chemicals. Respiratory tract allergies and increased rates for many cancers are also noted in people chronically exposed to chemical toxins.

Key Dietary Guidelines for Liver Support

The most important dietary guidelines for supporting good liver function are also those that support good general health and have been stressed earlier. In particular, avoid refined sugar; don't drink alcohol; drink at least 48 ounces of water each day; and consume plenty of high-fiber vegetables for a variety of reasons, especially their high water-soluble fiber content and rich supply of detoxifying enhancing phytochemicals. There are some specific foods that are particularly helpful because they contain the nutrients and phytochemicals your body needs to produce and activate the dozens of enzymes involved in the various phases of detox. Such foods include:

- Garlic, legumes, onions, eggs, and other foods with a high sulfur content
- Good sources of water-soluble fibers, such as pears, oat bran, apples, and legumes
- Cabbage-family vegetables, especially broccoli, Brussels sprouts, and cabbage
- Artichokes, beets, carrots, dandelion greens, and many herbs and spices such as turmeric, cinnamon, and ginger

Special Supplements for Liver Support

It is important to provide the liver with exceptional support to allow it to perform its vital detoxification role. Without proper support, detoxification can go awry and increase the risk for serious health issues. It begins with diet and lifestyle. That said, a few liver aids deserve special mention: N-acetylcysteine, SelenoExcell, and Siliphos. If you are looking for a formula that has all three and more, go with Liver Detox from Enzymedica.

N-acetylcysteine (NAC)

NAC can increase the manufacturer of glutathione. This amazing compound is the main intracellular antioxidant and is critical to detoxification of harmful chemicals throughout the body, but especially the liver. Glutathione is able to bind fat-soluble toxins like heavy metals, solvents, and pesticides to transform them into a water-soluble form allowing more efficient excretion via the kidneys. In fact, glutathione is the chief way that the body gets rid of persistent organic pollutants like pesticides, herbicides, and other man-made chemicals.

People who are exposed to chemical toxins, suffer from inflammatory conditions such as rheumatoid arthritis, or have chronic conditions such as diabetes experience a depletion of glutathione. It's a vicious cycle: toxins and health problems deplete the supply of glutathione, and reduced levels of glutathione increase the risk of worsening these issues or creating more problems. Fortunately, NAC can boost glutathione levels.

Siliphos

Siliphos is special form of milk thistle extract. Compared to regular milk thistle extracts, Siliphos exerts greater absorption and efficacy in protecting the liver and aiding its structure and function.

Like NAC, one of the key manners in which milk thistle extract enhances detoxification reactions is preventing the depletion of glutathione. The level of this valuable compound within the liver is critically linked to the liver's ability to detoxify. The higher the glutathione content, the greater the liver's capacity to detoxify harmful chemicals. Typically, when we are exposed to chemicals which can damage the liver including alcohol, the concentration of glutathione in the liver is substantially reduced. This reduction in glutathione makes the liver cell susceptible to damage. Milk thistle extract not only prevents the depletion of glutathione induced by alcohol and other toxic chemicals but has also been shown to increase the level of glutathione of the liver by up to 35%. Since the ability of the liver to detoxify is largely related to the level of glutathione in the liver, the results of this study seem to indicate that milk thistle extract can increase detoxification reactions by up to 35%.

Siliphos utilizes the Phytosome technology to bind silybin the key component of silymarin to phosphatidylcholine. This fatty substance is produced from sunflower oil and is also key component of our cellular membranes throughout the body. Phosphatidylcholine is not merely an emulsifier or carrier of the silybin, it has also been shown to promote liver health by helping to repair cell membranes. Hence, these two components of Siliphos work in a synergistic way to protect and repair liver cells. Scientific research indicates that Siliphos is better able to accomplish this goal than regular milk thistle extracts because it is better absorbed and has the added benefit of the phosphatidylcholine.

SelenoExcell

SelenoExcell is a special form of selenium that originates from a special strain of non-GMO baker's yeast (*Saccharomyces cerevisiae*). The particular yeast strain used in SelenoExcell is able to accumulate and incorporate selenium into proteins that enhance the absorption and utilization of selenium. The yeast is inactivated (dead) and cannot reproduce in the human body. Only the nutritional benefits remain.

SelenoExcell has shown greater antioxidant effects compared to other forms of selenium. For example, in a double blind, placebo-controlled trial, 69 healthy men were given a selenium as SelenoExcell (200 or 285 mcg/day) or selenomethionine (200 mcg/day) for 9 months. While blood selenium levels increased in all groups, only the men receiving the SelenoExcell demonstrated a decrease in oxidative stress. Levels of standard markers of oxidative damage (8-OHdG and 8-iso-PGF2α) were decreased 34% and 28%, respectively in the 285 mcg and 200 mcg SelenoExcell groups, versus no change in the selenomethionine group.

In addition to acting as an antioxidant, selenium-rich yeast helps in the detoxification of toxic compounds including heavy metals.

In light of the cumulative data on selenium supplementation, it is clearly apparent that high selenium content yeast in the form of SelenoExcell is the preferred form. In addition to selenomethionine, there are inorganic selenium salts like sodium selenite available in the marketplace. However, selenium salts are less effectively absorbed and are not as biologically active compared to organic forms of selenium, especially SelenoExcell.

The Kidneys

Let's now focus on the liver's detoxification partner—the kidneys. These paired organs located in the lower back just above the waist, on either side of the spinal column. The kidneys are responsible for filtering the blood and excreting waste products and excess water in the form of urine. The kidneys empty urine into the ureters—tubes that carry the urine from the kidney to the bladder.

In addition to eliminating waste products the kidneys regulate the body's acid-alkaline balance (pH) and fluid volume. It also secretes several important hormones like erythropoetin (EPO) that stimulates production of red blood cells in the bone marrow; and converts vitamin D into its most active form.

Assessing Detoxification Section B

Circle the number that best describes the intensity of your symptoms on the following scale:

0 = I do not experience this symptom
1 = Mild
2 = Moderate
3 = Severe

Some items are scored as either Yes or No. When adding your total, score 0 for each No answer and 10 for each Yes.

Section B: Kidney function

1.	Retain fluid in arms and legs	0	1	2	3
2.	Dry, itchy skin	0	1	2	3
3.	Rarely feel the urge to urinate	0	1	2	3
4.	Consume less than 48 ounces of water daily	0	1	2	3
5.	Cloudy urine	0	1	2	3
6.	Strong smelling urine	0	1	2	3

7.	Fatigue	0	1	2	3
8.	Metallic taste in the mouth	0	1	2	3
9.	Dark circles under the eyes	0	1	2	3
10.	High blood pressure (>140/90 mm Hg)	0	1	2	3

TOTAL _____

Scoring

- 8 or more: High Priority
- 3-7: Moderate Priority
- 1-2: Low Priority

Interpreting Your Score:

The questionnaire reflects the need to focus on supporting mild to moderate kidney dysfunction. Even with a score of 8 or more (high priority) it does not necessarily mean that you are experiencing a kidney "disease." The questionnaire contains several questions that indicate dehydration such as are you experiencing dry, itchy, skin; and strong or cloudy urine; or do you rarely feel the need to urinate. Fatigue with a metallic taste in the mouth may indicate uremia—the situation when components of urine back up into the blood. Uremia is also associated with fluid retention, high blood pressure, and dark circles under the eyes may indicate the kidneys are not doing a good enough job regulating fluid volume in the body. In fact, although we think of high blood pressure as being a cardiovascular disease it is really a disorder of the kidneys.

Following the guidelines for enhancing liver function go a long way in supporting proper kidney function too. When the liver does not properly detoxify, it leaves the kidney vulnerable to damage. My key recommendation for tuning up your kidneys is one that you probably have heard a thousand times. Drink at least six to eight glasses of water each day. Don't wait till your thirsty; schedule regular water breaks throughout the day instead. Drink a glass of water at least every two hours throughout the day and you will reach your goal.

Water is essential for life. The average person has a total body water level of about ten gallons. We need to drink at least 48 ounces of water per day to replace the water that is lost through urination, sweat, and expired through our lungs. If we don't, we are likely to become dehydrated.

Recent research also indicates that low fluid consumption in general and low water consumption in particular increases the risk of kidney stones; cancers of the breast, colon, and urinary tract; childhood and adolescent obesity; and heart disease.

Several factors are thought to increase the likelihood of chronic mild, dehydration, including a poor thirst mechanism, dissatisfaction with the taste of water, common consumption of the caffeine and alcohol, regular exercise increasing water lost through sweat, and living in a hot, dry climate. Surprisingly, if you drink two cups of water and two cups of coffee, cola or beer, you may end up with a net water intake of zero. Be aware of your "water budget." If you drink coffee or other dehydrating beverages, compensate by drinking an additional glass of water. That is great way to support your kidneys and hydration.

Fasting, Juice Fasting, and the Detox Diet

For centuries, many people have used fasting—the act of abstaining from all food and drink (except water) for a specified period of time—as a means of cleaning out the body. Fasts are part of many religious traditions. For example, Native Americans would fast during the Vision Quest, a days-long ritual involving the search for deep spiritual insight. Jews fast on Yom Kippur, the most solemn of holidays, as a sign of repentance.

Classically defined, fasting is the complete abstinence from all food and drink except water for a specific period of time, usually for a therapeutic or religious purpose. Fasting is one of the quickest ways to increase elimination of wastes and enhance the healing processes of the body. This process spares essential tissue (vital organs) while utilizing nonessential tissue (fatty tissue and muscle) for fuel.

Although therapeutic fasting is probably one of the oldest known therapies, it has been largely ignored by the scientific community until relatively recently. There is now considerable scientific support on the use of fasting in the treatment of obesity, chemical poisoning, arthritis, allergies, psoriasis, eczema, thrombophlebitis, leg ulcers, irritable bowel syndrome, impaired or deranged appetite, bronchial asthma, depression, neurosis, and schizophrenia.

One of the most encouraging studies on fasting was published in the *American Journal of Industrial Medicine* in 1984. This study involved patients who had ingested rice oil contaminated with polychlorinated biphenyls, or PCBs. All patients reported improvement in symptoms, and some observed "dramatic" relief, after undergoing seven-to-ten-day fasts. This research supports past studies of PCB-poisoned patients and indicates the therapeutic effects of fasting. Caution must be used, however, when fasting after significant contamination with fat-soluble toxins like pesticides. The pesticide DDT has been shown to be mobilized during a fast and may reach blood levels toxic to the nervous system. For this reason, I prefer juice fasts and detox diets. If you are going to water fast, I think it is critical to include those guidelines given below for supporting detoxification reactions while on a Juice Fast or 10-Day Detox Diet.

In addition to the release of stored toxins too rapidly, another concern that I have with water fasting is that you aren't getting the nutrients you need to keep the detoxification system running. Your liver needs a steady supply of protein, vitamins, and minerals to produce the substances that make detoxification happen. Without the nutritional support, you may not be detoxifying properly. Instead, you may simply be mobilizing the stored toxins to more delicate fatty tissues like the brain and kidneys. For these and other reasons, my feeling is that fasting should be done only under medical care and with caution.

The Juice Fast

By strict definition, during a fast it is only water that is consumed. If you are drinking fresh fruit or vegetable juice, this practice is technically known as an elimination diet rather than a fast, but let's just call it a "juice fast" for simplicity. In my opinion, most healthy people do not need to go on a strict water fast to aid in detoxification. Instead, a three-to-five-day fresh fruit and vegetable juice fast actually provides the greatest benefit. It is important to emphasize that only fresh fruit or vegetable juice be used.

Drinking fresh juice for cleansing reduces some of the side effects associated with a water fast, such as light-headedness, fatigue, and headaches. While on a fresh juice fast, individuals typically experience an increased sense of well-being, renewed energy, clearer thought, and a sense of purity.

Although a short juice fast can be started at any time, it is best to begin on a weekend or during a time period when adequate rest can be assured. The more rest, the better the results, as energy can be directed toward healing instead of toward other body functions.

Prepare for a fast on the day before solid food is stopped by making the last meal one of only fresh fruits and vegetables (some authorities recommend a full day of raw food to start a fast, even a juice fast).

Only fresh fruit and vegetable juices (ideally prepared from organic produce) should be consumed for the next three to five days, four 8- to 12-ounce glasses throughout the day.

Virtually any fresh juice provides support for detoxification; however, some of the better juices to consume during a fast include juice from lemons, beets, carrots, kale, celery, and sweet potatoes. You can sweeten if necessary, with apple and you can spice it up with ginger or turmeric. In addition to the fresh juice, pure water should also be consumed. The quantity of water should be dictated by thirst, but at least four 8-ounce glasses should be consumed every day during the fast.

10-Day Detox Diet

Instead of fasting or a juice fast for a quick detox, I recommend a 10-day detox diet (that ideally includes a 3-day juice fast in the middle). I think this strategy is actually the best approach as it allows for the proper detoxification and *elimination* of toxic compounds. If a person is particularly toxic, I don't recommend a longer time, I recommend successive cleanses separated by three weeks or so of following some basic dietary guidelines along with supporting detoxification through dietary supplementation. The diet should be at a caloric deficit. If you can keep the total daily calories near 1,200 that is ideal. We want fat cells to break down and release stored toxins, but we don't want to overwhelm our detoxification system. Here are the "do's and don'ts" of the detox diet.

Do's	Don't
Vegetables especially leafy greens	Refined processed foods
Legumes (beans and lentils)	High sugar foods and beverages
Whole fruit especially berries	Alcohol and diet sodas
Non-gluten grains	Wheat and gluten
Low mercury fish such as wild salmon, smaller species of ocean fish like sardines and herring, and rainbow trout	High mercury fish such as swordfish, marlin, orange roughie, shark, and larger tuna.
Organic, grass-fed meat and dairy (optional)	Grain fed and non-organic dairy
Nuts and seeds	Potato and corn chips
Good oils like olive, avocado, coconut, and flax	Bad oils like corn, safflower, soy, margarine, and shortening

Important Guidelines for a Juice Fast or 10-Day Detox Diet

It is extremely important to support detoxification reactions. This goal is partly done by electing to go on either a fresh juice fast or 1 10-day detox diet over a water fast, additional nutritional support is needed because during a fast, stored toxins in our fat cells are released into the system. Or, if you want to provide your own detoxification support, be sure and take the supplement recommendations given above.

- No coffee, soft drinks, sports drinks, or any other processed beverage should be taken. Herbal teas can be quite supportive of a fast, but they should not be sweetened with anything other than perhaps stevia or allulose.

- Drink plenty of pure, clean water.
- Follow the guidelines above for supplementation to support detoxification.
- Exercise is not usually encouraged while fasting. It is a good idea to conserve energy and allow maximal healing. Short walks or light stretching are useful, but heavy workouts tax the system and inhibit repair and elimination.
- Cleansing the skin with lukewarm water is encouraged, but extremes of temperature can be tiring. Deodorants, soaps, sprays, detergents, synthetic shampoos, and exposure to other chemicals should be avoided. These only hinder elimination and add to the body's detoxification and elimination burden.
- Rest is one of the most important aspects of a fast. A nap or two during the day is recommended. Less sleep will usually be required at night, since daily activity is lower.
- Body temperature usually drops during a fast, as do blood pressure, pulse, and respiratory rate—all measures of the slowing of the metabolic rate of the body. It is important, therefore, to stay warm.
- In breaking a juice fast, here is a good progression to eating healthfully again.

DAY 1

Breakfast	Lunch	Dinner
12 oz of one type of whole organic fresh fruit such as such as pears, berries, papaya, or citrus fruit	12 oz of another type of whole organic fruit such as pears, berries, papaya, or citrus fruit	Raw vegetable salad with leafy greens, tomato, celery, and cucumber or 2 pears, 2 apples, and ¼ avocado

DAY 2

Breakfast	Lunch	Dinner
Smoothie with 8 ounces of organic berries 20 grams of whey or some sort of plant protein.	Raw vegetable salad with leafy greens, tomato, celery, and cucumber or 2 pears, 2 apples, and ¼ avocado	Dinner salad and 8 oz of lean and clean protein. Choose organic and consider plant-based.

DAY 3
Resume healthy diet

Here are some specific recommendations to support a 10-day detox diet:

- Reduce calorie intake to approximately 1,200 calories per day to safely release stored toxins.
- Drink fresh vegetable juice. At least 8-12 ounces per day. If you can add one lemon to the mix it would be awesome as lemons contain incredible compounds that promote detoxification.
- If you elect to do a juice fast, make it for only 3 days out of the ten and do so in the middle of the cleanse to ease your way into and out of it.
- Include these foods during the cleanse as they contain the nutrients your body needs to produce and activate the dozens of enzymes involved in the various phases of detoxification:
  - Beets, celery, and carrots.
  - Cabbage-family vegetables such as broccoli, kale, Brussels sprouts, and cabbage.
  - Green foods like green leafy salads, wheat grass juice, dehydrated barley grass juice, chlorella, and spirulina.
- Again, follow the guidelines above for supplementation to support detoxification.

Longevity Lifestyle Tune-up #4—Boost the Dietary Intake of Antioxidants

One of my key dietary recommendations is to consume a "rainbow" diet. And, of course, I am not talking about eating more Skittles, Fruity Pebbles, or M&Ms. My recommendation is all about the need to focus on an increased intake of colorful fruits and vegetables. Regularly consuming colorful fruit and vegetables—red, orange, yellow, green, blue, and purple—provides the body the full spectrum of pigments with powerful antioxidant effects as well as the nutrients it needs for detoxification and protection against disease.

Fruits and vegetables are so important in the battle against cancer that some experts have said that cancer is a result of a "maladaptation" over time to a reduced level of intake of fruits and vegetables. As a study published in the medical journal *Cancer Causes and Control* put it, "Vegetables and fruit contain the anticarcinogenic cocktail to which we are adapted. We abandon it at our peril."

It is now well accepted that fruits and vegetable consumption is critical in the battle against cancer, but that was not always the case. I remember when I first started studying nutrition in the late 1970s that the American Cancer Society claimed there was no link between diet and most cancers. Then, in 1982 the National Academy of Sciences of the United States published a report on diet and cancer, emphasizing the importance of fruits and vegetables. The value of adding citrus fruits, carotene-rich fruits and vegetables, and cruciferous vegetables to the diet for reducing the risk of cancer was specifically highlighted.

This scientific view was extended to consumers in a 1989 a report from the National Academy of Sciences on diet and health recommended that Americans consume 5 or more servings of fruits and vegetables daily for reducing the risk of both cancer and heart disease. The Five-a-Day program was developed as a tool to increase public awareness of the health benefits of fruits and vegetable consumption. Has it been successful? Not really as surveys still show most Americans come nowhere near this level of intake.

We now know that 5 servings per day of fruits and vegetables is nowhere near the ideal. In the 2010 Dietary Guidelines for Americans it was recommended, based on a 2,000-calorie diet, that people should eat at least 9 servings of fruits and vegetables per day, or more precisely, 4 servings of fruits and 5 servings of vegetables. (Note: I recommend 7 servings of vegetables and 2 servings of fruit.)

Also, in 2010, a study found that the average consumption of fruits and vegetables in the United States is only 3.6 servings of fruits and vegetables (1.4 servings of fruits and 2.2 servings of vegetables) per person per day. It is even worse if the study would have eliminated commercial fruit juice and potatoes from the tally. The bottom line is that most Americans are not getting anywhere near the level of high-quality fruit and vegetables in their diet. Again, I recommend hitting the goal of 7 servings of vegetables and 2-3 servings of fruit each day. A serving is loosely defined as 1 cup uncooked or ½ cup cooked vegetable or fruit. This goal is easily reached with a little thought and effort.

Easy tips to reach your ten-a-day goal

- Buy many kinds of fruits and vegetables when you shop, so you have plenty of choices.
- Stock up on frozen vegetables for easy cooking so that you always have a vegetable dish with every dinner.
- Use the fruits and vegetables that go bad quickly (peaches, asparagus) first. Save hardier varieties (apples, acorn squash) or frozen goods for later in the week.
- Keep fruits and vegetables where you can see them. The more often you see them, the more likely you are to eat them.
- Keep a bowl of cut-up vegetables on the top shelf of the refrigerator.
- Make up a big tossed salad with several kinds of greens, cherry tomatoes, cut up carrots, red pepper, broccoli, scallions and

sprouts. Refrigerate in a large glass bowl with an airtight lid, so a delicious mixed salad will be ready to enjoy for several days.

- Keep a fruit bowl on your kitchen counter, table, or desk at work.
- Treat yourself to a fruit sundae. Top a bowl full of your favorite cut up fruits with vanilla yogurt, shredded coconut and a handful of nuts.
- Pack a piece of fruit or some cut-up vegetables in your briefcase or backpack; carry moist towelettes for easy cleanup.
- Add fruits and vegetables to lunch by having them in soup, salad, or cut-up raw.
- Use thinly sliced pears or apples in your next omelet.
- At dinner, serve steamed or microwaved vegetables.
- Increase portions when you serve vegetables. One easy way of doing so is adding fresh greens such as Swiss chard, collards or beet greens to stir fries.
- Choose fresh fruit for dessert. For a special dessert, try a fruit parfait with low-fat yogurt or sherbet topped with lots of berries.
- Add extra varieties of vegetables when you prepare soups, sauces, and casseroles (for example, add grated carrots and zucchinis to spaghetti sauce).
- Take advantage of salad bars, which offer ready-to-eat raw vegetables and fruits and prepared salads made with fruits and vegetables.
- Use vegetable-based sauces such as marinara sauce and juices such as low sodium v-8 or tomato juice.
- Freeze lots of berries. They make a great summer replacement for ice cream, popsicles and other sugary foods.

Table 4.1 - Examples of Anticancer Phytochemicals

Phytochemical	Actions	Examples of Sources
Carotenes	Antioxidants Enhance immune functions	Dark-colored vegetables such as carrots, squash, spinach, kale, tomatoes, yams and sweet potatoes; fruits such as cantaloupe, apricots, and citrus fruit
Coumarin	Antitumor properties Enhance immune functions Stimulate antioxidant mechanisms	Carrots, celery, fennel, beets, citrus fruits
Dithiolthiones, glucosinolates, and thiocyanates	Block cancer-causing compounds from damaging cells Enhance detoxification	Cabbage family vegetables—broccoli, Brussels sprouts, kale, etc.
Flavonoids	Antioxidants Direct antitumor effects Immune enhancing properties	Fruits, particularly darker fruits such as berries, cherries, and citrus fruits; also tomatoes, peppers, and greens; legumes
Isoflavonoids	Block estrogen receptors	Soy and other legumes
Lignans	Antioxidants Modulate hormone receptors	Flax seed and flax seed oil; whole grains, nuts, and seeds.
Limonoids	Enhance detoxification Block carcinogens	Citrus fruits, celery
Polyphenols	Antioxidants Block carcinogen formation Modulate hormone receptors	Green tea, chocolate, berries
Sterols	Block production of carcinogens Modulate hormone receptors	Soy, nuts, seeds

CHAPTER 5:

Tuning Up Your Metabolism

The term *metabolism* refers to all the chemical processes that take place in your body. Strictly speaking, everything I talk about in this book—digestion, detoxification, activity in the immune system, and so on—is all part of your metabolism. In this chapter, though, I'll focus mainly on the ways your body produces and uses energy

Each of us has a different rate of metabolism. Whatever your starting point, tuning up your metabolism will help you use energy more efficiently (This means you spend less energy to achieve the same level of function). A metabolic tune-up provides many benefits. You'll feel better, have more pep, control your weight, and sleep more soundly.

Understanding Your Basal Metabolic Rate

The rate at which these basic functions use energy when you are awake but not moving is known as the basal metabolic rate, or BMR. The BMR is sometimes referred to as the "energy cost of living." To calculate your approximate basal metabolism rate, determine your weight in kilograms.

Divide the number of pounds you weigh by 2.2. If you are a man, the result is your hourly BMR.

Example: John weighs 176 pounds (80 kilograms). His BMR is 80, which means he burns up 80 calories an hour, or 1920 calories per day, just staying alive. If you are a woman, you need to take an additional step. Multiple your weight in kilograms by 0.9. The result is your hourly Breamed: Mary weighs 121 pounds, or 55 kilograms. Her BMR is about 50 (55 x 0.9), which means she needs to consume at least 1200 calories per day to fuel her basic body functions.

People who do not get exercise spend about three fourths of their energy supply just maintaining their BMR. Any type of movement—getting up out of a chair, typing on a keyboard, scratching your nose—increases your energy expenditure. The more effort required, the faster the rate at which you use up energy. Even a few seconds of very intense activity can significantly increase your metabolic output. One reason for this increase is that skeletal muscles make up nearly half of your body's mass, and so they consume a proportionate amount of energy. When you exercise vigorously, even for only a few minutes, your metabolic rate increases to fifteen to twenty times normal. The rate remains high for several hours afterwards.

Table 5.1: Typical Energy Expenditure (kilocalories per hour)

Activity	Man (150 pounds)	Woman (120 pounds)
Sleeping	65	50
Sitting quietly	75	60
Walking	350	300
Cycling	450	350
Gardening	550	450
Jogging	600	450
Swimming	700	550
Running	900	700

Exercise raises your metabolic rate, not just during your workout but for a period of time afterwards. The impact on your metabolism depends on how intensely you exercise. A light workout might help you burn another five or ten calories after the session ends, while a moderate workout will use up another twelve to thirty-five. In contrast, strenuous exercise can increase post-exercise energy burning by up to 180 calories.

Factors Affecting BMR

Your BMR depends on many factors: the quantity and quality of food you eat (certain foods require more energy to digest than others, eating more food slows metabolism), adequate supplies of water and oxygen, the amount of heat your body produces. Genes play a major part in determining the BMR. Remember the concept of biochemical individuality: Each of us has a different energy requirement. Some people burn more calories to maintain body temperature and weight; others burn fewer calories to get the same result. Other important factors are:

- The body's general size and shape. As the ratio of body surface area to body volume increases, so does the rate of heat loss. The metabolism must work harder to make up for the lost heat. For this reason, a person who weighs 150 pounds and is five feet tall will have a lower BMR than one who weighs the same but who is six feet tall.

- The proportion of muscle (lean) tissue compared to fat tissue. Even at rest, muscles use up energy at a faster pace just to stay alive. The more muscle you have, the higher your energy needs. Build muscle!

- Gender. As a rule, women have proportionately more body fat and less lean tissue than men. Because of this, their BMR is five to ten percent lower.

- Age. As we get older, our muscle mass tends to decrease. This is partly due to natural body changes over time, but it is also the result of a decline in activity. Many older people put on weight because they do not decrease their calorie intake to compensate for their slowing metabolism.

- Stress. Physical or emotional stress activates the body's energy-producing system, known as the "fight or flight response," causing the BMR to soar. The longer stress continues, the more rapidly your body uses up its energy supply. This, in turn, leads to deep fatigue and leaves you vulnerable to infections and other illnesses.

- Growth rate. We need extra energy during growth periods, which is one reason why babies feed so often and why teenagers seem to be ravenously hungry all the time. During pregnancy and while breastfeeding, a mother's energy requirement increases by perhaps fifty percent, because she is sharing her body's energy supply with her developing baby.

- Environmental temperature. Your body works hard to maintain a steady temperature. To keep cool, people who live and work in tropical climates use about twenty percent more energy during the day than people in a temperate climate. Likewise, people in cold climates burn more energy to keep warm.

- Certain drugs, especially stimulants such as caffeine, nicotine, or amphetamines.

- Illness. If you develop an infection, your body's metabolism gears up to fight off the invading microbe. For each degree your body temperature rises, your BMR increases by ten to fifteen percent. Overall, an illness can increase your resting energy expenditure by up to forty percent. Recovery from surgery pushes the rate higher by a whopping fifty percent.

A NEAT Way to Boost Metabolism

In addition to exercise, increasing what is referred to as non-exercise activity thermogenesis or NEAT can also help with both boosting the metabolism and weight loss. Under the direction of James Levine, M.D., the Mayo Clinic conducted the most extensive investigation of NEAT and really believe it is an important missing link in the understanding of metabolism in overweight and obese people.

It is common sense that some people burn more calories than others in their daily occupation or activities of daily living. However, these Mayo Clinic researchers have discovered that there is a fundamental difference between normal weight and obese subjects in terms of how much energy they expend through NEAT in a given day.

Dr. Levine and his colleagues have shown that lean and obese individuals are different in the energy dedicated to the maintenance of posture, activities of daily living, and even fidgeting. For example, a person of normal weight typically sits 150 fewer minutes each day and burns 350 more calories per day from the collective impact of numerous small activities and movements. Burning 350 calories per day is equivalent to about 40 lbs. of fat in one year so this may be a very important factor in long-term weight control. Although this difference may be genetically preprogrammed to some extent, it can certainly be modified with some effort.

The Mayo Clinic researchers point out that long-term weight control may be easier to maintain by focusing more on increasing NEAT than by planned exercise. Certainly both are important, but the potential of NEAT is quite extraordinary. For instance, Dr. Levine's lab has set up a model office where workers each stand on treadmill with a special computer stand that allows them to type, talk on the phone and conduct their daily work while they walk at only .7 miles per hour.

People report that it is easy to get used to this very slow pace and they actually experience less fatigue, increased mental clarity and better work performance. Walking in this way burns an extra 100-150 calories per hour or up to 1000 calories per day! This is as many calories as an elite athlete might burn when training for an Olympic event.

Although the idea of treadmill desks or recumbent bikes built into computer workstations may be in our future, there are many things we can do to increase the calories we expend through NEAT. Increasing the amount of unstructured activity in your daily routine can potentially help you achieve a healthful weight as effectively as working out at the gym:

- Get out of your chair. Standing and doing nothing burns about two calories per minute, compared with one calorie for sitting and doing nothing. Stretch frequently while you stand to increase the calorie expenditure even further.
- Change your work environment. Although a treadmill with attached computer may not be practical, an adjustable-height worktable that allows you to stand and work is easy to find and is a surprisingly comfortable way to work for at least part of your day.
- Add activity wherever you can. Walk whenever you can, take the stairs instead of the elevator, do the dishes, work in the yard, etc. Remember, every little bit of activity adds to you daily calorie burn.
- Pace while handling phone calls. Use a headset or airbuds and pace when you talk on the phone. One minute of pacing burns three or more calories. Remember, every calorie burned is one less stored.

In general, sit rather than lie down, stand rather than sit, pace rather than stand, walk rather than pace. Even though the calories burned per hour from these kind of activities seems small, over days, months and years it can amount to hundreds of thousands of calories and many pounds of fat.

Why Most Diets Don't Work

If you've been struggling to lose weight on a low-calorie diet, I have an important tip for you: Eat more. Yes, in order to lose weight, you choose to eat well while reducing the number of calories, but you must eat to feed your metabolism. Instead of choosing high-calorie foods loaded with fats and sugars, choose high-fiber, low-calorie foods. These foods can help you achieve long-term results. What are high-fiber, low calorie foods? Vegetables, legumes (beans), most fruits, and whole grains.

The very act of eating and digestion requires a significant amount of energy. Eating breakfast, for example, can boost your resting metabolism rate by ten percent or more. On the other hand, dieting or fasting will cause your total energy expenditure to fall.

The biggest mistake people make when trying to lose weight is trying to starve themselves thin. It just doesn't work that way. Restricting food intake feeds into a phenomenon that too many Americans know too well - the yo-yo effect. They lose weight only to put it right back on and then some. When the body is not fed properly, it feels that it is starving. The result: metabolism will slow down and less fat will be burned. It is a natural response that our bodies have developed to help us survive famine and starvation. Even if a person is able to lose some weight initially, most often they will put it right back on and then some.

Diets do not work if the focus is on restricting food intake rather than on enhancing metabolism. If you need to get your weight under control, then your first step should be tuning up your metabolism.

The Thyroid: The Master Gland of Metabolism

The first step in tuning up metabolism is making sure the thyroid gland is functioning properly. The thyroid gland is located in the front of the neck below the voice box. It is just about the same size and shape—and is in the same location—as a small bow tie. The thyroid secretes two hormones that are crucial for regulating metabolism: triiodothyronine (T_3) and thyroxine (T_4). The numbers refer to the numbers of iodine atoms each molecule of hormone contains. T_4 is kind of a "prohormone" as it is not as potent as T_3. T_4 is the major thyroid in the blood and is delivered to cells where it can be converted into the more potent T_3 You need to have the right level and balance of these hormones to be healthy and have a good metabolism. Too little thyroid hormone causes BMR to plummet, leading to low body temperature, reduced heart rate, low blood pressure, intolerance to cold, decreased appetite, and weight gain. Low levels affect the brain and nervous system, causing such symptoms as depression, unusual sensations in the arms and legs, and lack of concentration. Because the digestive system slows down, constipation may result. The skin becomes pale, thick, and dry. The hair becomes course and thin, while the nails become hard and thick. In some cases, people who lack sufficient thyroid hormones become infertile.

Too much thyroid hormone can be equally troublesome but in opposite ways. The metabolism rate kicks into high gear, resulting in high body temperature, inability to tolerate heat, increased appetite, weight loss, and muscle weakness and atrophy. Rapid heartbeat and high blood pressure are common, posing a risk of heart failure. Effects on the brain and nerves include irritability, restlessness, insomnia, and bulging eyes. An overstimulated digestive system can lead to diarrhea and loss of appetite. The skin becomes flushed, thin, and moist, and the nails become soft and thin. Men often lose their ability to get an erection.

Assessing Thyroid Function

Circle the number that best describes the intensity of your symptoms on the following scale:

0 = I do not experience this symptom
1 = Mild
2 = Moderate
3 = Severe

Some items are scored as either Yes or No. When adding your total, score 0 for each No answer and 10 for each Yes.

1.	Thick skin and fingernails	0	1	2	3
2.	Dry skin	0	1	2	3
3.	Sensitive to the cold	0	1	2	3

		0	1	2	3
4.	Cold hands and feet	0	1	2	3
5.	Excessive menstrual bleeding	0	1	2	3
6.	Chronic fatigue	0	1	2	3
7.	Trouble waking up in the morning	0	1	2	3
8.	Depressed, apathetic	0	1	2	3
9.	Low sex drive	0	1	2	3
10.	Putty-like, wrinkled skin	0	1	2	3
11.	Sugar causes irritability and mood swings	0	1	2	3
12.	Premenstrual tension	0	1	2	3
13.	Constipation	0	1	2	3
14.	Thinning or loss of outside portion of eyebrow	0	1	2	3
15.	Gain weight easily	0	1	2	3
16.	Anemia unaffected by iron	0	1	2	3
17.	Slow reflexes	0	1	2	3
18.	Axillary (armpit) temperature below 97.6°F	NO	YES		
19.	Infertility	NO	YES		

TOTAL _____

Scoring

- 9 or more: High Priority
- 5-8: Moderate Priority
- 1-4: Low Priority

Thyroid Tune-Up

A low level of thyroid hormone is a common problem, affecting perhaps one out of five women and a smaller percentage of men. If your thyroid activity is reduced, your body may not respond as well as it should to nutritional or supplemental strategies. For that reason, a crucial step in tuning up your metabolism is to make sure your thyroid is working properly.

Your doctor can conduct blood tests that measure thyroid hormone levels. The test assesses the quantity of T_4 and T_3 hormones and determines how well the body's cells respond to the hormones. It also measures quantities of thyroid stimulating hormone (TSH), a chemical released by the pituitary gland. High levels of TSH indicate that the pituitary is in overdrive, frantically trying to signal the thyroid to step up its hormone output. However, in milder cases of thyroid hormone insufficiency, the blood test may show that hormone levels are within "normal" ranges, even if the person is experiencing symptoms. I usually suggest thyroid hormone therapy if the TSH value is greater than 2.5 IU/ml (International Units per milliliter) or if there are low levels of either T4 or T3. This recommendation is especially valid for patients suffering from depression—usually the first sign of low thyroid function.

Before rushing off to your doctor for a blood test, however, I suggest that you first determine your basal body temperature. Your body temperature reflects your metabolic rate, a rate that in turn is largely determined by thyroid hormone activity. When your thyroid is out of whack, your temperature often falls. Many experts agree that the basal body temperature is the most sensitive functional test of thyroid function. The test is simple: all you need is a thermometer.

Taking Your Basal Body Temperature

1. Plan to take the test first thing in the morning after you wake up, because it's important to measure temperature after you have had adequate rest.
2. Before going to sleep, shake down the thermometer to below the 95-degree mark and place it by your bed.
3. Immediately upon waking, place the thermometer in your armpit for a full 10 minutes if using a conventional thermometer (newer digital thermometers can give almost

immediate results). Hold your elbow close to your side to keep the thermometer in place.

4. Move as little as possible. Lying and resting with your eyes closed is best. Do not get up until the full 10 minutes have passed.

5. After 10 minutes, read and record the temperature and date.

6. Repeat the test for least three mornings (preferably at the same time of day). Give the information to your physician.

Note: Menstruating women must perform the test on the second, third, and fourth days of menstruation. Men and postmenopausal women can perform the test at any time.

Your basal body temperature, measured in the armpit, should be lower than the normal "under-the-tongue" temperature of 98.6 degrees Fahrenheit. The underarm temperature is more reflective of basal body temperature than the under-the-tongue method. The typical basal range is between 97.6 and 98.2 degrees. Lower than that may indicate a problem with hypothyroidism. If your basal body temperature is below 97.2 degrees, I recommend seeing your doctor for the blood test, playing close attention to the TSH level. If the temperature is between 97.2 and 97.6 degrees, try alternative methods to raise thyroid function (discussed below). I urge anyone with hypothyroidism, even mild cases, to take the appropriate steps to correct the problem. An underlying state of low thyroid function means that virtually every cell of your body is under performing. Conversely, restoring proper thyroid hormone levels can dramatically increase the metabolism within your cells.

Dealing with Low Thyroid

Severe hypothyroidism requires the use of supplemental thyroid hormone—available only by prescription. The medical treatment of most cases of low thyroid hormone levels involves the use of either desiccated thyroid (the dried form of natural thyroid from pork) or bioidentical synthetic versions of T_4 (for example, Synthroid).

Mild or subclinical hypothyroidism may respond to nutritional and herbal support. An important dietary recommendation is to avoid goitrogens. Some foods, especially when eaten raw, contain substances that interfere with your body's ability to absorb and use iodine. Because these foods can contribute to the risk of goiter, they are classified as goitrogens. Examples include turnips, cabbage, mustard, cassava root, soybean, peanuts, pine nuts, and millet. Because these foods contain many other valuable nutrients, I recommend that you avoid them only if low thyroid hormone levels are a problem for you. Cooking usually inactivates goitrogens, so don't be concerned about these items in your diet if you serve them cooked. Also, the BIG concern over soy isoflavones inhibiting thyroid function appears to be overstated as recent studies have shown no adverse effect on thyroid function.

Like other glands, the thyroid has special nutritional needs. Here are some key nutrients required for proper thyroid function:

- *Iodine.* The thyroid gland needs iodine to make its hormones. In fact, iodine's only role in your body is in making thyroid hormones. Too little iodine can cause impaired thyroid function, while too much iodine can actually interfere with the thyroid's ability to produce hormones. The dosage range for iodine supplementation is 300 to 400 mcg per day. Read the labels on your multivitamin supplement and on any thyroid preparations you are taking. Keep your intake of iodized salt to a bare minimum. Make sure that your total amount of iodine intake is within the recommended range—not too low or too high.

- *Tyrosine.* The other key ingredient in thyroid hormones is the amino acid tyrosine. Taking L-tyrosine alone or as a component as a nutritional supplement at a dosage of 250 to 500 mg daily may enhance thyroid function.

- *Copper and manganese*—low levels of these trace can contribute to hypothyroidism. Recommended levels for thyroid support are 500 to 1000 mcg daily.

- *Zinc and the vitamins A, B_2, B_3, B_6, C, and E* - A deficiency in any of these could cause or contribute to hypothyroidism. This is of special concern for people over the age of 65. Eating a balanced diet and taking a multiple vitamin and mineral supplement will ensure that you get adequate levels.

- *Exercise.* By speeding up your metabolism, exercise stimulates the thyroid gland to secrete hormones. Exercise also makes your other tissues more sensitive to the effects of thyroid hormones. Many of the general health benefits resulting from exercise are in fact directly due to its impact on thyroid function. Exercise is especially important if you are overweight and following a reduced-calorie diet, because exercise counteracts the drop in metabolic rate that occurs when you diet.

Case Study: More than a Weight-loss Problem

Danielle, age thirty seven, is the manager of a local flower shop. At five feet seven inches tall, she weighs 155 pounds—about twenty more than is healthy for her height and weight. She came to see me because of her depression. "I feel like crying all the time," she said. She also complained of fatigue and frustration over the fact that, no matter what she tried, she couldn't lose those twenty excess pounds. When I saw her, I noticed that the back of her arms and elbows were extremely dry. Tellingly, she was missing the outer third of her eyebrow. I commented that her skin looked red and irritated. "I itch like mad," she said. The problem—an allergic reaction called hives—had started about six months before. "Maybe it's some new plant in the shop," she mused. She had been taking constant doses of antihistamines to keep the hives under control. Her other symptoms had started four years earlier, after the birth of her second child.

Normally, when a patient presents with severe hives, I suspect allergies to foods or food additives. I suggested

Danielle undergo the standard food allergy study. I also felt that hypothyroidism was a likely diagnosis, especially when I saw that she had scored high on almost every question on the thyroid survey. Her dry skin and thinning eyebrows were other clues to hypothyroidism.

I ordered blood tests to measure her thyroid hormone levels (among other things) and to evaluate for food allergies. The results clearly showed she was suffering from hypothyroidism— her TSH was significantly higher than normal. I also told her to take her basal body temperature on the second and third day of her upcoming period. When she reported that her first basal body temperature reading was 96.2 degrees F, the diagnosis was confirmed. I had her start with one grain (65 mg) of USP thyroid daily.

Two weeks later Danielle came back to the office so we could discuss the results of her food allergy tests. To my surprise, she told me that her hives had cleared up. There are reports in the medical literature of patients whose allergic skin conditions clear up during thyroid hormone therapy, but I had not expected such treatment would help her. Happily, I was wrong. Still, Danielle's food allergy results indicated a significant allergy to milk, wheat, and peanuts. I instructed her to avoid these foods entirely.

After six weeks, during a routine recheck, Danielle's thyroid hormone levels were perfect, and her basal body temperature was up to 97.2 degrees F. Her hives vanished, her energy levels soared, her mood was brighter, and her crying spells had disappeared.

When I saw Danielle three months later, she was noticeably thinner. She had finally gotten rid of those extra pounds. I lowered her thyroid to ½ grain per day based upon her blood work. I will continue to monitor the dosage based upon half-yearly blood tests.

Blood Sugar Control

The body strives to maintains blood sugar levels within a narrow range through the coordinated effort of several glands and their hormones. If these control mechanisms are disrupted, hypoglycemia (low blood sugar) or diabetes (high blood sugar) may result. Often these control mechanisms are stressed through improper diet and lifestyle. As a result, poor blood sugar control is a common problem.

Assessing Blood Sugar Control

Circle the number that best describes the intensity of your symptoms on the following scale:

0 = I do not experience this symptom

1 = Mild

2 = Moderate

3 = Severe

Some items are scored as either Yes or No. When adding your total, score 0 for each No answer and 10 for each Yes.

A: Hypoglycemia

1.	Crave sweets	0	1	2	3
2.	Headaches relieved by eating sweets or alcohol	0	1	2	3
3.	Feel shaky	0	1	2	3
4.	Irritable if a meal is missed	0	1	2	3
5.	Wake up in middle of night craving sweets	0	1	2	3
6.	Feel tired or weak if a meal is missed	0	1	2	3
7.	Heart palpitations after eating sweets	0	1	2	3
8.	Tend to be impatient, moody, nervous	0	1	2	3
9.	Feel tired 1 to 3 hours after eating	0	1	2	3
10.	Calmer after eating	0	1	2	3

TOTAL _____

Scoring
- 12 or more: High Priority
- 6-11: Moderate Priority
- 1-5: Low Priority

B: Insulin resistance and/or type 2 diabetes

1.	Overweight	0	1	2	3
2.	Crave sweets, but eating sweets does not relieve craving	0	1	2	3
3.	Your waist measurement is larger than your hips	NO	YES		
4.	Elevated C-reactive protein	NO	YES		
5.	Waist is >35 inches in a woman and >40 inches in a man	NO	YES		
6.	Fasting blood sugar level greater than 125 mg/dl	NO	YES		
7.	Diagnosed with type 2 diabetes	NO	YES		

TOTAL _____

Scoring
- 10 or more: High Priority
- 3-9: Moderate Priority
- 1-4: Low Priority

For most people with hypoglycemia, the only step needed is to eliminate all refined carbohydrates from the diet, as well as food choices with a high glycemic load (discussed below). Foods rich in soluble fiber such as legumes and low-glycemic vegetables should be consumed regularly. Frequent, small meals may be more effective in stabilizing blood sugar levels. A deficiency in the trace mineral chromium can contribute to problems with blood sugar control. Your body needs chromium to use insulin effectively to control blood sugar levels. , For either hypoglycemia or diabetes, I recommend taking chromium in the form of either chromium picolinate or chromium polynicotinate. Both forms are well absorbed by the body. The daily dose is 200 to 400 mcg.

Research over the past 50 years has provided an ever-increasing amount of information concerning the roles that refined carbohydrates and faulty blood sugar control play in many disease processes. The term *metabolic syndrome* is used to describe a set of cardiovascular risk factors including blood sugar disturbances, high blood cholesterol and triglyceride levels, elevated blood pressure, and abdominal obesity. There is little doubt about that the key contributor the metabolic syndrome is an elevated intake of refined carbohydrates. An increased intake of high glycemic foods leads first to hypoglycemia and later to type 2 diabetes.

Insulin resistance is closely tied to abdominal obesity and type 2 diabetes. If your waist circumference is larger than your hips, there is an extremely strong likelihood that you suffer from insulin resistance. As the number and size of fat cells increase, they lead to a reduction in the secretion of compounds that promote insulin action, including a novel protein produced by fat cells known as adiponectin. Making matters even worse is that there is also an increase in the secretion of a substance known as resistin that dampens the effect of insulin.

How Do You Know if You Have Insulin Resistance?

One of the most useful clinical determinants of insulin resistance is simply measuring the waist to hip ratio. However, if the waist circumference for a man is greater than 40 inches, and for a woman greater than 30 inches, there is no need to do any further calculation because this measurement alone has been shown to be a major risk factor for both CVD and type 2 diabetes, two of the biggest consequences of insulin resistance, as well as high blood pressure and gout. A waist to hip ratio above 1.0 for men and above 0.8 for women is highly predictive of insulin resistance. To determine your waist to hip ratio,

1. Measure the circumference of your waist:_____
2. Measure the circumference of your hips:_____
3. Divide the waist measurement by the hip measurement:
    Waist/Hip _____. This is your waist/hip ratio.

How Big is the Problem of Insulin Resistance?

Here are some sobering facts: current estimates are that eight out of 10 adults in the United States are overweight, with about half of these people, 40% of our adult population, meeting the criteria of being obese. Insulin resistance and its consequences are crippling our health care systems and our productivity. Each year obesity-related conditions alone cost over $100 billion and cause an estimated 300,000 premature deaths in the U.S., making a very strong case that the obesity epidemic is the most significant threat to the future of the United States, as well as other nations.

Obese individuals have an average life expectancy 5–7 years shorter than that of normal-weight individuals, with a greater relative risk for mortality associated with a greater degree of obesity. Most of the increased risk for mortality is due to CVD, because obesity carries with it a tremendous risk for type 2 diabetes, elevated cholesterol levels, high blood pressure, and other risk factors for atherosclerosis (hardening of the arteries). The estimated annual medical spending due to overweight and obesity is now estimated at over $200 billion.

In addition to the epidemic of obesity there is a parallel epidemic of type 2 diabetes. Currently, 20 million Americans meet the criteria for type 2 diabetes and another 80 million suffer from prediabetes—a condition characterized by insulin resistance—and/or metabolic syndrome.

Insulin Resistance and Cardiovascular Disease

Insulin resistance is also linked to an increased risk for cardiovascular disease, cancer, and Alzheimer's disease. These are major killers. So, improving insulin action is critical to fight off these diseases and live longer. Let's take a look at how insulin resistance impacts cardiovascular disease:

- Elevated blood sugar levels are associated with increased attachment of glucose to receptor proteins, leading to loss of key feedback mechanisms. For example, if the receptor for low-density lipoprotein cholesterol (LDL; "bad" cholesterol) on the surface of a liver cell becomes damaged by the attachment of glucose, the liver cell does not get the feedback message that there is plenty of cholesterol. In fact, without the feedback the liver cell thinks that it needs to make more cholesterol.

- Elevated levels of blood sugar are also associated with increased oxidative stress leading to damage to LDL, as well as adding fuel to the fire of silent inflammation. In fact, insulin resistance is the key factor in causing silent inflammation and high levels of C-reactive protein (CRP), a blood marker of inflammation. Much of the inflammatory effect of insulin resistance is due to its negative effects on the endothelium, the lining of the blood vessel wall.

- Since there is a relative deficiency of glucose within cells because of insulin resistance, even though blood sugar levels are high, the pancreas begins dumping larger quantities of insulin into the blood. Higher blood insulin levels are now a well-established risk factor for heart disease. A high level of insulin in the blood promotes atherosclerosis by several mechanisms, including stimulating smooth muscle cell proliferation in the arterial wall, leading to thickening and stiffness of the arterial wall as well as narrowing of the artery.

- Insulin resistance is associated with high blood pressure. It not only contributes to more rigid and constricted blood vessels, it causes retention of sodium and water from the kidneys, which then leads to high blood pressure.

- Insulin resistance promotes greater fat breakdown, leading to a characteristic blood lipid pattern of elevated LDL and triglycerides with lower levels of high-density lipoprotein cholesterol (HDL; "good" cholesterol). In normal individuals, one of the functions of insulin is to suppress the breakdown of fat from the fat cells into the bloodstream. With insulin resistance this effect is blocked, leading to an exaggerated breakdown of fat from the fat cells and the release of free fatty acids into the blood. The liver takes up these free fatty acids and converts them into triglycerides in the form of very-low-density lipoprotein (VLDL), which ultimately lowers HDL levels. Insulin resistance also increases the formation of the smaller, denser LDL that is really damaging to arteries.
- Insulin resistance greatly increases the risk for clot formation. In addition, insulin resistance blocks the action of tissue plasminogen activator, a clot-busting compound produced by the cells that line the artery.
- Insulin resistance is associated with increased levels of the adrenal hormone cortisol.

Improving Insulin Sensitivity

Improving insulin sensitivity and blood sugar control is a major health goal for everyone, but even more so if someone has a goal of weight loss, reduction of risk factors for CVD, or prevention/treatment of type 2 diabetes. Improvement is most successfully done with a combination of lifestyle changes, such as increasing physical activity and improving diet and nutrition, and targeted nutritional supplementation.

Obviously, dietary carbohydrates play a central role in the cause, prevention, and treatment of insulin resistance and type 2 diabetes. In an effort to label carbohydrate sources as good or bad, one useful tool is the glycemic index (GI). It is a numerical scale used to indicate how fast and how high a particular food raises blood glucose levels compared with glucose. Refined sugars, white flour products, and other sources of simple sugars are quickly absorbed into the bloodstream, causing a rapid rise in blood sugar, severely stressing blood sugar control. It is important to avoid junk foods and pay attention to the GI of the food you eat.

Studies have shown that an elevated after-meal blood sugar level is a greater risk factor for heart disease that abnormal fasting plasma glucose. So even if you do not have insulin resistance it is critical to avoid high blood sugar levels at any time to prevent CVD.

Table 5.2 - Classifications of Foods by Glycemic Index Scores

Fruits and Non-starchy Vegetables			
Very High	High	Medium	Low
None	Bananas	Cantaloupe	Apples
	Raisins	Grapes	Apricots
	Beets	Oranges	Asparagus
		Orange juice	Broccoli
		Peaches	Brussels sprouts
		Pineapples	Cauliflower
		Watermelon	Celery
			Cherries
			Cucumbers
			Grapefruit
			Green beans
			Green peppers
			Lettuce
			Mushrooms
			Onions
			Plums
			Spinach

			Strawberries
			Tomatoes
			Zucchini

Grains, Nuts, Legumes, and Starchy Vegetables

Very High	High	Medium	Low
Refined sugar and flour products	Bagels	Brown rice	Lentils
Most cold cereals (e.g., Grape Nuts, corn flakes, Raisin Bran, etc.)	Bread (white flour)	Oatmeal	Nuts
Rice cakes	Pasta	Carrots	Seeds
Granola	Corn	Peas	
	Granola bars	Pita bread	
	Kidney beans	Pinto beans	
	Muffins (bran)	Rye bread	
	Potatoes	Whole-grain breads	
	Pretzels	Yams	
	White rice		
	Tortillas		

The GI is quite useful, but since it doesn't tell you how much carbohydrate is in a typical serving of a particular food, another tool is needed. That is where glycemic load comes in. The glycemic load (GL) is a relatively new way to assess the impact of carbohydrate consumption. It takes the glycemic index into account but gives a more complete picture of the effect that a particular food has on blood sugar levels based on how much carbohydrate you actually eat in a serving. A GL of 20 or more is high, a GL of 11–19 inclusive is medium, and a GL of 10 or less is low.

For example, let's take a look at beets, a food with a high GI, but low GL. Although the carbohydrate in beets has a high GI, there isn't a lot of it, so a typical serving of cooked beets has a very low GL, about 5. Thus, as long as you eat a reasonable portion of a low-glycemic-load food, the impact on blood sugar is acceptable, even if the food has a high GI.

Table 5.3 - Examples of Glycemic Index, Glycemic Load, and Insulin Stress Scores of Selected Foods

Food	Glycemic Index	Glycemic Load	Insulin Stress (Glycemic Impact)
Carrots, cooked, ½ cup	49	1.5	Low
Peach, fresh, 1 large	42	3.0	Low
Beets, cooked ½ cup	64	3.0	Low
Watermelon, ½ cup	72	4.0	Low
Whole-wheat bread, 1 slice	69	9.6	Low
Baked potato, medium	93	14	Medium
Brown rice, cooked, 1 cup	50	16	Medium
Banana, raw, 1 medium	55	17.6	Medium
Spaghetti, white, cooked, 1 cup	41	23	High
White rice, cooked, 1 cup	72	26	High

Grape Nuts cereal, ½ cup	71	33	Very high
Soft drinks, 375 ml	68	34.7	Very high

To help you design your diet, I recommend keeping the GL for any three-hour period to less than 20. I have provided a list of the GI, fiber content, and GL of common foods in Appendix B. In essence, foods that are mostly water (e.g., apple or watermelon), fiber (e.g., beet root or carrot), or air (e.g., popcorn) will not cause a steep rise in your blood sugar even if their GI is high, as long as you exercise moderation in portion sizes.

The Importance of Dietary Fiber in Improving Insulin Sensitivity

Population studies, as well as clinical and experimental data, show diabetes to be one of the diseases most clearly related to inadequate dietary fiber intake. Different types of fibers possess different actions. The type of fiber that exerts the most beneficial effects on blood sugar control is the water-soluble form. Particularly good food sources of water-soluble fiber are beans, peas, and other legumes; most vegetables; nuts; seeds; oat bran; citrus fruits; pears; and apples. These types of fiber-rich foods can help to slow down the digestion and absorption of carbohydrates, thereby preventing rapid rises in blood sugar.

A diet focused on non-grain, high-fiber foods, in particular, is associated with increasing the sensitivity of tissues to insulin and improving the uptake of glucose by the muscles, liver, and other tissues, thereby preventing a sustained elevation of blood sugar.

If you have type 2 diabetes or need to lose weight, I also recommend a taking PGX at all meals. PGX is a dietary fiber matrix that I helped develop with Dr. Michael Lyon when I worked at Natural Factors. It is a super soluble fiber in that it is able to bind more water than any other fiber source. It exerts a myriad of health benefits a clinical studies in humans show that it:

- Stabilizes blood sugar levels
- Reduces appetite and promote effective weight loss
- Increases the level of compounds that block the appetite and promote satiety
- Decreases the level of compounds that stimulate overeating
- Reduces after-meal blood glucose levels
- Reduces the GI of any food or beverage
- Increases insulin sensitivity and decreases blood insulin

PGX is available in capsules, but I prefer the granules. Take 2.5 to 5 grams of PGX before meals with 8-12 ounces of water. The granules mix easily in a water bottle or shaker. You can also add PGX to smoothies. I have made PGX a part of my diet for the last 15 years and it has paid huge dividends.

The Importance of Preventing Glycation

If you remember, one of the theories of aging is related to excessive attachment of blood sugar (glucose) molecules to cellular proteins. This process of glycation or glycosylation leads to tremendous disruption of cellular function. For example, cholesterol-carrying proteins that have been glycosylated do not bind to receptors on liver cells that halt the manufacture of cholesterol. As a result, there is a loss of that natural feedback and the liver cell thinks it needs to make more cholesterol because it is not getting the signal to stop.

Excessive glycation also leads to the formation of what are referred to as advanced glycation end-products (AGEs) has many adverse effects: inactivation of enzymes, damaging structural and regulatory proteins, impaired immune function, and increased likelihood for autoimmune diseases. Like free radical damage, AGEs are associated with many chronic degenerative diseases. Diets that promote glycation and poor glucose control lead to accelerated inflammation and cellular aging (inflammaging), obesity, and the development of chronic degenerative diseases like cancer, heart disease, Alzheimer's disease, and macular degeneration.

Obviously, we want to avoid excessive glycation. How is this done? Diet is the key. Keep blood sugar levels under control by consuming a low glycemic diet and if needed use special nutritional factors like PGX or other fiber sources. It is especially important to avoid high after meal elevations in blood sugar. That threshold is less than 140 mg/ml one or two hours after a meal. Diabetics are often told to keep the level below 180 mg/ml, but that is way too high for good health and will lead to excessive glycation.

After meal or post-prandial blood sugar level measurements can be performed by your doctor or you can use an at home glucose monitor. If you suspect insulin resistance or you have type 2 diabetes, make the investment in an at-home glucose monitor. Your health and even your life are at stake if you chronically go over that 140 mg/dl threshold. If you can get the number down most often through diet alone, but if you need additional support that is where PGX can prove very valuable.

Dietary Fat and Insulin Resistance

Dietary fat also plays a central role in insulin sensitivity. The type of dietary fat profile linked to insulin resistance is an abundance of saturated fat from animal foods and trans fatty acids (partially hydrogenated vegetable oils) along with a relative insufficiency of monounsaturated and omega-3 fatty acids. One of the key reasons appears to be the fact that because dietary fat determines cell membrane composition, such a dietary pattern leads to reduced membrane fluidity, which in turn causes reduced insulin binding to receptors on cellular membranes or reduced insulin action, or both.

The key focus is to rely on sources of monounsaturated fats and omega-3 fatty acids. They all improve insulin action. Clinical studies and population-based studies indicate that frequent consumption of monounsaturated fats such as olive oil, raw/ lightly roasted nuts and seeds, nut oils, and omega-3 fatty acids from fish protect against the development of type 2 diabetes. Healthy omega-3 fish include wild salmon, anchovies, sardines, and herring.

One of the most useful foods to reduce the risk of type 2 diabetes is nuts. Studies have shown that consumption of nuts is inversely associated with risk of type 2 diabetes, independent of known risk factors, including age, obesity, family history of diabetes, physical inactivity, smoking, and other dietary factors. In addition to providing beneficial monounsaturated and polyunsaturated fats that improve insulin sensitivity, nuts are also rich in fiber and magnesium and have a low GI. Higher intakes of fiber and magnesium and foods with a low GI have been associated with reduced risk of type 2 diabetes in several population-based studies. Eating mostly raw or lightly roasted fresh nuts and seeds rather than commercially roasted and salted nuts and seeds is advocated.

Summarizing to Keep Things Simple

Here is quick review: the most important dietary strategies for improving insulin sensitivity are (1) avoiding foods that quickly raise blood sugar levels like soft drinks, sources of refined sugar, and overconsumption of carbohydrates; and (2) increasing the amount of soluble dietary fiber, particularly from legumes and vegetables, as well as by supplementing with PGX. If you are trying to lose weight, my suggestion is to avoid grains, pasta, bread, rice, cereal, etc., as doing so will help you reestablish proper insulin sensitivity. Basically, what I recommend is the Mediterranean Diet Pyramid with the breads, pasta, and other starches crossed out. If that seems impossible to you, then it is very important that you exercise moderation in portion sizes with carbohydrate sources and keep your glycemic load for any three-hour period to less than 20.

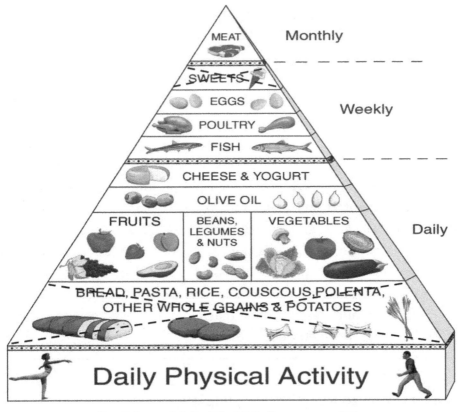

Dr. Murray's Modified Mediterranean Diet

A Key Target to Boost Metabolism

There are a lot of factors that influence metabolism, but there is one enzyme system that has the magical ability to burn fat and turn up our metabolism. The enzyme AMP-activated protein kinase (AMPk) is found inside every cell and serves as a "master regulating switch" in energy metabolism. Overall, the activity of this enzyme plays a major role in determining our body fat composition and especially the amount of visceral "belly" fat that we carry. Its activity is also tied to our life expectancy. When we are young, AMPk is more activate, but as we age the cellular AMPk activation decreases leading to belly (visceral) fat accumulation and loss of muscle mass.

The good news is that there are natural ways to enhance AMPk. Specifically, certain dietary strategies and food components greatly influence AMPk activity in a positive way. Not surprisingly, these natural approaches hold great promise in the goal of near effortless weight loss as a result. In addition, there are many other health benefits associated with activation of AMPk including a longer life.

Table 5.5 - Consequences of Low AMPk Activity
- Accelerated aging
- Chronic inflammation
- High blood cholesterol and triglycerides
- Increased visceral "belly" fat
- Insulin resistance
- Mitochondrial insufficiency and dysfunction
- Brain cell degeneration
- Obesity
- Poor blood sugar control

The first step in increasing AMPk activity is improving insulin sensitivity. When the body starts responding to insulin it leads to fat cells increasing the release of adiponectin and decreasing the release of resistin (discussed above). All of these effects are due to the influence these compounds have on AMPk activity. Adiponectin increases the activation of AMPk, while resistin impairs AMPk activity. So, while adiponectin is associated with improved insulin sensitivity and metabolism, resistin is associated with poor blood sugar control, increased blood lipids, and the development of atherosclerosis.

In addition to improving insulin sensitivity and a higher intake of soluble fiber, there are a number of other dietary factors that activate AMPk that you should take advantage of by including in your diet. Not surprisingly, many foods in the traditional Mediterranean diet and other diets associated with health activate AMPk such as olive oil, garlic, various flavonoids found in fruits and vegetables, and the omega-3 fatty acids EPA and DHA.

Table 5.5 - Factors that Influence AMPk

Inhibitors of AMPk

- Insulin resistance
- High fat diet
- Caloric excess
- Sedentary lifestyle
- Aging

Activators of AMPk

- Intense exercise
- Calorie restriction
- Intermittent fasting
- Thyroid hormone
- Adiponectin
- Dietary factors
  - Highly viscous dietary fiber (e.g., PGX)
  - Good oils
    - Olive oil (and polyphenols)
    - Fish oils (EPA+DHA)
    - Medium chain triglycerides (coconut oil)
  - Various plant pigments (e.g., flavonoids, polyphenols, carotenes, etc.)
    - Anthocyanins (blueberries and other berries)
    - Catechins (green tea)
    - Flavanols (cacao, cocoa, and dark chocolate)
    - Fucoidan (brown seaweed)
    - Genistein (soy)
    - Polymethoxylated flavones (citrus
    - Procyanidolic oligomers (grape seeds)
    - Resveratrol (red wine and Chinese knotwood)

- ○ Numerous spices, herbs, and herbal compounds
  - Berberine (from goldenseal, coptis, etc.)
  - Black pepper
  - Cayenne pepper
  - Cinnamon
  - Garlic and onions
  - Ginger
  - Green coffee bean extract
  - Mint family herbs including basil, oregano, rosemary, sage, and thyme
  - Mulberry leaf
  - Turmeric
- ○ Health-promoting bacteria (especially *Akkermansia muciniphila*)

My Recommendations on Intermittent Fasting

Intermittent fasting refers to various meal timing schedules that cycle between voluntary fasting over a given period and eating. The three methods of intermittent fasting are alternate-day fasting, periodic fasting (e.g., every Sunday or two days fasting per week), and time-restricted feeding. It is interesting to note that it could be interpreted that certain religions employ forms of intermittent fasting exist in their practices, e.g., Vrata in Hinduism, Ramadan fasting (Islam), Yom Kippur fasting and other Jewish fasts (Judaism), Orthodox Christian fasting, Fast Sunday (The Church of Jesus Christ of Latter-day Saints), and Buddhist fasting.

Recently, intermittent fasting has become quite a fad, but I think one form of it can promote health. I like the idea of a restricted feeding window. The intermittent fast will activate AMPk but I think the biggest value for a lot of people is that it promotes a reduced calorie intake. The most popular technique is the 16/8 method whereby a person will fast for 16 hours each day and eat during an 8-hour window. That can be accomplished by skipping breakfast and not eating anything after dinner.

The 16/8 method can be tough, so I modify it a bit from a strict no food intake outside of the window. In particular, I don't like going to sleep hungry. If my weight in the morning when I wake up is above 182 pounds two days in a row, I will employ my modified intermittent fast strategy. I restrict my breakfast to a low-caffeine energy drink (e.g., Bai, Celsius, or just hot or cold green tea) along with my vitamins. I then go workout and will not eat my typical breakfast protein smoothie until at least 9:00 am. I eliminate my mid-morning snack and proceed with my typical daily routine except that I eat a bit earlier dinner at 5:00 or 6:00 pm. Later in the evening I will have my hot cacao brew (recipe given on page 352). I think a later evening snack is 100% O.K. as long as it is not anything that will raise your blood sugar levels. I don't see a problem drinking water, tea, and other non- or low-caloric beverages during the fast. They can help reduce hunger levels. I have found my modified approach is effortless and when needed keeps me in the weight range I like best for me (i.e., between 178-182 lbs.).

The real key to successful intermittent fasting is what you eat during your eating window. Obviously, it doesn't work if you binge on excess calories or unhealthful food. If you employ all of the other principles of healthful eating during your window and intermittent fasting can be very effective.

Additional Recommendations that Help with Weight Loss

The first recommendation is to track your food intake. It can help. In August 2008, a Kaiser Permanente study published in the American Journal of Preventative Medicine found that participants in a weight-loss program lost twice as much weight when they kept a food diary compared with when they did not. Keep track of what you eat as well as your calories burned really helps create awareness and reinforces change.

Though I am not a big fan of strict calorie counting, I do think it is important to have an idea of the general range of calories that you need and consume on average. Calculating your calorie intake has never been easier; your smartphone can do the work for you. There are a number of apps available to choose from. The most popular is probably is Lose It! This free app features a barcode scanner, a recipe builder, and a comprehensive database of foods.

In helping you answer the question, "how many calories should I consume to lose weight?" it is important first to point out that the basic equation for losing weight never changes. In order for you to lose weight, your calorie intake must be less than the calories you burn. This goal can be achieved by decreasing caloric intake or by burning more calories through exercise. Obviously, the best results are achieved by doing both.

To lose one pound, a person must consume 3500 fewer calories than he or she expends. The loss of one pound each week requires a negative caloric balance of 500 calories/day. This can be achieved by decreasing the number of calories ingested by 250 calories a day and by increasing physical activity. And, if you reduce daily caloric intake by 500 calories and burn an additional 500 calories a day with exercise (accomplished by a 45-minute jog, playing tennis for an hour, or a brisk walk for 1.25 hours) that will result in a weight loss of 2 pounds per week. Hence, the most sensible approach to weight loss is to both decrease caloric intake and increase energy expenditure through exercise.

To determine your daily calorie needs there are now a lot of websites with free calculators where you enter your height, weight, sex, age, and activity level to help you determine your approximate calorie needs. That said, here is a simple calculation that I use to create an estimate of daily calorie needs based upon a little different criteria—How much do you want to weigh? Now, take this number and add a zero at the end. For example, if you want to weigh 120 pounds, your number would be 1,200. If it is 180 pounds, the number would 1,800. To reach either weight goal your number reflects the number of calories that I recommend that you consume on a daily basis until you reach your weight goal. Of course, if you burn that extra 500 calories a day through exercise and achieve both targets, you should be losing about 2 pounds per week on average. More than likely, it will be closer to 2.5-3 pounds at the start and slow down a bit as you come closer to your goal. Use your body composition scale to make sure that it is fat loss and adjust either your calorie intake or your exercise level to hit that 2 pounds per week goal.

Once you reach your goal weight, you can try increasing your calorie intake a little bit, but I think it is important to make no big adjustments for at least 3 months. Body weight is closely tied to what is referred to as the "set point"—the weight that a body tries to maintain by regulating the amount of food and calories consumed. The key to overcoming the fat cell's set point is increasing the sensitivity of the fat cells to insulin. We have been focused on that goal. But something else is required to help reset the set point—TIME! If you hit your goal and relax a bit, it will likely lead to rebound eating. You don't want to do that. So, it is critical that once you achieve your goal weight that you keep fighting against the internal mechanisms that want to rob you of your success, especially insulin resistance.

Focus on Body Fat, Not Body Weight

The number on a typical scale represents your total weight, not the relationship of fat to muscle or body composition. While being overweight is a risk factor for early mortality and type 2 diabetes, it is not the critical risk factor. Correctly stated it is increased body fat that is associated with type 2 diabetes, not increased body weight. While there is a strong correlation between body weight and body fat content, people of normal body weight can develop Type 2 diabetes if they have an increased body fat percentage, especially if that excess fat is collecting around the waist or gut. That spare tire accumulation of fat can lead to what is referred to as "metabolic obesity."

To more accurately determine body composition, I recommend using a scale that utilizes a safe, low level amount of electricity to determine body fat percentage, known as bioelectrical impedance. Since fat does not conduct much bioelectricity, a higher degree of impedance of the electrical charge is associated with higher body fat percentage. The most popular scales of this sort are manufactured by Tanita and start as low as $44. The one that I have is the Yunmai Premium Smart Scale. It is a bit more money ($69.95), but I really like the extra features.

Smart scales track your weight, body fat percentage, and BMI, painting a picture of your long-term progress. It wirelessly syncs your stats with your cell phone, and I think that helps with motivation and staying on track.

Ideally, women should strive to keep their body fat percentage below 25 percent and men below 20 percent.

Table 5.6–Body Fat Rating Chart for Use with a Body Fat Measuring Scale

MALE

Age	RISKY	EXCELLENT	GOOD	FAIR	POOR
19-24	<6%	10.8%	14.9%	19.0%	23.3%
25-29	<6%	12.8%	16.5%	20.3%	24.4%
30-34	<6%	14.5%	18.0%	21.5%	25.2%
35-39	<6%	16.1%	19.4%	22.6%	26.1%
40-44	<6%	17.5%	20.5%	23.6%	26.9%
45-49	<6%	18.6%	21.5%	24.5%	27.6%
50-54	<6%	19.8%	22.7%	25.6%	28.7%
55-59	<6%	20.2%	23.2%	26.2%	29.3%
60+	<6%	20.3%	23.5%	26.7%	29.8%

FEMALE

Age	RISKY	EXCELLENT	GOOD	FAIR	POOR
19-24	<9%	18.9%	22.1%	25.0%	29.6%

25-29	<9%	18.9%	22.0%	25.4%	29.8%
30-34	<9%	19.7%	22.7%	26.4%	30.5%
35-39	<9%	21.0%	24.0%	27.7%	31.5%
40-44	<9%	22.6%	25.6%	29.3%	32.8%
45-49	<9%	24.3%	27.3%	30.9%	34.1%
50-54	<9%	26.6%	29.7%	33.1%	36.2%
55-59	<9%	27.4%	30.7%	34.0%	37.3%
60+	<9%	27.6%	31.0%	34.4%	38.0%

Fill Up on "Free" Foods

One of my theories for explaining the epidemic of obesity in America is that the shortage of compounds from plant foods in our body is creating a short circuit in our brain that results in overeating. One way to combat that and promote satiety is to fill up on what I refer to as "free" foods. This designation represents that certain vegetables are termed "free foods" when dieting for weight loss because they can be eaten in any desired amount because the calories, they contain are offset by the number of calories your body burns in the process of digestion. If you are trying to lose weight, these foods are especially valuable as they help to keep you feeling satisfied between meals. Consider the following vegetables as free foods that may be consumed in any amount and as often as desired in their raw, uncooked form:

Alfalfa sprouts
Bell peppers
Bok choy
Cabbage
Chicory
Celery
Chinese cabbage
Cucumber
Endive
Escarole

Lettuce
Parsley
Radishes
Spinach
Turnips
Watercress

Drink Water to Lose Weight

Can drinking more water help you lose weight? Absolutely. In fact, it is well-established medical fact that water consumption before a meal can acutely reduce meal caloric intake, especially among middle-aged and older adults.

In one recent study, 48 overweight adults age 55-75 years were assigned to one of two groups: (1) low calorie diet + 500 ml water prior to each daily meal (water group), or (2) low calorie diet alone (non-water group). Weight loss was approximately 4 pounds greater in the water group than in the non-water group, and the water group showed a 44% greater decline in weight over the 12 weeks than the non-water group. Thus, when combined with a low-calorie diet, consuming 500 ml water prior to each main meal leads to greater weight loss than a low-calorie diet alone in middle-aged and older adults.

Four Key Tips to Increase the Consumption of Water

- Set a specific target. This tip may be the most effective. Setting a goal creates awareness. Drinking at least a 3 liters of water a day is an excellent goal.
- Get an app for your smart phone. There are several free apps out there that help you reach your daily water intake goals. These apps allow you to set reminders at scheduled or random intervals to drink water and keeps track of how well you are meeting your daily water drinking goals. Waterlogged is the most popular.

- Have a glass of water before every meal and snack. For weight loss, this practice is something that you want to make a habit. It is easy, affordable, and really does help (especially when mixed with PGX!).
- Make it more "interesting." Personally, I do not drink much plain water, but I do drink a lot of tea, flavored water, fresh juice, protein shakes, and other healthy beverages. I just find plain water a bit boring. Just squeezing some lemon or lime juice is enough to liven things up for me and get me to drink more water. Or, make your own infused water by getting a gallon container and adding fresh fruit or sliced vegetables. Strawberries, lemons, cucumbers, mint, ginger, and watermelon are some of my favorites.

Add Spices and Herbs to Rev Up Metabolism and Activate AMPk

It seems that every culinary herb and spice that has actually been examined for their effect on AMPk have found them to be activators. Some examples tested and shown to have this activity to date include the components of curry (turmeric, cayenne pepper, garlic, and ginger), mint family herbs or their components (basil, oregano, rosemary, sage, and thyme), aromatic herbs (cinnamon, clove, and black pepper), and garlic. The key takeaway message is that adding some herbs and spice to your life can help you boost your metabolism and fight inflammaging even something as simple as red or black pepper.

Spicy foods, in particular curries, may help people lose weight. The principle spices used in curry all contain compounds that activate AMPk. Most of the research on weight loss effects of these ingredients has focused on animal studies with results being quite impressive. There are a few human studies, mainly with cayenne pepper that focused on its capsaicin content—the compound that give red pepper its hot and spicy character. These studies have shown that cayenne pepper intake increases the basal metabolic rate while reducing appetite and caloric intake. However, there are other components in red pepper that seem to also help activate fat-burning actions. So, even liberal use of paprika can help you lose weight.

Dietary Supplements and Herbal Products to Activate AMPk

There are a lot of dietary supplements and herbal products that activate AMPk that may be useful in helping people lose weight. I have already stressed the importance of PGX for promoting improved insulin sensitivity. It is also a great strategy for increasing AMPk activity.

In regard to dietary supplements, compounds that enhance the function of the mitochondria, the energy producing factories in our cells, such as alpha-lipoic acid creatine, carnitine, and coenzyme Q10 may be helpful. Of these substances, I would rate alpha-lipoic acid the best choice.

Alpha-lipoic acid (ALA) is a naturally occurring and necessary biological factor in our cells. Although it has some vitamin-like functions, as it can be synthesized in the body, it is not classified as a vitamin. The medical use of ALA has focused on its positive effects in patients with diabetes. Double-blind clinical trials in humans have demonstrated that it improves insulin sensitivity, blood sugar control, cardiovascular health, nerve function and lipid levels, and reduces symptoms of diabetic neuropathy.

Recent pre-clinical studies indicated that ALA may help to boost metabolism, promote the burning of fat as energy, reduce food intake, and therefore, potentially aid in weight loss. In one double-blind study, ALA at a dosage of 300 mg per day contributed to approximately 3 pounds of extra weight loss over the course of 10 weeks. That is a pretty good effect!

In regard to herbal products to activate AMPk, three really stand out: berberine, mulberry leaf extract, and green coffee bean extract. I mentioned berberine earlier in Chapter 3 for its effects on digestive health. It is a yellow pigment found in many medicinal plant species worldwide. These plants include barberry (*Berberis vulgaris*) and goldenseal (*Hydrastis canadensis*). Berberine is a potent activator of AMPk and has shown impressive results in improving blood sugar control, enhancing insulin sensitivity, and lowering blood pressure in overweight subjects with modest benefits in weight loss as well. For example, is one double-blind study subjects taking berberine at a dosage of 500 mg three times daily before meals for 3 months compared to a placebo showed a significant decrease in waist circumference as well as improvements in blood pressure, triglycerides, blood sugar levels, and insulin sensitivity. In a pilot study, the same dosage of berberine for twelve weeks produced an average weight loss of over 10 pounds. So, the effects of berberine can be quite significant.

The mulberry plant (*Morus alba*) is probably best known as the food for silkworms, but it has also been highly regarded in traditional Chinese and Japanese medicine. Recently, human clinical studies have confirmed the benefits of mulberry leaf extract in helping to improve blood sugar control, promote weight loss, prevent and treat type 2 diabetes as well as exerting favorable actions against the metabolic syndrome and cardiovascular disease. Many of these effects of mulberry leaf extract are due to it positively influencing AMPk activity. The daily dosage is generally equivalent to 3,000 mg of dried mulberry leaves. Extracts are generally used. The dosage for a 10:1 extract is 300 mg daily.

Another popular dietary supplement for weight loss that activates AMPk is green coffee bean extract. The extract is rich in chlorogenic acid, a compound that has been shown to improve glucose metabolism, inhibit the accumulation of fat, and decrease the absorption of glucose in the intestines. Roasting coffee beans destroys most of the chlorogenic acid, so drinking a cup of coffee will not yield these benefits. Only raw green coffee beans contain a significant amount of this health-promoting compound. Clinical studies indicate that green coffee bean extract can promote weight loss, as well as reduce blood pressure in people with hypertension. The typical dosage recommendation is 400 mg three times daily.

The Human Microbiome, Insulin Resistance, and AMPk

The role of gut microorganisms in determining our health is enormous. Just consider that we have more microbial cells in our intestinal tract than we have human cells in our entire body. The modern term for our gut flora is referred to as the human microbiome. This field of study is finally taking off and looks like it could revolutionize medicine. It may be that weight loss could be as simple as making sure a person has the right intestinal flora.

A possible link to gut flora and obesity was first discovered by comparing intestinal bacteria in obese and lean individuals. There were significant differences. That led to studies in animals that found that switching the bacterial flora from the colons of fat and skinny mice would reverse their condition. In other words, when skinny mice were inoculated with the bacteria flora of the fat mice, they became fat mice themselves and vice versa.

A large body of emerging science indicates that having the right type of bacteria and yeast in the microbiome plays a significant role in insulin activity, AMPk activation, and satiety. Foremost in promoting a microbiome that helps with insulin sensitivity and weight loss is following the recommendations given on in Chapter 3 on how to increase the levels of the beneficial organism *Akkermansia muciniphila*.

Oleoylethanolamide

Oleoylethanolamide (OEA) is a naturally occurring substance found in olive and safflower oil, avocadoes, nuts, and seeds. It is also made in the human body from oleic acid, the main monounsaturated fatty acid in these very same foods. OEA has a high affinity to bind to a receptor in the nucleus of cells that stimulates the production of a compound known as PPAR-α—an important regulator of many cellular processes including inflammation. OEA also exerts important physiological and metabolic action through the endocannabinoid system including appetite and satiety. It also stimulates the breakdown of fat cells and promotes the burning of fat as energy. The satiety-inducing effects occur by activating specific areas in the brain and the release of oxytocin (the "love hormone").

OEA as a Dietary Supplement for Weight Loss

As a dietary supplement, OEA has been shown to exert significant effects in regulating calorie intake, fat cell metabolism, and helping promote effective weight loss in overweight subjects. In a fasted state OEA levels are low, but with a meal the level of OEA rises especially if the meal is high in oleic acid, which acts as a precursor for OEA synthesis. Genetics, stress, and exercise also influence the level of OEA. Supplementing with OEA mimics the body's natural production of OEA and through several mechanisms promotes decreased caloric intake and fat breakdown.

Pre-clinical studies have shown OEA regulates appetite and promotes weight loss by reducing meal size as well as increasing the time interval between meals. These effects have been confirmed in double-blind, placebo-controlled studies. For example, in one study of 56 obese people (BMI = 30 to 40), those that received 250 mg OEA daily for 60 days experienced decreased appetite and BMI at the end of the study, the most impressive effect was the loss of nearly two inches off the waist circumference. The OEA treated subjects are experienced significantly increased peroxisome proliferator-activated receptor-α (PPAR-α) gene expression (signifying improved fat breakdown to energy and improved metabolism).

Table 5.7 Results from Double-blind Study with OEA vs. a Placebo

Variables	OEA group (n = 27)	Placebo Group (n = 29)
Weight (kg)		
Before	93.0	91.2
After	91.8	91.7
BMI (kg/m2)		
Before	34.7	35.1
After	34.4	35.4
Waist circumference (cm)		
Before	105.3	102.5
After	100.6 (14.5)	103.0

OEA Promotes the Growth of Beneficial Bacteria

OEA also stimulates the growth of *Akkermansia muciniphila*. As previously mentioned this beneficial bacterium is particularly exciting as it plays a key role in the health of the gut lining as well as promotes improved insulin action to help fight obesity and diabetes.

Without sufficient *A. muciniphila* the gut barrier is compromised, and it leads to the absorption of gut-derived toxins that overstimulate the immune system as well as produce a lot of inflammation. These gut-derived toxins can also lead to a condition known as non-alcoholic fatty liver disease (NAFLD) as well as produce systemic inflammatory effects that can lead to arthritis, skin disorders, cardiovascular disease, and brain disorders.

OEA promotes the growth of *A. muciniphila*. In a randomized, double-blind, controlled clinical trial, 60 obese people were selected and divided randomly into two groups: an OEA group (received two capsules containing 125 mg of OEA daily) and a placebo group (received two capsules containing 125 mg of starch daily). The treatment lasted for 8 weeks. The abundance of *A. muciniphila* bacterium increased significantly in OEA group compared to placebo group ($p < 0.001$). In addition, the OEA group experienced reduced total calorie and carbohydrate intakes. Calorie intake at baseline was 2714.30 (and decreased significantly to 2379.07 after 4 weeks ($p < 0.001$). That calorie difference means a fat loss of about one pound every ten days. In the OEA group, the amount of carbohydrate intake was reduced from 422.25 at baseline to 368.44 per day after 8 weeks. These results provide clear evidence of OEA's weight loss promoting effects as well as an ancillary mechanism, i.e., promoting the growth of *A. muciniphila*.

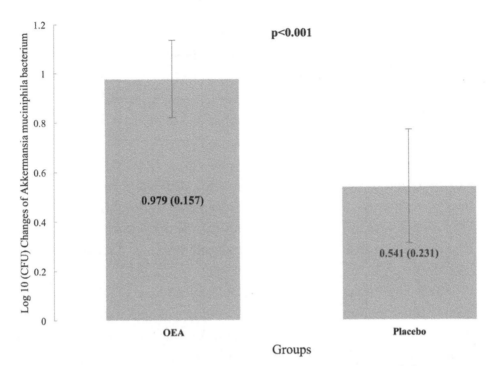

Effect of OEA on the growth *Akkermansia muciniphila*

OEA in Non-alcoholic Fatty Liver Disease (NAFLD)

When the liver is damaged it leads to the depositing of fat within the liver. This process can occur with liver damage caused by alcohol, but there is a new epidemic form called non-alcoholic fatty liver disease (NAFLD). It ranges in severity from a rather benign impairment of liver function to an inflammation of the liver referred to as non-alcoholic steatohepatitis (NASH), which may advance to cirrhosis and eventually liver failure. The biggest cause is being overweight. NAFLD occurs in over 70% of patients who are 10% above ideal body weight and nearly 100% of those who are obese.

OEA exerts significant benefits in protecting against NAFLD via several mechanisms including the promotion of the growth of *A. muciniphila*. When the muco-protective lining of the gut is impaired it leads to increased absorption of gut-derived toxins that play a major role in the development of NAFLD. Other actions of OEA against NAFLD include reducing inflammation and oxidative stress, enhancing energy metabolism within liver cells, and also improving fat metabolism. OEA is so impressive in these effects that it has been referred to as a "molecular target" in the treatment of NAFLD. Preliminary evidence points to impressive results with OEA in improving NAFLD.

OEA and Oxytocin

OEA may have some additional benefits beyond appetite control and weight loss through promoting the release of oxytocin—the "love hormone." Oxytocin is a hormone produced by the pituitary gland that plays a key role in social bonding, sexual reproduction, childbirth, and the period after childbirth. For example, during childbirth oxytocin is released into the bloodstream in response to stretching of the cervix and uterus during labor. Release also occurs with stimulation of the nipples from breastfeeding. This released oxytocin is crucial for not only mother-baby bonding, but also in milk production.

Oxytocin exerts effects beyond social and mother-child bonding. For example, intranasal administration of oxytocin is associated with significant weight loss as well as improvements in insulin sensitivity. Oxytocin also produces significant antidepressant effects. And it promotes socialization, empathy, and feelings of trust. Some of these effects are noted through measurement of urine levels in both human and animal models, while others are based upon the effects of administering oxytocin intranasally. Women, in particular, appear to be more sensitive to oxytocin, especially with responding to important social and relationship stimuli. This may be the result of testosterone blocking oxytocin effects while estrogen enhances oxytocin effects. It makes sense from an evolutionary standpoint. With testosterone suppressing oxytocin, feelings of empathy are also reduced. This would allow less mental conflict for men during activities such as hunting or protecting the tribe against attack. Nonetheless, empathy in healthy males has been shown to be increased after intranasal oxytocin.

Although oxytocin has a multitude of effects on feelings and mood, it is its role in love that it is most associated with. Higher levels of oxytocin have been correlated with feelings of love and romantic attachment. Oxytocin is thought to aid romantically attached couples by decreasing their feelings of anxiety and depression when they are separated. In animal studies, oxytocin evokes feelings of contentment, reductions in anxiety, and feelings of calmness and security when in the company of the mate. It is safe to assume the same occur in humans.

Oxytocin has also received a lot of attention as it relates to sexual intimacy. It is well established that oxytocin release is increased during sexual arousal. However, men and women are wired a little different here with most men showing no increase in oxytocin during orgasms while women show a surge in oxytocin at orgasm that lasts for up to 5 minutes after. This oxytocin surge at orgasm in women is thought to play a role in all of the bonding effects described above.

Lastly, there is growing interest in the oxytocin system as a potential therapeutic target for the treatment of alcohol and substance use disorders. Accumulating preclinical evidence suggests that oxytocin may aid in reversing some of the damage and neuroadaptations that occur as a result of chronic alcohol or drug exposure. Some clinical studies with oxytocin administration have shown some positive effects improving behavior in alcohol- and drug-dependence suggesting a possible beneficial effect.

How this entire oxytocin discussion relates to OEA is that OEA is an endogenous enhancer of oxytocin. As such, it may help promote improved oxytocin release resulting in improved mood, feelings of empathy, enhanced relationships, and even improved behavior. Preclinical evidence exists for all of these applications with OEA. In particular, OEA exerts significant effects in not only potentially being effective in alcohol abstinence, it has shown tremendous effects in blocking alcohol-induced brain inflammation and toxicity.

The Real Danger of Artificial Sweeteners

The common belief is that consumption of artificial sweeteners like aspartame, sucralose, and saccharin will lead to a reduction in the calories consumed. This, in turn, will lead to weight loss or prevention in weight gain. Unfortunately, this is not what happens, as detailed studies have not shown these artificial sweeteners reduce the number of calories consumed or to have any significant effect on body weight. In fact, some studies have actually shown artificial sweeteners, may actually increase appetite.

Another interesting line of research shows that artificial sweeteners can actually create insulin resistance via alterations in the gut microbiome. This effect has been now shown in both mice and humans. Think about it. Many people who are overweight, obese, or with type 2 diabetes are reaching for diet drinks and other artificially sweetened foods and beverages thinking it will help their blood sugar control. In actuality, artificial sweeteners add fuel to the fire.

If that is not enough reason to stay away from artificial sweeteners, let me give you another—they increase the risk of depression. A study conducted by researchers at the National Institutes of Health (NIH) showed that adults who drink artificially sweetened beverages—diet drinks in particular— were 30% more likely to develop depression compared to those who do not drink such beverages. The study was huge as it involved 263,925 people between ages 50 and 71 years at enrollment. The risk for depression was greatest among those people who drank more than 32 ounces per day of diet soda or other diet beverages. Drinking 4 cans/cups per day of regular soda or sweetened beverage was also associated with a greater risk for depression.

The bottom line is that consumers need to be staying away from all artificial sweeteners and look to nature for low-calorie sweeteners instead such as:

- Stevia - a natural sweetener extracted from the *Stevia rebaudiana* plant. Some stevia compounds are 300 times sweeter than sugar and stevia has an excellent safety profile.
- Monk fruit or luo han guo extract is not as popular as stevia, but it may actually be a little sweeter without the bitter aftertaste.
- Sugar alcohols or polyol sweeteners like erythritol, xylitol, sorbitol, mannitol, and maltitol are extremely safe at moderate dosages. However, because they are poorly absorbed at higher dosages

(e.g., greater than 10 grams daily) they can cause gastrointestinal symptoms ranging from mild discomfort to severe diarrhea especially in children because of their smaller size.

- Allulose is a naturally occurring sugar that may be the "Holy Grail" of sweeteners. Allulose is about 80% as sweet as sugar but has only 1/10th the calorie level of sucrose or fructose.

Allulose is absorbed from the gastrointestinal tract, so it does not cause the gas and bloating that sugar alcohols do. Even though allulose is absorbed, it is not utilized by the body has an energy source. About 70% of the allulose that is ingested is excreted in the urine. What I really like about allulose and why it is my favorite sweetener is that it actually exerts positive effects on blood sugar control and may actually help promote weight loss. A sweetener that promotes weight loss is a major nutritional breakthrough.

One double-blind, placebo-controlled trial found that the people who consumed 5 g of allulose with their meals had a significantly reduced blood sugar response compared with those who ate the same meal, minus the allulose. The effect was more pronounced in those with pre-diabetes than in the healthy subjects. This data supports some of the studies in animals with allulose where it showed an ability to both improve blood sugar control and promote fat loss.

Allulose is made through a natural enzymatic reaction or through a GMO process. Obviously, look for the non-GMO version such as my Doctor Murray Superfoods AllSweet Plus Sweetener available at iHerb. com. Allulose is safe and does not appear to influence the microbiome as it is absorbed quickly and not metabolized by gut bacteria.

Longevity Matrix Lifestyle Tune-Up #5—Develop and Write Out Your Daily Routine

If you made it this far, your head may be spinning a bit trying to figure out how to incorporate all of this incredible information into your daily routine. Don't worry, in this tune up you are going to work on starting to put it all together.

One of my key recommendations when trying to help people improve their health is make a plan and write it all down. I think one big reason why so many people have found themselves overweight is that they don't take the time to actually plan out their daily meals in advance. Instead, they end up eating on impulse. What eating on the run and grabbing food on impulse promotes is usually wrong food choices that can easily pack on extra calories. Trust me, if you don't have a plan, you will not get where you want to go. When it comes to eating with health in mind, you absolutely must plan out your meals and general calorie intake each day.

Meal planning is neither difficult nor time consuming. Even the busiest people can find that time to do a bit of planning and add some structure to their eating habits. You can do it in 20 minutes for the entire week or you can do it before you go to bed for the next day. A simple menu plan with breakfast, lunch and dinner along with healthy snacks is not a tough chore. Write it down, commit to it, and do it. I like doing it for the whole week because you can then create a grocery list as well. Write down all the supplements that you are taking and be sure to plug into your plan when it is you are actually going to take them.

Preparing nutritious delicious meals don't need to take a lot of time. There are thousands of recipes that require only minutes of preparation and little culinary skill. As well, part of your planning can include cooking more than you need and freezing portions for other meals or keeping the extra for leftovers. To help you, I am featuring some of my favorite recipes on the resources section on www.thelongevitymatrix.com.

The point is that if you plan properly, your chance for success increases dramatically. You also have to have things on hand as quick snacks to keep you on track, especially low-calorie foods like carrots, celery, cucumbers, daikon radish, and others that can add to your daily quota of servings of vegetables. If you are engaged in a regular exercise program, it is important to have a whey-protein or other high protein shake as a snack or meal to meet your protein needs. For me, always having high protein bars, or ingredients for healthy high protein smoothies is important to fill in for any quick urge for more calories or satisfaction. I have some great options in phenomenal tasting protein bars (whey and vegan) and protein powders that are available exclusively through iHerb.com.

Menu Guidelines of the Longevity Matrix

The basic dietary principles that promote health and longevity broken down to the following seven keys:

1. Eat to support blood sugar control by eating a low glycemic load diet.
2. Eat a "rainbow" assortment of fruits and vegetables.
3. Eat the right types of fats.
4. Focus on eating whole, organic foods (avoid processed foods, food additives, and artificial sweeteners).
5. Keep salt intake low, potassium intake high.
6. Drink sufficient amounts of water each day.

What I want to do next is offer some very specific suggestions for constructing a healthy breakfast, lunch, and dinner as well as snack options.

Breakfast

An old adage is that breakfast is the most important meal of the day. I agree with that entirely. It really does set the stage for how the day is going to unfold in many ways. Here are my recommendations for breakfast:

- Focus on high quality protein. This recommendation is important for a lot of reasons. For example, I think focusing on protein for breakfast is a critical tool for weight loss. Protein has been well demonstrated to be vital in the maintenance of healthy appetite control. Starting the day with a high-protein breakfast can promote prolonged satiety. My day general start with either a whey protein-based smoothie or a mixture of 1 or 2 organic eggs and one cup egg whites. I try to get 25 to 50 grams of high-quality protein at breakfast. Twenty-five grams on the days I am working out in the morning usually from a protein shake or smoothie; fifty grams when I am not working out (off days), usually in the form of my one or two organic egg and egg whites. On the days I am working out, after my workout I usually have a protein bar that provides another 15 to 20 grams of protein.

- If your breakfast is a whey protein smoothie, add some frozen berries. If it is an omelet or scrambled eggs, add lots of fresh herbs, or black or red pepper, or other spices; and also have a side of either berries, fresh or sautéed tomatoes, or other non-starch vegetable (e.g., asparagus is an awesome choice!).

- Mix one cup unsweetened, non-fat Greek yogurt with berries or cut up fresh fruit two tablespoons of ground flaxseeds.

- Avoid grains and sugar. I know that many people are in the habit of cereal and oatmeal. But I think it really sets you up for straining your blood sugar control later in the day. If you are going to eat oatmeal or other healthy whole grain cereal, please use PGX to reduce the glycemic load.

- Do not be afraid to try non-traditional breakfast choices. Poached salmon with grilled vegetables, grilled chicken with vegetables, or scrambled tofu with vegetables.

- If you are going to have any toast, make it whole grain and limit it to one slice. If you are trying to lose weight, avoid it entirely. You don't need the calories.

- Drink green tea or coffee (regular if you can handle it, otherwise decaf).

Mid-morning snack

In order to meet the desired intake of health promoting foods, snacking is an absolute must. Otherwise, you are just putting too much stress on your digestive system and physiology. Better to spread your nutrition and calories throughout the day with balanced meals and snacks rather than loading up when your hunger kicks into full gear.

Here is the key, snacking is a very good habit as long as you keep the portion size small and calorie count low. There are lots of choices for healthy snacks: cut up vegetables, fruit, fresh juice, green tea, nuts, seeds, and other whole foods. For me, on my workout days, I will usually have a protein bar and a mug of my special hot cacao brew (see page 352). On my non-workout days, I just have my special brew. I admit that I am hooked on this health habit, but the key thing is that it is a habit that promotes health. So, it is a good one. Find your own mid-morning habit that will help you achieve your goals. Just a reminder, it is important when you first start making dietary changes to journal your dietary intake including snacks and beverages.

Lunch

Lunch is a perfect time to take advantage of high volume, low calorie soups and salads. You can see some excellent suggestions on the Longevity Matrix website (www.longevitymatrix.com/resources).

Mid-afternoon snack

Again, just like the morning snack, there are endless health promoting possibilities here. For me, it is usually a low-calorie fresh juice break mid-afternoon, especially in the summer. It is also a great time to fill up on the "free foods" listed on page 152. Remember, you can eat as much of these foods as you want without fear of weight gain because it costs you just as many calories to digest the foods as they contain.

Dinner

Here are some simple, but important guidelines in constructing your main meal of the day:

- Create volume. To help you feel full, fill up on non-starchy vegetables. These are considered "free" since they are high in fiber and very low in calories. Avoid large amounts or big portions of root vegetables such as potatoes, parsnips, and squash since these contain more starch and more calories.

- Go for low-glycemic index foods. Choose fruit and starches that have a lower glycemic index so it will not cause your blood sugar level to spike. These low GI foods will give your body better blood sugar control and sustained energy.
- Aim for balance. When creating a balanced meal, include three or four food groups.
- Lower the fat. When cooking, try baking, broiling, grilling, poaching, roasting, sautéing with little oil, steaming, and stir-frying
- Use nonstick cookware: This will allow you to reduce calories by cooking with less or no fat.
- Use spices liberally. Skip gravy and rich sauces and enhance the flavor of foods by cooking with spices and herbs.
- Trim away any fat on meat and go skinless with poultry before cooking.

Evening Snack

Do you need an evening snack? Not necessarily, but I think some of us can benefit from it. What changed my philosophy on this matter was seeing the effect of a nighttime feeding on my kids. They seemed to sleep much better on a full stomach. I think the same is true for many adults. The key is to avoid eating high glycemic foods that are going to promote a blood sugar roller coaster.

For many years I tried not to eat after dinner but was not too successful at that goal. I had a bit of a "nighttime eating disorder." In the most classic form, people with this disorder are able to stick to their diet goals during the day, but when they start eating dinner it triggers a hormonal reaction that leads them to feel like the more they eat, the hungrier they get. For me, PGX was a Godsend. I now regularly have a nighttime snack of PGX in instant oatmeal (see above) or mixed in with Greek yogurt and ground flaxseed or berries along with some of my AllSweet Plus to sweeten it up. Again, this habit supports my health and helps me achieve my dietary goals. And, I also find it really helps me sleep through the night soundly.

I also have gotten into the habit of having some sort of relaxing or caffeine-free herbal tea at night. I think this habit is just another way to give your body (and mind) some additional support. Variety is a key for me here. I like many different types of teas at night including rooibos, peppermint, chamomile, ginger, and decaffeinated English breakfast.

Some Recommendations When Eating Out or Traveling

When you eat out or travel, it is critical to plan ahead. I don't want to eat the food and snacks served on a plane. So, when I fly, after passing through security I buy my own water and drinks that I can mix some PGX or whey protein packets into easily on the plane. If it's a long flight, I will buy a salad or healthy wrap if they are available before I board the plane and I always have some of my favorite protein bars in my carryon.

When I eat out, I simply follow some basic guidelines. I love food, so you can be assured that I enjoy eating at fine restaurants. But even lower priced establishments these days don't mind modifications. Here are some of my basic tips when eating out.

- For me, the first step is to take PGX before I leave for the restaurant or as soon as I get there. That gives me tremendous control over my appetite and portion sizes.
- Next, for me the biggest rule that I work hard not to break is avoiding the breadbasket. Now, if it is whole grain bread that looks too good to pass up, I take one piece or maybe just a half, and then ask them to take the bread away.
- When I go out to eat with my family or friends, I just make them keep the bread away from me. It's tempting, but I know that I would rather spend my calories on other choices.
- Next, I order a salad with no croutons and the dressing on the side that way I can add it myself and use just a little. One way to do this is to just dip your fork in the dressing before you pick up a bite of the salad. This adds enough flavor to make the salad enjoyable and you will only go through a small amount of dressing by the time you finish the salad. My strategy is to always try to

"spoil my appetite" with something healthy before my main entrée so that I will feel very satisfied.

- Since the main course is usually more than you need, eat only half your meal and take the other half for lunch the next day. As an alternative, split a main course with a friend or have a low fat, low calorie main course like broiled fish and only eat a small portion of the rice or potatoes.

- I am assertive in asking if menu items can be altered. For example, recently I was at a restaurant and I really liked the looks of one item featuring scallops, but the scallops were wrapped in bacon. Well, I don't eat bacon for a lot of reasons. So, I simply asked if the chef could prepare the dish without it. It was no problem and the meal was absolutely fantastic. Frankly, I think the bacon would have ruined the item.

- As well, be sure to ask for substitutions on the side dish as well. For example, ask for steamed vegetables instead of French fries, extra salad instead of rice, etc. Be sure to ask for all sauces, butter, dressings, and gravy on the side and use them very sparingly.

- You can probably figure out my last rule—saying no to dessert. If the restaurant offers fresh berries, I will generally enjoy them. I love this quote from my friend David Snow, "nothing tastes as good as healthy feels". I think that applies to many desserts out there. That said, an occasional treat or reward certainly has its place in our diet, just keep the portion size small.

CHAPTER 6:

Enhancing the Immune System

The immune system plays a central role in any longevity plan. It is complex, but the immune system is involved in many facets that impact aging. In particular, the immune system not only protects against infection and cancer, it is involved in inflammation—a key factor in increasing the effects of aging. Remember inflammaging? It is influenced by the immune system, especially immune cells known as macrophages.

When working properly, the immune system has a remarkable arsenal of weapons to fight off microorganisms that have the capacity to infect us and do us harm. At all times, day and night, we are constantly exposed to various "bugs" –bacteria, viruses, fungi, and other invisible invaders. They are in the food we eat and the air we breathe. They're in everything we touch or smell. Despite this onslaught, many of us rarely catch a cold or get sick because of the strength or our immune system. I am proud of the fact that despite my travel schedule, constant exposure to people who are obviously dealing with a cold, and a high stress workload, that I went 22 years without a cold. I am in my new streak of 2 years without a cold and my goal is to NEVER have a cold again. Is it possible? Absolutely.

With a strong immune system, you are safe from attack by all but the most virulent microorganisms. Even if infection does gain a foothold, it's usually just a matter of time before your immune system mounts an effective counterattack.

The immune system is not only fending off infections, it is on constant surveillance for cancer cells. When found, the scout cells send out powerful chemical messages that call troops of white blood cells to the area to bombard and destroy the cancerous cells. Low immune function sets the stage not only for constant struggles with infections, but also for cancer.

While many people may be aware of the consequences of low immune function, what they may not know is that for many people the immune system is a double-edged sword—it protects them on one hand, but on the other it literally destroys them. What I am referring to are conditions where the immune system is hyperactive and out of control such as allergies (especially asthma) and autoimmune conditions like rheumatoid arthritis, lupus, and multiple sclerosis where the immune system literally starts attacking the body.

The principles involved in tuning up your immune system are basically the same whether you are suffering from low immune function or an immune system that is out of control. The first goal is to make sure that you provide the immune system with a constant steady stream of high-quality nutrition. Next is following a healthy lifestyle. These two simply steps can go a long way in supporting central control mechanisms to keep the immune system in proper balance. The bottom line is that by tuning up your immune system you'll not only increase your resistance to colds and flu and other infections but also protect yourself against cancer and other potentially deadly diseases.

Key Components of the Immune System

The immune system is composed of white blood cells and the organs that produce immune cells, or that play a role in their activity, including the bone marrow, thymus, lymph nodes, spleen, and tonsils.

The infantry of the immune system are white blood cells. Amazingly, every minute of your life, your body is making about *twelve million* new white blood cells to replace an equal number that have just worn out. At the same time, each living immune cell is busy making its own special mix of chemical messengers or antibodies. These rates increase during infection or disease. As you can imagine, your body devotes a tremendous amount of its resources to keeping your immune system running. By providing your body with the nutrients and energy it needs to keep up with this challenging task, you are taking a huge step in tuning-up your immune system.

The *thymus* deserves some special mention as it is the "master gland" of the immune system. It is composed of two soft pinkish-gray lobes that lie in bib-like fashion in the upper chest area. To a great extent, the health of the thymus determines the health of the immune system. Without a healthy and well-functioning thymus, your immune system cannot function effectively. Inside the thymus, immature white blood cells mature to form T lymphocytes (the *T* stands for "thymus-dependent"). People with low thymus function are prone to frequent or chronic infections, allergies, migraine headaches, and rheumatoid arthritis. The thymus gland also produces hormones that regulate many immune functions. A low level of these hormones can reduce your immune response and leave you more vulnerable to disease. Common causes of low thymus hormone levels include advancing age, stress, and nutrient deficiencies. Chronic viral or yeast infections or the presence of cancer are signs that your thymus gland desperately needs support. That support is best offered through diet, lifestyle, and supplement strategies. Most importantly, since the thymus is sensitive to the effects of poor nutrition, stress, or exposure to environmental toxins, it is critical to eat a diet rich in antioxidant nutrients and to supplement your diet with key nutritional antioxidants especially vitamins C and E, selenium, and zinc.

Another important tissue in immune function is the *interstitium*. It refers to the space between cells and represents approximately one sixth of the entire. The interstitial fluid contains primarily waste products that result from activity inside your cells and flows as *lymph* into the *lymphatic vessels.* As the lymph travels along these vessels, it passes through the *lymph nodes.* The lymph nodes filter the lymph to remove impurities. Inside the nodes, *macrophages* ("big eaters") engulf and destroy the particles of debris, foreign cells, and other impurities. In chapter 2, the role that macrophages play in inflammaging was described. If the lymph is full of impurities or during an infection, macrophages have to work overtime as the garbage collector and eliminator. Sometimes macrophages get overwhelmed. That's why the nodes often swell during an illness. And, overwhelming macrophages on a chronic basis is a big factor in inflammaging.

Lymph fluid flows in one direction, so that the fluid leaving the node is always cleaner than the fluid that enters it. The lymphatic vessels generally run alongside the blood vessels. At a point just below the neck, major lymph ducts drain into two major veins. In this way, lymph fluid, now filtered of its impurities, is put back into circulation as part of the liquid portion of blood. There is no real "pump" that forces lymph to circulate through your body, the way the heart pumps blood. Instead, lymph circulation depends on breathing and movement by your body. Muscular contractions pump lymph out of the arms and legs into larger lymphatic vessels in the chest and abdomen. But the main mechanism of lymph circulation is breathing. Inhaling expands the diaphragm, which puts pressure on the large lymphatic vessels in the abdomen and chest. In turn, this eventually forces lymph to empty into the heart, so it can then be distributed through the blood circulation. This is another reason why exercise and breathing exercises are so important for your tune-up: Body movement and deep breathing with the diaphragm speeds up the rate at which the lymph nodes filter out impurities. There is no direct data currently to support it as far as I know, but I believe that exercise, body movement, and breathing are the key factors that keep macrophages functioning properly. The circumstantial effects of the anti-aging and life extending effects of these activities certainly provide some evidence.

Nearly 70% of the immune system is found in the "*gut-associated lymphoid tissue* or GALT." It encompasses a huge area of nearly 1,000 square feet. In order to maximize the surface area for absorption of nutrients, the intestinal lining is made up of finger-like projections (villi), covered by a single layer of intestinal epithelial cells. Because this surface is highly absorptive while also being such an important barrier, it is clearly important for the immune system to be part of this interface with the intestinal contents. The health and integrity of the GALT is a key factor in the health of the overall immune system as well as to protect the body from invasion in the gut. Poor digestive function, an altered microbiome, and gastrointestinal inflammation all interfere with the GALT functioning properly. The reason why there was such a focus on digestive health previously, is that if digestion is incomplete or the intestinal barrier is disrupted or there is a disturbance in the microbiome it leads to the absorption of unwanted compounds into the body and accelerated inflammaging.

The *spleen*, located in the upper left abdomen behind the lower ribs, plays several roles in the immune system. It produces some white blood cells, destroys and removes bacteria, and cleans up debris from worn-out cells such as old red blood cells. The spleen also serves as a reservoir of red blood, which it can release in case of emergency such as injury. The spleen produces several compounds that enhance immune system activity and is particularly important in fighting off bacterial infections.

The *tonsils* are a pair of oval-shaped masses of tissue located at the back of the throat. The tissue contains small cul-de-sacs, called crypts, which trap bacteria and particles that enter from your nose and mouth. Immune cells living in the tonsils then destroy the invaders. Tonsils often become infected and swollen as a result of this activity, especially during childhood. But there's a payoff: The immune cells are able to "remember" what invaders they meet, which helps your body fend off attacks later in life. Forty or fifty years ago doctors were quick to recommend removing a kid's tonsils if they got infected frequently. We now realize that such tissue serves a purpose and that usually the tonsils should be left in place to carry out their natural immune function.

Types of White Blood Cells

There are several types of white blood cells including neutrophils, eosinophils, basophils, lymphocytes, and monocytes.

- *Neutrophils:* These cells actively phagocytize - engulf and destroy - bacteria, tumor cells, and dead particulate matter. Neutrophils are especially important in preventing bacterial infection.

- *Eosinophils and basophils*: These cells are involved in allergic conditions. They secrete histamine and other compounds which are designed to breakdown antigen-antibody complexes, but also promote allergic mechanisms.

- *Lymphocytes*: There are several types of lymphocytes, including - T cells, B cells, natural killer cells.

  - T cells stand for thymus derived lymphocytes. These cells orchestrate many immune functions and are the major components of cell-mediated immunity (discussed above). There are different types of T cells including helper T cells which help other white blood cells to function; suppressor T cells which inhibit white blood cell functions; and cytotoxic T cells which attack and destroy foreign tissue, cancer cells, and virus infected cells.

  - B cells are responsible for producing antibodies which are large protein molecules which bind to foreign molecules (antigens) on bacteria, viruses, other organisms, and tumor cells. After the antibody binds to the antigen it sets up a sequence of events that ultimately destroys the infectious organism or tumor cell.

  - Natural killer cells or NK cells received their name because of their ability to destroy cells that have become cancerous or infected with viruses. They are the body's first line of defense against cancer development. The level or activity of natural killer cells in chronic fatigue syndrome, cancer, and chronic viral infections is usually low.

- Monocytes: These large white blood cells are circulating macrophages responsible for cleaning up cellular debris after an infection. They are the garbage collectors of the immune system. Monocytes are also responsible for triggering many immune responses.

Special Chemical Factors

There are a number of special chemical factors produced by the immune system that play a huge role in both immunity and inflammation. These compounds are produced by various white blood cells, e.g., interferon is produced primarily by T cells, interleukins are produced by macrophages and T cells, and complement fractions are manufactured in the liver and spleen. These special chemical factors are extremely important in activating the white blood cells to destroy cancer cells.

Low Immunity Assessment

Circle the number that best describes the intensity of your symptoms on the following scale:

0 = I do not experience this symptom
1 = Mild
2 = Moderate
3 = Severe

Some items are scored as either Yes or No. When adding your total, score 0 for each No answer and 10 for each Yes.

1.	Inflamed or bleeding gums	0	1	2	3
2.	Runny nose	0	1	2	3
3.	Get boils or sties	0	1	2	3
4.	Fatigue	0	1	2	3
5.	Throat infections	0	1	2	3
6.	Cold sores, fever blisters	0	1	2	3
7.	Poor wound healing	0	1	2	3
8.	Swollen lymph nodes	0	1	2	3

9.	Slow to recover from cold or flu (lasts more than 4 days)	0	1	2	3
10.	Catch colds or flu easily (more than two colds per year)	0	1	2	3
11.	1uffering from chronic infection	NO	YES		
12.	History of cancer	NO	YES		

TOTAL _____

Interpreting Your Score

If you are suffering from recurrent infections, the importance of tuning up your immune system was probably known prior to taking the assessment for low immune function. Just how important it is can be prioritized based on your score. If your score is: 12 or more it is a high priority; 6-11 a moderate priority; and 1-5 a low priority. Sometimes a person can be suffering from hyperimmunity and signs of low immune function at the same time. The reason is that chronic allergies or the use of drugs such as prednisone can suppress the body's ability to fight infections.

Your Immune System Tune-Up

Now let's discuss the practical steps you can take to improve immune system function. The first is to take a look some common causes of low immune function:

- Chronic or severe stress
- Too much simple sugar in the diet
- Small intestinal bacterial overgrowth (SIBO) and a "leaky gut"
- Excessive consumption of alcohol
- Exposure to environmental toxins
- Cigarette smoke
- Obesity
- Lack of exercise
- Food allergies

Once you've identified any harmful influences, of course, the next step is to do what you can to correct them.

Stress and Immunity

For most people, the biggest factor for an immune disturbance is stress. When a person comes to see me complaining of chronic infections or a flare-up of their allergies, most often we can pinpoint stress as the underlying factor. When you are stressed out, your adrenal glands pump out more adrenaline and corticosteroids. These hormones inhibit white blood cell formation and function and cause the thymus gland to shrink. Stress suppresses immunity by stimulating the *sympathetic nervous system*. This is a part of the autonomic nervous system that is responsible for the fight-or-flight response.

Good immune function requires being under the control of the other "arm" of the autonomic nervous system, the *parasympathetic nervous system*. This system automatically assumes control during periods of rest, relaxation, visualization, meditation, and sleep. But, if we stay relaxed and calm during our waking hours, it can balance out the negative effects the sympathetic nervous system exerts. During the deepest levels of sleep, potent immune-enhancing compounds are released, and many immune functions are greatly increased. At least seven hours of sleep per day is essential for helping the immune system function at its peak.

If you want a properly functioning immune system, it is absolutely vital that you reduce the amount of stress in your life as well as learn to better control it. Because stress exerts so many body systems, I have focused several Longevity Matrix Lifestyle Tune-Up Tips to help you deal with stress more effectively.

The basic strategy for stress reduction is to find positive, relaxing ways of releasing excess tension and help your autonomic nervous system function under parasympathetic control. Stress reduction does not mean that you have to give up the high-energy lifestyle that you really enjoy. Find a routine that works for you. Doing so will not only help your immune system but will also improve your relationships and free up energy and focus. So you can actually accomplish more—without sacrificing your health.

Nutrition and Immunity

A deficiency of virtually any single nutrient can significantly impair immunity. Throughout the world, nutrient deficiency is by far the most common cause of poor immune function. This fact is by no means limited to people whose diets are restricted by poverty. In America, many people are overfed but undernourished. They choose foods that have a lot of calories, but little real nutritional value. Every week I see people in my practice who are suffering from poor immune function. They benefit tremendously by following these simple guidelines:

- Eat a diet that is rich in a variety of vegetables (especially the green leafy ones), fresh fruits, whole grains, beans, nuts, and seeds. These plant foods are rich in essential nutrients and immune boosting chemicals.

- Cut out refined carbohydrates. Sugar makes your white blood cells sluggish. Studies show that eating 100 grams of sugar (about 3.5 ounces) reduces the ability white blood cells known as neutrophils to engulf and destroy bacteria by as much as forty percent within two hours after ingestion. Since neutrophils account for about sixty to seventy percent of your white blood cells, interfering with them can seriously impair your immune function.

- Decrease the intake of saturated fats and cholesterol. A diet high in saturated fat suppresses immunity. Many of my patients initially presenting with high levels of cholesterol and triglycerides also report more frequent colds and flu. When cholesterol and triglyceride levels are normalized, proper immune function is restored.

- Eat sufficient, but not excessive amounts of protein. Adequate protein intake is critical in the making of white blood cells, antibodies, and chemical messengers such as interferon. You also need protein to make antioxidant enzymes such as glutathione, which is found in abundance in white blood cells. Elevated glutathione levels are associated with better immune function.

Patients with low immune function can benefit from eating more protein from fish, lean poultry, and lean cuts of meats. I have seen many vegetarians who are suffering from low immunity solely as a result of not consuming enough protein. In these patients, I recommend either supplemental vegan protein powder if they eat absolutely no animal products, or whey protein if they eat dairy. An additional 40 to 50 grams per day for one month will boost protein stores back to normal. After the month is up, I would still recommend 20 grams of either choice daily.

- Take a high-potency, high-quality vitamin and mineral supplement. Doing so will increase your intake of the key nutrients for immune function that I will discuss below. Not long ago, a study of adults found that those who took a multi vitamin and mineral supplement had a fifty percent decrease in the number of days of illness due to infection compared to the group that took a placebo. Those taking the supplement were also showed improvement on eight out of twelve objective measures of immune function. Pretty good results for such little effort!

The Magnificent Seven Nutrients in Immune Support

Vitamin A is necessary for maintaining the cells of the skin and the mucous membranes that act as the first lines of defense against infection. In addition, vitamin A is a necessary for proper white blood cell function and enhances many of your immune system's activities, including thymus function, tumor-fighting activity, and antibody response. Vitamin A is especially important for fighting off viruses. For example, it has been found that children with lower vitamin A levels are much more prone to measles and viral respiratory tract infections. It also reverses immune suppression resulting from such conditions as high levels of stress hormones (glucocorticoids), severe burns, or surgery.

Carotenes are important in protecting your thymus gland because of their antioxidant effects. Studies back in the 1940s showed that the higher a child's carotene intake the fewer the number of school days missed due to infections. More recent research has documented that carotenes enhance many aspects of immune function. Carotenes are found in green leafy vegetables, carrots, and other colorful vegetables.

B vitamins, especially B_1, B_6, and B_{12}, are required for making disease-fighting antibodies. In addition, B vitamins are essential to normal cell division. Therefore, low levels of B vitamins prevent your body from manufacturing new white blood cells. What's more, the lymphoid tissues (such as the thymus and spleen) shrink if they don't get enough B vitamins.

Vitamin C literally turns on white blood cells to attack intruders and also boosts interferon levels, antibody levels and response, and secretion of hormones from the thymus. Vitamin C acts directly against viruses, which is one reason it is used to fight off colds. When you have an infection or are under stress, your need for vitamin C increases.

Vitamin D offers important in protection against viral or bacterial upper respiratory infection. It has been shown to produce a wide range of immune enhancing effects including an ability to:

- Up-regulate anti-microbial peptides, to enhance clearance of bacteria at various barrier sites and in immune cells.
- Modulate the immune system by direct effects on T cell activation.
- Protect against the development of autoimmune diseases (e.g., Crohn's disease, juvenile diabetes mellitus, multiple sclerosis, asthma, and rheumatoid arthritis).
- Reduce the frequency of viral upper respiratory infections.

Zinc is directly involved with immune function on many levels. Like vitamin C, zinc can act against certain viruses, such as those that cause the common cold (see Box). When zinc levels are low, the number of T cells plummets, thymus hormone levels fall, enzyme production and activity declines, and certain white cell functions shut down. What's more, zinc is crucial for proper absorption of nutrients by the intestinal tract.

Selenium is involved in important antioxidant mechanisms that protect the thymus gland. People who are low in selenium have reduced levels of cellular and humoral immunity and lower antibody levels. It appears that selenium works, in part, by enhancing the ability of white blood cells to produce interleukin-2, a chemical that stimulates white blood cells to proliferate and attack foreign cells. One study found that people who took supplements of 200 micrograms (mcg) per day showed a nearly doubling in the activity and ability of white blood cells to kill tumor cells. The typical American diet does not contain enough selenium, supplementation is essential.

Cold Facts About Zinc

A double-blind clinical trial found that lozenges containing zinc significantly reduced the average duration of the common cold. The lozenges used in the study contained 23 mg of elemental zinc, dissolved in the mouth every waking hour after an initial double dose. After seven days, eighty-six percent of the patients were symptom-free, compared to only forty-six percent of those treated with placebo. Apparently, zinc works in two ways: by reducing the ability of viruses to reproduce, and by boosting other aspects of immune function. This study led to an explosion of interest in the use of zinc as a strategy for reducing the severity of colds.

Not all studies on zinc have produced positive results. It appears that, to be effective, zinc lozenges must be free of sorbitol, mannitol, and citric acid. These compounds bind with the zinc and reduce its effectiveness. The best lozenges are those that utilize the amino acid glycine as a sweetener. Use lozenges that supply 15 to 25 mg of elemental zinc. If you feel a cold coming on, take a double dose, then take one tablet every two hours. Let the tablet dissolve in your mouth. Continue for up to seven days.

Remember not to overdo it. Too much zinc can have the undesired effect of lowering immune function. For treatment of colds, I recommend that you take a total dose of no more than 150 mg a day for no more than a week.

Special Natural Products for Immune Support

One of my favorite immune enhancing products is ImmunoPro-LP, a well-defined, clinically tested stabilized product using a special strain of the probiotic organism *Lactobacillus plantarum* common to fermented foods. ImmunoPro-LP is not technically a probiotic as the organism is not viable as it has been heat stabilized. It is referred to as an "immunobiotic" or "paraprobiotic." Compounds known as lipotechoic acids on the cell surface of this organism are responsible for effects. Human clinical studies show systemic effects in boosting production of an important immune system regulator: interleukin-12. This compound exerts significant activity in fighting against infection, particularly viral infections. ImmunoPro-LP also increases the ratio of T helper cells to T suppressor cells (Th1 to Th2 ratio), thereby producing a balancing effect on immune function making it useful in both infections and allergies. Double-blind, placebo-controlled studies have shown ImmunoPro-LP to reduce the incidence, duration and severity of upper respiratory tract infections. It is also fantastic in promoting oral health by reducing pocket depth in periodontal disease. Here are the benefits noted with ImmunoPro-LP:

- Exceptional clinical documentation of immune enhancement
- Exerts a balancing effect on immune function
- Improves immune function in low states
- Improves immune function in allergies
- Reduces incidence of upper respiratory tract infections
- Reverses age-related decline in immune function
- Increases the production of anti-viral compounds

Another ingredient I am a big fan of is Wellmune, a special preparation of baker's yeast containing immune enhancing compounds known as beta-glucans. Medicinal mushrooms like maitake (*Grifola frondosa*), shitake

(*Lentinus edodes*), reishi (*Ganoderma lucidum*), and *Cordyceps sinensis* also contain beta-glucans, but they are a bit different in structure to those in Wellmune. Nonetheless, numerous experimental and clinical studies have shown that yeast extracts and mushroom beta-glucans activate white blood cells by binding to receptors on the outer membranes of neutrophils, macrophages, natural killer (NK) cells and cytotoxic T-cells. Just like a key in a lock, the binding of the beta-glucan to cellular receptors literally flips white blood cells on and triggers a chain reaction leading to increased immune activity. In addition to increasing the ability of the neutrophils and macrophages to engulf and destroy microbes, cancer cells, and other foreign cells, the binding stimulates the production of important signaling proteins of the immune system, such as interleukin-1, interleukin-2, and lymphokines. These immune activators ramp up defenses by activating immune cells.

Wellmune is by far the best researched beta-glucan sources. It is a whole glucan particle composed of 1,3-1,6-beta-glucan derived from the cell walls of a highly purified, proprietary baker's yeast (*Saccharomyces cerevisiae*). Once absorbed, Wellmune is taken up by macrophages and digested into smaller fragments and slowly released over a number of days. The fragments bind to neutrophils, enhancing their activity. As of 2011, six double-blind clinical studies have been conducted with Wellmune demonstrating positive results in reducing the signs, symptoms, frequency, and duration of upper respiratory infections. In a study in marathon runners (who experience increased infections after long runs like marathons), Wellmune significantly reduced symptoms of upper respiratory tract infection (e.g., sore throat, stuffy nose, etc.) in the test subjects. Furthermore, the Wellmune group reported 22% higher scores in vigor, 48% reduction in fatigue, 38% reduction in tension and a 38% reduction in confusion over the control groups.

In a double-blind study during the cold and flu season, compared with the placebo group, the Wellmune group reported: (1) No incidence of fever compared with 3.5 incidences over a 90-day period. (2) No need to take a "sick day" from work or school, compared with 1.38 days of work/

school missed for the placebo group. (3) An increase in general health, including physical energy and emotional well-being.

In the latest study of 122 healthy volunteers, participants taking 250 mg of Wellmune daily for 12 weeks reported a 58% reduction in upper respiratory tract infection symptoms, compared with individuals taking a placebo. These subjects also experienced improvement in energy levels compared to the placebo group.

Eating a good diet and taking extra doses of vitamins and minerals, especially antioxidants, are important steps for boosting immunity. Herbs can provide extra immune support. As a rule, such herbal products should be used only for short periods of time (up to two months)—for example, to stimulate the immune system during an acute infection, to help cure a chronic infection, or just to bring your system back up to normal.

For boosting general immune function, choose one of the following:

Astragalus membranaceus
- Dried root (or as decoction): 1-2 g three times daily
- Tincture (1:5): 2-4 ml three times daily
- Fluid extract (1:1): 2-4 ml three times daily
- Solid (dry powdered) extract (0.5% 4-hydroxy-3-methoxy isoflavone): 100-150 mg

ImmunoPro-LP
- 10 mg daily providing over 12 billion cells of the probiotic organism *Lactobacillus plantarum* L137

Wellmune
- 250 to 500 mg daily.

Herbs for the Common Cold and Upper Respiratory Infections

I want to mention three herbs for use to deal with common upper respiratory infections: *Astragalus membranaceus, Echinacea sp.* and umka (*Pelargonium sidoides*). These two botanicals have exceptional scientific support for the common cold, bronchitis, sinusitis, and sore throat.

Astragalus membranaceus

Many herbs have been shown to have antibacterial, antiviral, and immunostimulatory effects. As far as an herb to produce overall immune enhancing effects during a cold or other viral infection, a good choice is the root of *Astragalus membranaceus*. Clinical studies in China have shown it to be effective when used as a preventive measure against the common cold. It has also been shown to reduce the duration and severity of symptoms in acute treatment of the common cold as well as to raise white blood cell (WBC) counts in persons with chronic low levels of WBCs.

Research in animals has shown that *Astragalus* apparently works by stimulating several factors of the immune system, including enhancing phagocytic activity of monocytes and macrophages, increasing interferon production and natural killer cell activity, improving T-cell activity, and potentiating other antiviral mechanisms. Astragalus appears particularly useful in cases in which the immune system has been damaged by chemicals or radiation. In immunodepressed mice, Astragalus has been found to reverse the T-cell abnormalities caused by an immune suppressing drug (cyclophosphamide), radiation, and aging.

Echinacea

There have been over 300 scientific investigations on the immune enhancing effects of echinacea—one of the most popular herbs in the treatment of the common cold. Mixed results from clinical studies with echinacea are most likely due to lack of or insufficient quantity of active compounds. The axiom for effectiveness of any herbal product is its ability to deliver an effective dosage of active compounds. If the product, had sufficient levels of active compounds, it would be effective. If not, it would likely be no more effective than a placebo. For example, in one double-blind study 160 subjects were given either echinacea or placebo and then exposed to a common cold virus. Infection occurred in 44 and 57% and illness occurred in 36 and 43% of the echinacea- and placebo-treated subjects, respectively. However, the preparation contained no echinacosides or alkamides and contained only 0.16% cichoric acid. In other words it lacked the active components of echinacea.

In contrast, in a clinical trial using a well-defined echinacea extract containing alkamides, cichoric acid, and polysaccharides at concentrations of 0.25, 2.5, and 25 mg/ml, respectively, prepared from freshly harvested *E. purpurea* plants (commercially available as Echinilin or Echinamide), showed excellent results. In this randomized, double-blind, placebo-controlled trial, 282 subjects 18 to 65 years old with a history of two or more colds in the previous year, but otherwise in good health, were randomized to receive either echinacea extract or placebo. They were instructed to start the echinacea or placebo at the onset of the first symptom related to a cold, consuming 10 doses the first day and four doses per day on subsequent days for 7 days. Severity of symptoms (10-point scale: 0, minimum; 9, maximum) and dosing were recorded daily. A nurse examined the subjects on the mornings of days 3 and 8 of their cold. A total of 128 subjects contracted a common cold (59 echinacea, 69 placebo).

The total daily symptom scores were found to be 23.1% lower in the echinacea group than in the placebo group. Throughout the treatment period, the response rate to treatments was greater in the echinacea group. This study indicated that early intervention with a standardized formulation of echinacea (as Echinilin or Echinamide) resulted in reduced symptom severity in subjects with naturally acquired upper respiratory tract infection.

Pelargonium sidoides (South African Geranium or Umcka)

P. sidoides is a medicinal plant in the geranium family that is native to South Africa. *Umckaloaba,* its common name, is a close approximation of the word in the Zulu language that means "severe cough" and is a testimony to its effect in bronchitis. In addition to showing significant benefits in bronchitis and sinusitis, it has also shown benefit in treating the common cold. In one study, 103 adult patients with at least two major and one minor or with one major and three minor cold symptoms (maximum symptom score of 40 points), present for 24 to 48 hours, and who gave provision of informed consent were randomized to receive either 30 drops (1.5 mL) of an extract of *P. sidoides* (EPs 7630 or Umcka) or placebo three times a day. From baseline to day five, the average symptom intensity differences (SSID) of the cold intensity score (CIS) improved by 14.6 points in the EPs 7630 group compared with 7.6 points in the placebo group. After 10 days, 78.8% EPs 7630 versus 31.4% in the placebo group were clinically cured (CIS equals zero points or complete resolution of all but a maximum of one cold symptom). The mean duration of inability to work was significantly lower in the EPs 7630 treatment group (6.9 days) than in the placebo group (8.2 days). EPs 7630 significantly reduces the severity of symptoms and shortens the duration of the common cold by a little more than a day compared with placebo.

Stopping a Cold-Cold

The common cold is caused by a variety of viruses that infect the oral and nasal passages and the sinuses. The symptoms of a cold are well known fever, headaches, nasal congestion, sore throat, a general "blah" feeling (more technically known as malaise).

If you are an adult and you get more than one or two colds a year, or if your cold lasts more than four or five days, you probably have a weakened immune system. Kids have a tendency to get more colds because of increased exposure to cold viruses, but any more than 3 or 4 per year is excessive.

As is true of all health concerns, prevention is the smartest strategy. By boosting your immunity, you'll have a better chance of keeping colds from developing in the first place. When you do get a cold, follow these recommendations:

Be sure to:

- Rest
- Drink plenty of liquids (water, diluted vegetable juices, soups, or herb teas). Try to drink eight ounces of water every hour.
- Avoid sugar (including natural sugars such as honey, orange juice, and fructose), because sugar depresses the immune system.
- Eat a healthy balanced diet.
- Use the "wet sock treatment" (see below).

And take:

- High potency multivitamin-multimineral supplement
- Vitamin C: 500 mg every hour that you are awake with a glass of water. If excessive gas or diarrhea is produced reduce dosage to 500 mg every two hours.
- Choose one of the following
  - Echinilin or Echinamide: Fluid extract of the fresh aerial portion of E. purpurea (1:1): 2 to 4 ml (1/2 to 1 tsp) three times daily
  - *Pelargonium sidoides.* Dosage recommendations for EPs 7630 (Umcka) or equivalent preparation:
    - Adults: 1.5 ml three times daily or 20 mg tablets three times daily for up to 14 days.
    - Children: age 7-12 years, 20 drops (1 ml) three times daily; age 6 years or less, 10 drops (0.5 ml) three times daily.

The Wet Sock Treatment

Please, if you are suffering from a cold or flu here is a treatment prescribed by physicians at Bastyr Center for Natural Health that you absolutely must try. It may seem strange, but it is based on principles of hydrotherapy that have stood the test of time. It involves putting on ice-cold socks and ... are you ready for this? ... sleeping in them! The process rallies the body's defenses. This sort of treatment is known as a "heating compress," meaning that it's up to the body to heat the cold, wet socks. The body reacts to the cold socks by increasing blood circulation to the head as well as the feet. It not acts to reflexively increase the circulation in the head, it also can decrease congestion in the upper respiratory passages, head and throat. It also has a sedating action, and many patients report that they sleep much better during the treatment. It's best to start the wet sock treatment on first day of an illness, ideally repeating it for three nights in a row if necessary.

Supplies:
- 1 pair of very thin socks, liner socks or polypropylene socks
- 1 pair of thick wool socks or thick polypropylene socks
- 2 sets of sweats or pajamas
- 1 bowl of ice water

Directions:
1. Soak the pair of thin socks in the bowl of ice water. Then wring the socks out thoroughly so they do not drip.
2. Take a hot bath for 5-10 minutes. This is very important for the effectiveness of the treatment. In fact, it could be harmful if your feet are not warmed first.
3. Dry off feet and body with a dry towel.
4. Place ice-cold wet socks on feet. Then cover with thick wool socks. Put on the first set of pajamas. Go directly to bed. Place the second set of pajamas next to the bed. Avoid getting chilled.
5. Wear the socks overnight. During the night, you may wake up with your whole body wet from sweat. If so, change into the dry pajamas, but leave on the socks. You will find that the wet cotton socks will be dry in the morning.

Exercise and Immune Function

Regular exercise has been shown to lead to improved immune status. However, there is an important distinction that needs to be made. Although more strenuous exercise is required to benefit the cardiovascular system, light to moderate exercise may be best for the immune system. In particular, studies have shown that immune function is significantly increased by the practice of Tai Chi exercises. Tai Chi is a martial art technique that features the movement from one posture to the next in a flowing motion that resembles dance. Interestingly, the same sort of improvement was also noted with ballet. The research thus far suggests that light to moderate exercise stimulates the immune system, while intense exercise (e.g., training for the Olympics) can have the opposite effect. Excessive exercise (leading to painful exhaustion two or more times a week) actually depresses the immune system for several hours after exertion, thus increasing the risk of infection during that time. One reason is that by stepping up metabolic activity, exercise results in a more rapid production of free radicals. If you exercise—and you should—be sure to eat a diet high in antioxidants and take adequate doses of nutritional antioxidants as detailed throughout this book.

Special Topic: COVID-19 and the SARS-Cov2 Virus

The worldwide COVID-19 pandemic brought focus to prevention of viral infections—both in terms of reducing risk through good hygiene as well as measures to bolster the immune system. But even before our immune system comes in contact with a coronavirus or any microorganism, there are natural barriers to infection. As it relates to the respiratory viruses, the first line of defense is the lining of the airways or respiratory tract—nasal cavity, sinuses, throat, trachea, and bronchi.

The Health of the Mucous membrane is Critical in Fighting Respiratory Infections

In order for any virus to infect the throat, sinuses, airways or lungs it must first pass through or enter the body through the mucous membranes or mucosa. It is the first barrier to infection; the immune system is the second line of defense. There are two routes for respiratory tract viruses like influenza and coronavirus to enter the lungs and cause serious damage. The primary route is through the respiratory tract, the other route is through the gastrointestinal tract.

The respiratory tract mucous membrane that lines the airways is the first line of defense. It consists primarily of cells known as ciliated epithelial cells. These cells have their external surface covered by hair-like structures called cilia. The cilia are formed into bundles and act like brushes to move the respiratory tract secretions, microorganisms, and debris up and eventually out the nose or mouth. On top of the ciliated epithelial cells are two layers of mucus. The mucus is produced by another type of epithelial cell called a goblet cell. A thinner version of mucus lies intermixed with the cilia bundles while a thicker layer sits on top of that layer. The mucus is composed of mucin, which refers to a network of proteins complexed with sugars.

The mucous membrane and mucus are specially designed to protect against any microorganism or particles from getting into the lungs. Inside the lungs is composed of specialized epithelial cells that do not have cilia. Nor are there goblet cells in the lungs. In the lungs there are only very thin epithelial cells, connective tissue, and blood capillaries all designed to perform the function of delivering oxygen to the blood and exchanging it for carbon dioxide that is then exhaled through the airways. When particulate matter or microorganisms make it to the lungs it is a very serious situation as there is very little protection there. The importance of the health of the mucus and the lining of the airways in preventing COVID-19 infection cannot be overstated ass conditions associated with poor functioning of this line of defense is associated with an increased risk of more serious infection.

The secondary route of infection for many respiratory tract viruses like SARS-CoV2 entering the body is through the gastrointestinal tract. Within the GI tract, there are a number of protective factors beyond the mucus lining. The most notable additions are digestive secretions such as stomach acid and digestive enzymes. The immune system structure in the gut is also much larger. If a virus is able to avoid these protective factors and infect the GI tract it is able to enter the bloodstream and also infect the lungs. Interestingly, this ability of coronaviruses to travel from the gut to the lungs was confirmed with Middle East respiratory syndrome coronavirus (MERS-CoV) by increasing the gastrointestinal replication of the virus by infecting animals with viruses orally while at the same time giving them an acid-blocking drug known as a proton pump inhibitor. Obviously, this begs an answer to the question "Does taking a proton pump inhibitor increase the risk for viruses that can attack the lungs by increasing the secondary route of access to the lungs." The answer is yes.

Another factor that greatly increases the risk of the secondary route of infection is a lack of digestive enzymes. It is well established that pancreatic enzyme insufficiency is a major risk factor for all viral respiratory infections. In fact, enzyme replacement therapy is the key medical approach to reduce the risk of lung infections in these patients. Enzymes that digest protein, proteases, are able to digest not only proteins in food but also the proteins on the cell walls of the virus. Viruses contain proteins protruding from their cell membranes that play critical roles in the infection process. Without these proteins, the virus simply cannot enter human cells. Supplemental proteases are also effective in supporting the mucus barrier in the airways as well (discussed below).

Support the First Line of Defense?

From the above discussion it should be clear that the first step in supporting our host defenses against COVID-19 or any organism that targets the respiratory tract is to support the production of an effective mucosal barrier. Here are some key strategies useful for added protection against infection:

- Adequate hydration.
- Supply key nutrients for epithelial function and the production of mucin (the components of mucus).
- Utilize protease enzyme formulas.

- Take N-acetylcysteine.

Adequate Hydration is Very Important to the Mucous Membranes

Water is critical to the health of the mucous membranes for several reasons. The mucin that the epithelial cells make is made "dry" otherwise there would not be enough space in the cell itself. Mucins are able to bind 1,000 times their weight in water. Without sufficient water they are not able to grow. Remember grow toys? Those cheap little toys that get bigger after you leave them in water. That is how mucus is formed. So, sufficient water is critical to mucus function. Humidifiers may help keep the airways moist but ensuring sufficient hydration from the inside out is critical to proper barrier function.

What are the Key Nutrients for Epithelial Function and the Production of Mucin?

A deficiency of any essential vitamin and mineral can lead to an altered mucosal barrier. The epithelial cells need a constant supply of nutrients in order to replicate properly as well as perform both their structural role as well as manufacturing role. It is not just mucin that these cells manufacture, they also manufacture many other protective substances critical in fighting off viruses and harmful organisms. Taking a multiple vitamin and mineral formula is crucial. Take one that provides at least the recommended dietary intake level for key nutrients like vitamin A, C, and D; B vitamins; and zinc as these nutrients are especially important. Since most multiples now contain beta-carotene as the vitamin A source, I would also recommend taking additional vitamin A in the form of retinol during a virus outbreak or increased exposure to particularly virulent forms of respiratory tract viruses. This form of vitamin A has more direct anti-infective action.

Vitamin A was the first fat-soluble vitamin to be discovered, but that is not the only reason why it was called "A"—it was given the name to signify its "anti-infective" properties. Vitamin A is absolutely critical to the health and function mucous membranes. Vitamin A deficient individuals are more susceptible to infectious diseases, in general, but especially viral infections. Vitamin A supplementation has been shown to produce significant benefits in improving immune function during viral infections, especially when fighting respiratory tract viruses in children.[2]

Dosage ranges for vitamin A reflect intent of use. During the cold and flu months to support the health of the mucosa and immune system, a dosage of 3,000 mcg (10,000 IU) for men and 1,500 mcg (5,000 IU) for women is safe. During an acute viral infection, a single oral loading dosage of 15,000 mcg or 50,000 IU is safe as long as there is ZERO chance of pregnancy. Because high doses of vitamin A during pregnancy can cause birth defects, women of childbearing age should not supplement with more than 1,500 mcg (5,000 IU) of vitamin A per day. The same warning applies during lactation.

Vitamin D is also important to take a little extra of than what is typically found in a multiple vitamin and mineral formula. There is a growing body of science that show low levels of vitamin D increase the risk for viral respiratory infections. Since we can make vitamin D in our skin when it interacts with sunlight, there is obviously a natural tendency for many people to make less vitamin D during the winter months. Supplementing the diet with additional vitamin D can help prevent this winter-time drop in vitamin D levels. Beyond that it appears that vitamin D functions in the body in a way that prevents viruses from infecting cells. Research has shown that vitamin D supplementation prevents respiratory infections in adults and children. During the winter months, most vitamin D experts recommend taking 5,000 IU per day for adults and children over 10 years of age. For children under the age of 1 year the dosage is 1,000 IU; for children between the ages of 2-4 years 2,000 IU; and for children between the ages of 4 through 9 the suggested dose is 3000 IU daily. During an acute viral infection, a single loading dose of up to ten times these suggested dosages is appropriate.

Protease Enzyme Formulas Fight Infection

Certain protease enzymes have shown benefits in improving the composition, physical characteristics, and function of mucus. Proteases are often used in digestive formulas to aid in the breakdown of dietary protein. When taken on an empty stomach away from food, these proteases are absorbed into the bloodstream to exert systemic effects including beneficial effects on mucus composition and function.

The best studied protease is mucolase - a special fungal protease with confirmed actions on respiratory tract mucus. One clinical study looked at the effect of mucolase on mucus in patients with chronic bronchitis. The patients were randomly assigned to receive either the protease or a placebo for ten days. While the placebo had no effect on the mucus, mucolase produced significant changes in both viscosity (thickness) and elasticity (stretchiness) at the end of treatment. In fact, the improved mucus structure and function was apparent up to eight days after the end of treatment.

In another ten-day double-blind study, mucolase was shown not only to improve the viscoelasticity of mucus, but also reduce airway inflammation. Key benefits in fighting any sort of respiratory tract infection. Other proteases like bromelain, nattokinase, and serratia peptidase have shown similar effects. All of these proteases decrease the thickness of the mucus while at the same time increasing mucus production as well as dramatically increasing the ciliary transport of the mucus. The net effect is the production of much more mucus that is effective in neutralizing microbes and moving them out of the body. In addition to enhancing the mechanical effects of mucus, proteases may enable special protective factors within mucus to more effectively neutralize invading organisms. Some of the protective factors secreted in mucus are secretory IgA, various white blood cell-derived protease inhibitors that block viruses, nitric oxide, and lactoferrin.

For best results during times of need, I recommend using protease formulas that contain mucolase from well-respected brands. Be sure to take these enzymes away from food and follow label dosage instructions.

Protease Enzymes Exert Antiviral Activity

While proteases are capable of attacking and digesting proteins on viruses within the digestive tract, within the body and along the respiratory tract any antiviral action of supplemental proteases is likely much more complex than simply taking out their proteins that attachment to epithelial cells. In fact, the most significant antiviral effect may be mediated by just the opposite effect—protease inhibition. When proteases are taken into the systemic circulation or interact with our immune system, it results in an increase in the production of protease inhibitors being produced by the body, particularly white blood cells as a compensatory mechanism. Protease inhibitors secreted by our own white blood cells as well as in drug form are known antiviral agents. In particular, white blood cells within the lining of the mucosa of the respiratory secrete a protease inhibitor that protects the epithelial cells from microbial proteases that promote infection and spreading. This not only protects the cells from infection, but also exerts antimicrobial effects as well. More technically, secretory leukocyte protease inhibitor (SLPI) is particularly important in airway secretions because of its broad-spectrum antibiotic activity including its antiviral effects. And, the protection of SLPI goes even further by blocking viral attachment and also protecting the lungs against attack by our own immune system.

One of the hallmark features of severe COVID-19 infection is massive destruction to lung tissues caused not so much by the virus, but rather by our immune system. Much of this damage is caused by the release of proteases from our own white blood cells. SLPI is one of the major defenses against the destruction of the lungs by our own immune system. My feeling is that people most susceptible to the lung damage in COVID-19 infection is the result of lower levels of SLPI. Studies with influenza virus shows that when there is a decrease in respiratory tract protease inhibitors it leads to increased activation and replication of the influenza virus. The same scenario is likely happening with COVID-19 pneumonia.

How N-Acetylcysteine Supports the Respiratory Tract

N-acetylcysteine (NAC) is a sulfur containing amino acid that has an extensive history of use as a mucus modifying agent to support the respiratory tract. It is also used in the body to form the glutathione—the major antioxidant for the entire respiratory tract and lungs. People who are exposed to smoke or other respiratory toxins, who suffer from conditions associated with inflammation such as diabetes, obesity, and other chronic conditions have lower levels of glutathione. Low levels of glutathione may be responsible for these conditions also being risk factors for more severe outcomes with COVID-19. NAC supplementation can boost glutathione levels and help protect the lungs and respiratory tract.

NAC is also a mucus modifying agent. It has been used orally with great success as well as in hospitals through breathing tubes to help people dealing with inefficient or thick mucus in acute and chronic lung conditions such as emphysema, bronchitis, chronic asthma, and cystic fibrosis. NAC helps to reduce the viscosity of bronchial secretions. NAC has also been found to improve the ability of cilia in the respiratory tract to clear mucus, increasing the clearance rate by 35%. As a result of these effects NAC improves bronchial and lung function, reduces cough, and improves oxygen saturation in the blood when the respiratory tract is being challenged. For protection and boosting glutathione levels in the lung the dosage is generally 500 to 1,000 mg daily. For use in reducing mucus thickness, the typical dosage is 200 to 400 mg three times daily.

Take Protease Enzymes and/or NAC During an Active Respiratory Tract Infection

The mucus modifying effects of supplemental proteases and NAC are well-displayed during an acute respiratory infection. By decreasing the viscosity, ciliary action is improved leading to less mucus congestion thereby not only reducing symptoms of congestion, but also the likelihood of a secondary bacterial infection. Thick mucus is a breeding ground for disease-causing bacteria. NAC and formulas that contain protease enzymes like mucolase, bromelain, or serratia peptidase should be used whenever mucus is thick or viscous to reduce the risk of infection.

Hyperimmunity Assessment

Circle the number that best describes the intensity of your symptoms on the following scale:

0 = I do not experience this symptom

1 = Mild

2 = Moderate

3 = Severe

Some items are scored as either Yes or No. When adding your total, score 0 for each No answer and 10 for each Yes.

1.	Entire body aches or is painful to touch	0	1	2	3
2.	Swollen joints	0	1	2	3
3.	Food sensitivity or allergy	0	1	2	3
4.	Certain foods make you sick, depressed, jittery	0	1	2	3
5.	Chronic pain or inflammation	0	1	2	3
6.	Painful stomach and/or intestine	0	1	2	3
7.	Hay fever symptoms (eyes itch, nasal discharge)	0	1	2	3
8.	Puffiness or dark circles under eyes	0	1	2	3
9.	Chronic sinusitis/rhinitis	0	1	2	3
10.	Use cortisone, prednisone, or antihistamines	NO	YES		
11.	Eczema	NO	YES		
12.	Asthma/bronchitis	NO	YES		
13.	Autoimmune disease (rheumatoid arthritis, lupus, etc.)	NO	YES		

TOTAL _____

Interpreting Your Scores

If you are suffering from asthma, rheumatoid arthritis or some other clear-cut condition linked to an overactive immune system, you will definitely need to make tuning up your immune system a top priority. Based upon the assessment, if your score is: 12 or more it is a high priority; 6-11 a moderate priority; and 1-5 a low priority. As noted above, a person can be suffering from hyperimmunity and signs of low immune function at the same time. The reason is that chronic allergies or the use of drugs such as prednisone can suppress the body's ability to fight infections. Likewise, all of the nutritional recommendations above in regard to boosting your immune system apply here as well, however, I would not go with the herbal approaches. I will give different recommendations for support below. I do want to stress that for people suffering from allergies, autoimmune disease, or any other sign of hyperimmunity the importance of eating an allergy free diet that is also free of animal foods (with the exception of fish because of their omega-3 fatty acids) must not be underestimated. These simple dietary approaches have shown remarkable effectiveness in these conditions.

Food Allergies

Food allergies are an underlying factor in many cases of poor immune function. It's essential that you identify, and deal with, any food allergies especially if you scored high on the hyperimmunity assessment. Strange as it sounds, the biggest source for antigens in the body (substances that trigger an immune response) is the food we eat.

If you are allergic to a food, your body reacts to it as if it were a dangerous invader. The white blood cells migrate in large numbers to the mucous membranes and the lining of the intestinal tract. There they release allergic and inflammatory compounds in an attempt to kill the false invader. All this inflammation causes the intestinal tract to become more permeable. The "leaky gut" can allow large, harmful molecules to be absorbed into the bloodstream. The immune system rightfully recognizes these large molecules as foreign and develops antibodies against them. The result of this immune response can be a range of unpleasant conditions, from asthma, eczema, psoriasis, and even severe inflammatory conditions like rheumatoid arthritis (see Table 6.1).

Table 6.1 - Symptoms and Diseases Commonly Associated with Food Allergy

System	Symptoms and Diseases
Gastrointestinal	Canker sores, celiac disease, chronic diarrhea, duodenal ulcer, gastritis, irritable bowel syndrome, malabsorption, ulcerative colitis
Genitourinary	Bed-wetting, chronic bladder infections, nephrosis
Immune	Chronic infections, frequent ear infections
Mental/emotional	Anxiety, depression, hyperactivity, inability to concentrate, insomnia, irritability, mental confusion, personality change, seizures
Musculoskeletal	Bursitis, joint pain, low back pain
Respiratory	Asthma, chronic bronchitis, wheezing
Skin	Acne, eczema, hives, itching, skin rash
Miscellaneous	Arrhythmia, edema, fainting, fatigue, headache, hypoglycemia, itchy nose or throat, migraines, sinusitis

The Elimination Diet

Many nutritionally oriented physicians perform blood tests to diagnose food allergies. However, in most cases such tests are not really necessary. I think trying a simple elimination diet first is a good idea to see if their symptoms improve. If there is only partial or little improvement and I still think food allergy is a significant factor, then I will perform a blood test to identify food allergies. Often, however, we are able to see the foods that trigger the symptoms when they are re-introduced into the diet. Start by eliminating the most common allergens:

- Milk and all dairy products

- Wheat
- Corn
- Citrus
- Peanuts and peanut butter
- Eggs
- Processed foods containing artificial food coloring

The standard elimination diet consists of lamb, chicken, potatoes, rice, banana, apple, and a cabbage-family vegetable (cabbage, brussels sprouts, broccoli, etc.). There are variations of the elimination diet that are suitable. However, it is extremely important that no allergenic foods be consumed.

The individual stays on the elimination diet for at least one week, and up to one month. If the symptoms are related to food sensitivity, they will typically disappear by the fifth or sixth day of the diet. If the symptoms do not disappear, it is possible that a reaction to a food in the elimination diet is responsible. In that case, an even more restricted diet must be utilized.

After the elimination-diet period, individual foods are reintroduced every two days. Methods range from reintroducing only a single food every two days, to reintroducing a food every one or two meals. Usually, after the one-week "cleansing" period, a person will develop an increased sensitivity to offending foods.

Reintroduction of allergenic foods will typically produce a more severe or recognizable symptom than before. A careful, detailed record must be maintained, describing when foods were reintroduced and what symptoms appeared upon reintroduction. It can be very useful to track the wrist pulse during reintroduction, as pulse changes may occur when an allergenic food is consumed.

Will you be able to eat that food again? That depends on whether the allergy is cyclic or fixed:

Cyclic allergies develop slowly and result from repeatedly eating a certain food. After avoiding the allergenic food for a period of time (typically three to four months), it may be reintroduced. Usually the food won't cause symptoms again unless you eat it too frequently or in high amounts. Cyclic allergies account for roughly eighty to ninety percent of food allergies.

Fixed allergies occur whenever a food is eaten, no matter how much time has passed. If you have a fixed allergy, you will remain allergic to the food for life.

Rheumatoid Arthritis (RA) and Other Autoimmune Diseases

Autoimmune diseases refer to conditions where the body's immune system literally attacks body tissues. What triggers the autoimmune reaction is not clear but genetic abnormalities, dietary factors, food allergies, bacterial overgrowth, the "leaky gut syndrome", and immunizations have all been suggested as possible causes. The most well-known autoimmune disease is rheumatoid arthritis (RA)—a condition where primarily the joints come under attack. Diseases similar to RA that affect connective tissue (collagen structures which support internal organs as well as cartilage, tendons, muscles, and bone) include systemic lupus erythematosus (lupus or SLE), ankylosing spondylitis, scleroderma, polymalgia rheumatica, and mixed connective tissue disease. There is tremendous overlap among these diseases in terms of underlying causes, symptoms, and treatment. They share many common features with RA, but the autoimmune and inflammatory process is a bit different in each of these other diseases. There are many treatments available to relieve the symptoms of RA and these other autoimmune diseases, but rather than simply mask the symptoms I recommend addressing some of the underlying causes. The two primary factors that I recommend that you focus on if you have RA or any other autoimmune disease is to identify and eliminate food allergies along with changing the type of fatty acids in body tissues by eliminating animal products (with the exception of fish) from the diet.

The most common food allergies in RA are wheat, corn, dairy products, beef, and plants of the nightshade family (tomatoes, eggplants, peppers, etc.). I recommend an elimination diet to identify your food allergies.

Case History: Kim's Miracle

Kim was a 22-yearold student who had already been struggling with severe rheumatoid arthritis for more than ten years. The disease—and the twenty-one different medications that she was taking—were crushing body, mind, and spirit. She wanted to be rescued both from the ravages of this cruel disease and from its dangerous treatment.

Since Kim was taking prescription medications for her condition, I could not administer a blood test for food allergies. Instead I began her treatment with a low-allergy diet for two weeks. I restricted her dietary intake to fresh carrot juice, pineapple juice, herbal teas, vegetable broths, and three servings of a hypo-allergenic meal replacement formula. My goal was to decrease the absorption of allergic food components. After the two weeks, I would evaluate her symptoms and joint swelling. If she was better, it would suggest that food allergies were likely responsible for her symptoms. I also started Kim on the following supplements:

- High potency multiple vitamin and mineral formula
- Vitamin C: 1000 mg three times daily
- Vitamin E: 800 IU daily
- Fish oils: 3,000 mg EPA+DHA daily
- Bromelain: 400 mg (1800 to 2000 mcu [milk clotting units]) between meals three times daily
- Curcumin: 400 mg between meals three times daily

At her return visit two weeks later, she was noticeably improved, so we moved to Phase 2. Kim reintroduced a "new" food item every second day. If she noticed an increase in pain, stiffness, or joint swelling within two to forty-eight hours, she omitted his item from her diet for at least seven days before reintroducing it a second time. If the food caused worsening of symptoms after the second time, it was omitted permanently.

We identified some real problem foods for Kim: corn, wheat, milk and dairy products, oranges, strawberries, and peanuts. Those foods were permanently removed from her diet. I also recommended that she stay away from beef, chicken, turkey, and other meats. The only animal foods that I approved for her were fish and wild game such as venison, elk, or buffalo (these meats have lower overall fat with a higher percentage of omega-3 fatty acids). I also urged Kim to drink up to twenty-four ounces of fresh vegetable and fruit juice each day.

After three months, I started weaning her off some of her drugs. After one year, Kim reduced the number of drugs she was on from twenty-one down to three: prednisone, methotrexate, and Plaquenil. Her dosage of prednisone had been as high as 15 mg per day; anything less and she suffered excruciating pain. Three years after first seeing me, Kim was able to only be on prednisone at a dosage of 5 mg per day. She no longer takes the 20 other drugs she was taking. Her symptoms have cleared up, her disease is in remission (permanently, it seems). Most important, she has gone from someone who was being ravaged to a ravishing young woman full of life.

Once you've identified any foods that trigger allergies, you should eat a diet that is rich in whole foods, vegetables, complex carbohydrates, and fiber, and that is low in sugar, meat, refined carbohydrates, and animal fats. It's especially important to take flaxseed oil and eat lots of cold-water fish, such as mackerel, herring, halibut, and salmon. These provide omega-3 fatty acids, which promote healthy cells and suppress production of inflammatory compounds. They also reduce your body's response to allergens. I also recommend taking a fish oil to supply a dosage of 3,000 mg per day of EPA+DHA.

Also make sure your antioxidant intake is up to par. In addition to taking extra vitamin C and E, I strongly recommend that you increase

your intake of fresh fruits and vegetables by consuming fresh j.
below). Autoimmune diseases such as RA and lupus are associated \
tremendous amount of inflammation, much of which is due to free radical
damage. Since antioxidants protect against oxidative damage, low levels of
antioxidants in the diet appear to increase the risk for these inflammatory
diseases. A recent study, which followed patients for fifteen years, found
that those most at risk of developing autoimmune diseases were those who
had lower levels of vitamin A, beta-carotene, and selenium.

During flare-ups, fresh pineapple juice along with some fresh ginger
root may help to relieve symptoms of RA due to their anti-inflammatory
activity. Ginger possesses anti-inflammatory action by inhibiting the
manufacture of inflammatory compounds and by the presence of an anti-
inflammatory enzyme similar to bromelain, which is found in pineapple.
In one clinical study, seven patients with RA in whom conventional drugs
had provided only temporary or partial relief were treated with ginger.
One patient took 50 g/day of lightly cooked ginger while the remaining
six took either 5 g of fresh or 0.1-1 g of powdered ginger daily. All patients
reported substantial improvement, including pain relief, joint mobility,
and decrease in swelling and morning stiffness.

I also recommend for severe inflammatory conditions like RA to take
curcumin along with proteolytic enzymes:

- *Proteolytic Enzymes* (or proteases) include bromelain (pineapple
  enzyme), papain (papaya enzyme), fungal proteases, and
  Serratia peptidase (the "silk worm" enzyme). Preparations of
  proteolytic enzymes have been shown to be useful in RA and
  other inflammatory conditions. For anti-inflammatory effects,
  proteolytic enzyme products should be taken on an empty
  stomach. Take two capsules of a high potency complex twice daily
  between meals. I recommend Repair Gold from Enzymedica.
- *Curcumin* is the yellow pigment of Curcuma longa (*turmeric*).
  It exerts excellent support for the body's anti-inflammatory and
  antioxidant systems. In models of acute inflammation, curcumin
  is as effective as either cortisone or the potent anti-inflammatory

drug phenylbutazone. However, while phenylbutazone and cortisone are associated with significant toxicity, curcumin is without side effects. In human studies, curcumin has demonstrated some beneficial effects that are comparable to those of standard drugs in clinical trials in arthritis. Theracurmin and Meriva are the most biovailable and well-researched forms of curcumin. In RA, the dosage I recommend for Theracurmin is 180 mg daily, for Meriva it is 2000 mg daily.

Tune-Up Tip: Turn on the Juice

One of the best things you can do for health is to drink fresh juice, the liquid extracted from fresh fruits and vegetables. Fresh juice provides high-quality nutrition that is easily absorbed. It also provides a wide assortment of compounds that are extremely beneficial to health, including enzymes; pigments such as carotenes, chlorophyll, and flavonoids; and numerous other antioxidant components. Here is my all-time favorite recipe for relief of rheumatoid arthritis and other autoimmune diseases:

- Juice the following: 1/2 medium-sized pineapple cut into slices (skin and all if your juicer can handle it); 1/2 cup of blueberries; and a half-inch slice of fresh ginger.
- The blueberries offer benefit because of their high flavonoid content. Fresh pineapple contains bromelain, an anti-inflammatory enzyme. Fresh ginger possesses significant anti-inflammatory action.
- In order to juice you are going to need two things: fresh organic produce free from pesticides and surface sprays, and a good juicer.

DHEA for RA and Lupus

Defective manufacture of testosterone and dehydroepiandrosterone (DHEA) has been proposed as a potential predisposing factor for lupus as well as rheumatoid arthritis. Studies at Stanford Medical Center have shown that supplementation with DHEA offers moderate therapeutic benefits in patients with lupus. In the most recent double-blind study, 21 patients with severe lupus received DHEA (200mg/day) or a placebo for six months. Both patient groups continued conventional treatment with corticosteroids and/or drugs that suppress the immune system. Significant improvements were noted in seven of the nine patients on DHEA. DHEA supplementation also protected against the bone loss (osteoporosis) so typical of long-term corticosteroid use. Although the dosage of DHEA was very high, mild acne and disruption of normal menstrual cycles were the only side effects noted.

Since these studies were done at Stanford, your physician will feel comfortable supervising a trial of high dosage DHEA if you have lupus or RA. In my own clinical experience, I have found that dosages of 50 mg per day are usually sufficient in cases of RA or lupus in people less than 50 years of age; higher dosages are usually required in older subjects.

Longevity Matrix Lifestyle Tune Up Tip #6: Laugh Hard and Often

Our mood and attitude have a tremendous bearing on the function of our immune system. When we are happy and optimistic, our immune system functions much better. Conversely, when we are depressed or pessimistic, our immune system tends to be depressed. It was easily accepted by conventional medical authorities that negative emotional states adversely affect the immune system, but for some reason the medical community initially scoffed at the notion that positive emotional states can actually enhance immune function.

By the end of the 1970s, several studies had shown that negative emotions suppress immune function. But in 1979, Norman Cousins' popular book Anatomy of an Illness caused a significant stir in the medical community. Cousins' book provided an autobiographical anecdotal account that positive emotional states can cure the body of even a quite serious disease (he had scleroderma, an autoimmune disease). Cousins' watched Candid Camera, Marx brothers' films, and read humorous books.

Originally physicians and researchers scoffed at Cousins' account. Now, however, it has been demonstrated in numerous studies that laughter and other positive emotional states can in fact enhance the immune system. In addition, the use of guided imagery, hypnosis and other meditative states have been shown to enhance immune system function.

Obviously, if you want to have a healthy immune system, you need to laugh often, view life with a positive eye, and put yourself in a relaxed state of mind on a regular basis. By laughing frequently and taking a lighter view of life, you will find that life is much more enjoyable and fun. Here are seven tips to help you get more laughter in your life:

Tip #1. Learn to laugh at yourself. Recognize how funny some of your behavior really is - especially your shortcomings or mistakes. We all have little idiosyncrasies or behaviors that are unique to us that we can recognize and enjoy. Do not take yourself too seriously.

Tip #2 - Inject humor anytime it is appropriate. People love to laugh. Get a joke book and learn how to tell a good joke. Humor and laughter really make life enjoyable.

Tip #3. Read the comics to find a comic that you find funny and follow it. Humor is very individual. What I may find funny, you may not, but the comics or "funny papers" have something for everybody. Read them thoroughly to find a comic strip that you find particularly funny and look for it every day or week.

Tip #4. Watch comedies on television. With modern cable systems, I am amazed at how easy it is to find something funny on television. When I am in need of a good laugh, I try to find something I can laugh at on TV. Some of my favorites are the old-time classics like Andy Griffith, Gilligan's Island, Mary Tyler Moore, etc.

Tip #5. Go to comedies at the movie theater. I love to go to the movies with friends and family, especially a comedy. If we see a funny movie together, I find myself laughing harder and longer than if I had seen the same scene by myself. We feed off each other's laughter during and after the movie. Laughing together helps build good relationships.

Tip #6. Play with kids. Kids really know how to laugh and play. I am truly blessed with two great kids that I find hilarious to play with. If you do not have kids of your own, spend time with your nieces, nephews, or neighborhood children with whose families you are friendly. Become a Big Brother or Sister. Investigate local Little Leagues. Help out at your church's Sunday School and children's events.

Tip #7. Ask yourself the question - "What is funny about this situation?" Many times in life we will find ourselves in seemingly impossible situations, but, if we can laugh about it, somehow, they become enjoyable or at least tolerable experiences. So many times, I have heard people say, "This is something that you will look back on and laugh about." Well, why wait - find the humor in the situation and enjoy a good laugh immediately.

CHAPTER 7:

The "Heart" of Extending Life

The heart and all of the blood vessels compose the cardiovascular system. Its primary functions are to deliver oxygen and vital nutrition to cells throughout the body as well as aid in the removal of cellular waste products. Basically, blood flow is critical to all body tissues. And, improving the health of any tissue, whether it is the brain or the heart itself, involves improving blood flow to that tissue.

Our heart is truly amazing. Each day, it beats 100,000 times, pumping 2,500 to 5,000 gallons of blood through the 60,000 miles of blood vessels within our bodies. In an average lifetime, the heart will beat 2.5 billion times and pump 100 billion gallons of blood! These numbers fill me with awe.

Obviously, we need to support the heart in its near tireless efforts. Unfortunately, as a nation we are doing a very poor job of keeping our hearts healthy. Heart disease and strokes are our nation's number one and four killers, respectively. All together, these two conditions are responsible for at least 40% of all deaths in the United States. Both are referred to as "silent killers" because the first symptom or sign in many cases is a fatal event. The cause of both conditions is often due to the process of atherosclerosis - hardening of the artery walls.

Arteries carry blood away from the heart, and veins carry blood toward the heart. Atherosclerosis also contributes to high blood pressure, which is a major risk factor for a heart attack or stroke. Blood pressure refers to the resistance produced each time the heart beats and sends blood coursing through the arteries. The peak reading of the pressure exerted by the heart's contraction is the systolic pressure. Between beats the heart relaxes, and blood pressure drops. The lowest reading is referred to as the diastolic pressure. A normal blood pressure reading for an adult is: 120 (systolic) / 80 (diastolic). Readings above this level are a major risk factor for heart attack and stroke. High blood pressure readings can be divided into the following levels:

- Prehypertension (120-139/80-89)
- Borderline (120-160/90-94)
- Mild (140-160/95-104)
- Moderate 140-180/105-114)
- Severe (160+/115+)

Case History: The Breath of Health

My new patient was near tears as she told me why she had come. Anna was 74 years old. Her medical doctor had recently told her that her blood pressure was way too high—190 over 140—and prescribed a drug to bring it down. She told me she absolutely didn't want to take a drug, when I measured her pressure again, I found it had soared to 210 over160—dangerously high. I told her I agreed with her previous doctor that something had to be done and explained that sometimes drug therapy is the best approach if the benefits outweigh the risks.

She protested tearfully that I didn't understand. Her mother had been in perfect health except for high blood pressure well into her 80's. When her mother finally started taking blood pressure medication, her health started a very fast downward spiral. She died soon afterward. Anna associated her death to the medication. Not surprisingly, she was deathly afraid of taking drugs for blood pressure herself.

It was then I noticed how fearful Anna was, near a full-on panic attack. Her breathing was especially shallow and rapid. I knew that I had to help her get herself calm and under control. I started asking her questions about her life: What are the things you really enjoy? Do you have grandchildren? Where is the most peaceful place you have ever been? Her breathing started to slow down, but she was still breathing shallowly, using only her upper chest. I spent the next few minutes teaching her diaphragmatic breathing. It took a while, but finally she started to engage her diaphragm and truly breathe. Then, as I continued to ask questions that conjured up peaceful and relaxed images in her mind's eye, I took her blood pressure. It had fallen to 160/110 mm Hg. I explained to Anna that we could keep her off blood pressure medication, but only if she agreed to do everything that I asked of her.

My first prescription was for her to perform diaphragmatic breathing for five minutes every waking hour. The second task was to walk down to her local fire station for a free blood pressure check every afternoon. And finally, I prescribed a nutritional supplement to lower blood pressure, extra potassium, and a high-quality garlic product. It was Wednesday, and I asked Anna to call me on Saturday morning to give me a report.

Saturday at seven AM my phone rang. (I learned a valuable lesson here: always specify the time for a patient to check in!) Anna told me that her blood pressure had dropped to 140 over 90. A few days later in my clinic I was pleased to find Anna's blood pressure a normal 120/80 mm Hg.

Was it the pills I had given her? Honestly, I don't think so. I really think it was simply that she had learned how to breathe deeply again. There is actually an FDA approved breathing apparatus that is clinically proven to lower blood pressure. It is called Resperate. It is a portable electronic device that promotes slow, deep breathing by using chest sensors to measure your breathing. A computerized unit creates a melody for you to use to synchronize your breathing. It is available without a prescription. If you need help learning to really breathe and relax, I highly recommend it.

Assessing Your Cardiovascular System

Circle the number that best describes the intensity of your symptoms on the following scale:

0 = I do not experience this symptom
1 = Mild
2 = Moderate
3 = Severe

Score 0 for each No answer and 10 for each Yes.

Section A: Heart and blood pressure

1.	Shortness of breath	0	1	2	3
2.	Chest pain while walking	0	1	2	3
3.	Heaviness in legs	0	1	2	3
4.	Calf muscles cramp while walking	0	1	2	3
5.	Heart pounds easily	0	1	2	3
6.	Feel jittery	0	1	2	3
7.	Heart misses beats or has extra beats	0	1	2	3
8.	Swelling of feet and ankles	0	1	2	3
9.	Rapid beating heart (>80 beats per minute)	0	1	2	3
10.	Feel exhausted with minor exertion	0	1	2	3

11.	Do you snore or suffer from sleep apnea	0	1	2	3
12.	Do you have male-patterned baldness	NO	YES		
13.	Presence of diagonal ear lobe crease (wrinkle)	NO	YES		
14.	Is your blood pressure high (>140/90 mm Hg)?	NO	YES		
15.	Total cholesterol level above 200?	NO	YES		

TOTAL _____

Scoring
- 11 or more: High Priority
- 7-10: Moderate Priority
- 1-6: Low Priority

Section B: Circulation

1.	Cold hands and feet	0	1	2	3
2.	Slurred speech	0	1	2	3
3.	Calf muscles cramp while walking	0	1	2	3
4.	Headaches	0	1	2	3
5.	Numbness in extremities	0	1	2	3
6.	Poor concentration	0	1	2	3
7.	Ringing in ears	0	1	2	3
8.	Dizziness	0	1	2	3
9.	Ringing in the ears	0	1	2	3
10.	History of stroke	NO	YES		

TOTAL _____

Scoring
- 9 or more: High Priority
- 5-8: Moderate Priority
- 1-4: Low Priority

Interpreting Your Score

The questions in Section A assess the overall condition of your heart. Symptoms such as shortness of breath or swelling of the feet may indicate that your heart isn't pumping efficiently enough to remove fluid. Heaviness in the legs or muscle cramping may mean not enough blood is reaching the muscles, especially during work or exercise. Abnormal heart rhythms result from problems with electrical signals that regulate the beat, due to damaged or constricted blood vessels, stress, or hormonal imbalance. In most cases, heart disease results from the buildup of cholesterol-containing plaque in the blood vessels.

Section B reflects the state of your circulation. For example, if your blood pressure is not high enough to propel blood to your hands and feet, your fingers and toes may feel cold or numb all the time. In contrast, high pressure can cause vessels to burst, leading to stroke.

You May be Wondering . . .

What does the presence of a diagonal earlobe crease have to do with heart disease? The answer: plenty. More than thirty studies have shown that the presence of a diagonal ear lobe crease is more predictive of the risk for having a heart attack than an angiogram (a procedure where dye is injected into the coronary arteries to determine blockage). The earlobe is richly veined, and a decrease in blood flow over a period of time is believed to result in collapse of the vascular bed. This leads to a diagonal crease. Other interesting findings are that the presence of hair in the ear canal, male-pattern baldness, and snoring are also very strong predictors of heart disease and strokes.

A Brief Guide to Cardiovascular Disorders

The term "heart disease" is most often to describe atherosclerosis (hardening of the artery walls due to a buildup of plaque containing cholesterol, fatty material, and cellular debris) of the blood vessels supplying the heart—the coronary arteries. Atherosclerosis is one main cause of heart attacks and strokes. Atherosclerosis results from the buildup of a cellular debris called plaque along the walls of the blood vessel. Normally your arteries are very flexible, like a rubber tube. Plaque, especially when it becomes calcified, causes them to become stiff and can even block blood flow.

The plaque can also lead to the formation of blood clots - thickened clumps of blood that form when disk-shaped particles called platelets collect at the site of blood vessel damage. The platelets are held in place by stringy protein strands called fibrin, which is made from smaller particles called fibrinogen. Usually what happens is that the clot forms in a large vessel, where it may slow down—but not stop—blood flow. But if a piece of the clot breaks off, it will eventually circulate into a vessel that is too small to allow it to pass. As a result, blood flow to that part of the body stops, and the nearby organ or tissue can die. The bigger the clot, the bigger (and more important) the vessel it can block. The technical term for this condition is thrombosis (from the Greek word for clot.) A thromboembolism indicates that the clot has traveled away from its site of origin (*embol-* comes from the Greek meaning "to throw").

A *heart attack* (also called a myocardial infarction) occurs when something blocks the flow of blood to the heart—it can be a clot, a spasm of a coronary artery; or accumulation of plaque. Like each of your other organs, the heart needs its own supply of blood. This hard-working pump requires a steady supply of oxygen and other nutrients. The coronary arteries feed the heart. If something interrupts the blood supply, the starved muscle tissue begins to die very rapidly. The longer the blockage lasts, the greater the risk that the heart attack will be fatal.

A *stroke* is brain damage that occurs when the blood flow is interrupted or when a vessel bursts, causing blood to spurt into the surrounding tissue. While attacks involve coronary arteries, while strokes involve arteries feeding to the brain (carotid arteries). When the supply of blood is shut off, nerves in the brain die almost immediately. Sometimes the pressure of blood gushing through a ruptured vessel slices through the delicate nerves, severing their millions of connections. Depending on which part of the brain is affected, damage can include loss of movement, speech, memory, or virtually any function of the body. Strokes are fatal in about one case out of three.

High blood pressure can play a critical role in the development of heart disease and strokes. In fact, it is generally regarded as the most serious risk factor for a stroke. The higher the pressure, the greater the stress on the arteries and the more rapid buildup of plaque leading to atherosclerosis. Your blood contains lots of different chemicals and particles besides red and white cells. Pressure forces these substances past the cells that line the blood vessels, possibly leading to cell damage due to friction, irritation, or inflammation. If the vessel has a weak spot, high pressure can cause the spot to bulge or, in the case of some of the small blood vessels in the brain, possibly burst, resulting in a stroke.

Understanding Atherosclerosis

Your blood vessels have three major layers. The innermost layer is known as the intima or the endothelium. The cells of this layer are exposed to constant friction as blood and the various particles in contain flow by, often at high pressure. Molecules known as glycosaminoglycans (GAGs) line the cells, protecting them from damage and promoting repair. Beneath the surface of endothelial cells is a protective membrane, which also contains GAGs.

The middle layer, or media, is mainly muscle that allows the vessel to widen (dilate) or shrink in diameter, depending on your circulation needs of the moment. The outer layer, the adventitia, is an elastic membrane consisting of connective tissue. These layers also contain GAGs and other substances that provide support and elasticity.

Atherosclerosis begins when something happens to damage the GAG layer that protects the inner lining of the blood vessel. That "something" might be the presence of a pathogen, such as a virus; a drug or environmental toxin; physical damage due to a spasm or high blood pressure; or an overeager immune response.

Like a leak in a dike, even a small amount of damage to the inner lining can set a deadly chain of events in motion. One critical thing that happens is that fat-carrying proteins (lipoproteins), always circulating in the blood, start attaching themselves to the GAGs, like unwanted bystanders at a traffic accident. The low-density lipoproteins (LDL) carry cholesterol. Thus, their arrival causes cholesterol to build up. When LDL binds to the site, it begins to break down, or oxidize. This releases free radicals, which further damage nearby cells. This is why dietary cholesterol is such a major risk factor for heart disease. The more you have in your blood, the more it can pile up at the site of damage to the blood vessel.

Vessel damage sets off alarms in the immune system, spurring your body's repair mechanism into action. The damaged cells secrete a chemical called growth factor, which stimulates cells to reproduce and replace damaged cells. The cells also release fibrinogen, the sticky stringy protein that collects platelets so a clot can form to prevent blood from leaking out of the vessel. White blood cells, ever helpful, arrive at the site and attach themselves to the vessel wall, turning into macrophages. These cells are on duty to destroy any harmful particles, such as oxidized LDLs. But once they become stuffed with LDL, they change into useless blobs called foam cells and lose their scavenging ability.

Macrophages also contribute their own supply of growth factor. All this growth factor causes a weird thing to happen: Cells from the smooth muscle layer of the vessel start migrating toward the inner layer. Once there, they begin replicating. They too turn into foam cells. In the process these cells dump cellular debris such a fiber-like proteins into the intima, adding more trash to the heap. Soon a kind of scar tissue, called a fibrous cap, appears in the surface of the artery lining. This combination of lipoprotein, cholesterol, fibrous protein, and biological litter forms a stiff patch called plaque. Over time the plaque continues to grow until eventually it either ruptures and a clot breaks off or it blocks the entire artery.

Your blood flow can be reduced by up to ninety percent before you feel any symptoms of atherosclerosis. By then it may be too late. You are a heart attack waiting to happen.

Keeping Blood Vessels Clear–Natural "Clot Busters"

The plaque formed in atherosclerosis can lead to the formation of blood clots—thickened clumps of blood that form when disk-shaped blood platelets collect at the site of blood vessel damage. The technical term for clot formation is thrombosis (from the Greek word for clot.) A thromboembolism indicates that the clot has traveled away from its site of origin *(embol-* comes from the Greek meaning "to throw").

If a piece of the clot breaks off to form a thromboembolism, it will eventually circulate into a vessel that is too small to allow it to pass. As a result, blood flow to that part of the body stops, and the nearby organ or tissue can die.

The bigger the clot, the bigger (and more important) the vessel it can block. If the thromboembolism blocks a blood vessel in the heart, it leads to a heart attack (also called a myocardial infarction). If it happens in the brain, it can cause a stroke. And, if it happens in the lungs it causes a pulmonary embolism. Any one of these events can result in death.

Inhibiting Excessive Platelet Aggregation

Excessive platelet aggregation is an important part of the process of atherosclerosis and is an independent risk factor for heart disease and stroke. Once platelets aggregate, they release potent compounds that dramatically promote the formation of the atherosclerotic plaque, or they can form a clot that can lodge in small arteries and produce a heart attack or stroke.

The adhesiveness or "stickiness" of platelets is largely determined by the type of fats in the diet and the level of antioxidants. While saturated fats and cholesterol increase platelet aggregation, omega-3 fatty acids from fish oils and monounsaturated fats from olive oil, and nuts and seeds have the opposite effect. Particularly useful for decreasing platelet aggregation are the long-chain omega-3 fatty acids EPA and DHA form fish oil. In fact, the beneficial effects of fish oils on platelet aggregation is one of the key reasons why higher levels of EPA and DHA in the body are associated with a 38% reduced risk of having a stroke or heart attack.

In addition to the omega-3 fatty acids there are a number of other nutritional and herbal supplements that impact platelet aggregation. Most notable is nattokinase, the clot-busting enzyme derived from natto - a traditional Japanese food prepared from fermented soybeans by the bacterial *Bacillus subtilis*. Blood clots and platelets are held in place in the atherosclerotic plaque by stringy protein strands called fibrin, which are made from smaller particles called fibrinogen. Blood levels of fibrinogen is a major determinate of cardiovascular death. In fact, there is a stronger association between cardiovascular deaths and fibrinogen levels than there is for cholesterol levels. There are a number of other natural therapies designed to promote the breakdown of fibrin (fibrinolysis) including the Mediterranean diet, exercise, omega-3 fatty acids, niacin, garlic, and ginger, but nattokinase appears to be the most potent.

Several clinical studies have confirmed the ability of nattokinase to reduce the level of fibrinogen in the blood. As stated above, since elevated fibrinogen levels are another clear risk factor for a heart attack or stroke, the results from these studies are extremely significant. Two capsules of nattokinase (100 mg or 2000 fibrinolysis units per capsule) for 2 months:

- Drops the level of fibrinogen by 7-10%
- Dissolves excess fibrin in blood vessels to which improves circulation, causes clot dissolution, and reduces risk of severe clotting to prevent strokes and heart attacks
- Reduces LDL (bad) cholesterol and increases HDL (good) cholesterol
- Reduces blood viscosity, improves blood flow and lowers blood pressure

Nattokinase should be used with caution when taking Coumadin or anti-platelet drugs (including aspirin, but especially drugs like clopidogrel, ticlopidine, ticagrelor, prasugrel, and cangrelor) as it may increase bleeding tendencies.

Speaking of aspirin. While low-dose aspirin (e.g., 80 to 325 mg/day) is a popular recommendation for preventing a heart attack, it is flat out not as effective as dietary, supplement strategies, and a health promoting lifestyle. Furthermore, in studies in patients who have had a heart attack, low dose aspirin is not effective and doses of aspirin ranging from 325 to 1500 mg per day have NOT been shown to reduce mortality and are associated with significant side effects, especially ulcers and bleeding episodes. Several studies have shown that dietary modifications are not only more effective in preventing recurrent heart attack than aspirin but can also reverse the blockage of clogged arteries. The research is strongest for using the Mediterranean diet, and a diet rich in nuts and fish sources of omega-3 fatty acids.

Precautions with Coumadin and Other Anticoagulant Drugs

Coumadin has been a mainstay in the medical prevention of clot formation, but it has many issues with breakthrough bleeding and other side effects plus patients must be constantly monitored by routine blood tests. The problem with bleeding while on these drugs is that relatively minor trauma—a fall or being hit - can cause severe internal bleeding, which can be deadly.

In the last few years, FDA has approved four new oral anticoagulant drugs—Pradaxa (dabigatran), Xarelto (rivaroxaban), Edoxaban (Savaysa), and Eliquis (apixaban). These drugs also cause bleeding, but do not require monitoring.

While the new oral anticoagulant drugs are touted as producing better results than Coumadin in preventing strokes, it may come at a price. And, not just its nearly $6,000 a year cost to the patient vs. the $200 per year for generic Coumadin, but the fact that they can cause serious spinal cord complications leading to permanent paralysis as well inflammation of the blood vessels (vasculitis), which can be minor or can cause serious problems such as blood clots, blindness, and organ damage.

The drug coumadin works by blocking the action of vitamin K. The newer drugs are direct inhibitors of clotting factors and vitamin K has no impact on their function. In people taking Coumadin, they need to avoid vitamin K supplements and foods such as green leafy vegetables, green tea, and natto. Alternatively, a person can usually eat the same levels they are accustomed to as long as they just don't increase their consumption. Physicians monitor the effects of Coumadin using a test known as the International Normalized Ratio (INR) and will adjust the dosage up or down as needed. In addition to high vitamin K-containing foods, other natural remedies may interact with coumadin. It's likely that you can continue using these products, but don't change the dosage from what your body is accustomed to. INR values must be monitored appropriately. For example:

- Coenzyme Q10 and St. John's wort (*Hypericum perforatum*) may reduce coumadin's efficacy
- Proteolytic enzymes, such as nattokinase and bromelain, and several herbs, including Panax ginseng, devil's claw (*Harpagophytum procumbens*), and dong quai (*Angelica sinensis*), can increase coumadin's effects.
- Garlic (*Allium sativum*) and ginkgo (*Ginkgo biloba*) extracts may reduce the ability of platelets to stick together, increasing the likelihood of bleeding. However, neither appears to interact directly with coumadin. Generally people taking coumadin should avoid taking these products at higher dosages (more than the equivalent of one clove of garlic per day for garlic or more than 240 mg per day of ginkgo extract) but not to worry if they are just on the typical support dose.

- Iron, magnesium, and zinc may bind with coumadin, potentially decreasing its absorption and activity. Take coumadin and iron/magnesium/zinc-containing products at least two hours apart.

  Here is a key recommendation to reduce the likelihood of bleeding and easy bruising with Coumadin, take 150 to 300 mg of either grape seed or pine bark extract daily. It will not interfere with coumadin, but it will definitely help prevent the easy bruising.

Risk Factors for Cardiovascular Disease

Risk factors are divided into two primary categories: major risk factors and other risk factors. Keep in mind that some of the other risk factors have been shown to actually be more important than the so-called major risk factors. For example, a strong argument could be made that insulin resistance and elevations in C-reactive protein (CRP), a marker for inflammation, are much more important than elevated cholesterol levels. It is also important to point out that the risk for a heart attack increases exponentially with the number of risk factors.

Table 7.1 - Risk Factors for Atherosclerosis

Major Risk Factors:
- Smoking
- Elevated blood cholesterol levels (especially oxidized LDL known as oxLDL)
- High blood pressure
- Diabetes
- Physical inactivity

Other Risk Factors for Atherosclerosis:
- Elevations of high sensitivity C-reactive protein
- Insulin resistance

- Low thyroid function
- Low antioxidant status
- Low levels of essential fatty acids
- Increased platelet aggregation
- Increased fibrinogen formation
- Low levels of magnesium and/or potassium
- Elevated levels of homocysteine
- "Type A" personality

If two or more of these major factors apply to you, your risk increases significantly. For example, if you smoke, have high cholesterol, and have high blood pressure, you are more than 700 times likelier to have heart disease—and you will probably die twenty to thirty years sooner—than someone without any of these factors.

Table 7.2 - Compounding Risk

Condition	Increased Risk of Heart Disease
Presence of 1 major risk factor	30%
High cholesterol + high blood pressure	300%
High cholesterol + smoking	350%
High blood pressure + smoking	350%
Smoking + high blood pressure + high cholesterol	720%

To calculate your risk, complete the risk assessment for men or women below. You'll need to ask your doctor for some of the information required. You should also undergo a thorough clinical examination if you have a personal or family history of heart disease.

Men: Determining Your Risk for Heart Disease and Strokes

Answering the questions below will help you calculate your risk of having a heart attack within the next ten years. Circle your score for each section, add your total points, and find your risk. Then compare your risk with the average risk for other people your age.

1. Age

Age	Points
30-34	-1
35-39	0
40-44	1
45-49	2
50-54	3
55-59	4
60-64	5
65-69	6
70-74	7

2. Total cholesterol

Less than 160	-3
160-199	0
200-239	1
240-279	2
280 or more	3

3. HDL cholesterol

Less than 35	2
35-44	1
45-49	0
50-59	0
60 or more	-2

4. Blood pressure

Find the point on the chart where your systolic and diastolic blood pressure readings intersect. For example, if your reading is 130 (systolic) over 80 (diastolic), your point score is 1.

Systolic	Diastolic				
	79 or less	80-84	85-89	90-99	100 or more
Less than 120	0	0	1	2	3
120-139	0	0	1	2	3
130-139	1	1	1	2	3
140-159	2	2	2	2	3
160 or more	3	3	3	3	3

5. Have diabetes

No   0

Yes   2

6. Smoker

No   0

Yes   2

7. 10-year heart disease risk
Add your total points: _____

Total points	Risk
Less than 0	2%
0	3%
1	3%
2	4%
3	5%

4	7%
5	8%
6	10%
7	13%
8	16%
9	20%
10	25%
11	31%
12	37%
13	45%
14 or more	53% or more

Compare with average and low risk by age

Age	Average risk	Low risk
30-34	3%	2%
35-39	5%	3%
40-44	7%	4%
45-49	11%	4%
50-54	14%	5%
55-59	16%	7%
60-64	21%	9%
65-69	25%	11%
70-74	30%	14%

Women: Determining Your Risk for Heart Disease and Strokes

1. Age

Age	Points
30-34	-9

35-39	-4
40-44	0
45-49	3
50-54	6
55-59	7
60-64	8
65-69	8
70-74	8

2. Total *cholesterol*

Less than 160	-2
160-199	0
200-239	1
240-279	1
280 or more	3

3. HDL cholesterol

Less than 35	5
35-44	2
45-49	1
50-59	0
60 or more	-3

4. Blood pressure

Find the point on the chart where your systolic and diastolic blood pressure readings intersect. For example, if your reading is 130 (systolic) over 90 (diastolic), your point score is 2.

	Diastolic				
Systolic	79 or less	80-84	85-89	90-99	100 or more
Less than 120	-3	0	0	2	3

120-139	0	0	0	2	3
130-139	0	0	0	2	3
140-159	2	2	2	2	3
160 or more	3	3	3	3	3

5. Have diabetes

No   0

Yes   4

6. Smoker

No   0

Yes   2

7. 10-year heart disease risk
Add your total points: _____

Total points	Risk
-2 or less	1%
-1 to 1	2%
2 to 3	3%
4	4%
5	4%
6	5%
7	6%
8	7%
9	8%
10	10%
11	11%
12	13%
13	15%
14	18%

15	20%
16	24%
17 or more	27% or more

Compare with average and low risk by age

Age	Average risk	Low risk
30-34	Less than 1%	Less than 1%
35-39	Less than 1%	1%
40-44	2%	2%
45-49	5%	3%
50-54	8%	5%
55-59	12%	7%
60-64	12%	8%
65-69	13%	8%
70-74	14%	8%

A Closer Look at Risk Factors

Insulin Resistance

In Chapter 5 Tuning Up Your Metabolism, the subject of insulin resistance was discussed. A very strong argument can be made that insulin resistance is much more important than elevated cholesterol levels as a risk factor for atherosclerosis and cardiovascular disease (CVD). In fact, if we look at the big picture it's easy to conclude that insulin resistance is the biggest factor contributing to an increased risk of heart disease in most North Americans, especially if they do not smoke. So, the strategies detailed in Chapter 5 to improve insulin sensitivity are critically important here as well in reducing the risk for CVD.

Smoking

Cigarette smoking is a huge risk factor for CVD, as statistical evidence reveals smokers have a 70% greater risk of death from CVD than nonsmokers. The more cigarettes smoked and the longer the period of years a person has smoked, the greater the risk of dying from a heart attack or stroke. Overall, the average smoker dies 7 to 8 years sooner than the nonsmoker.

Tobacco smoke contains more than 4000 chemicals, of which more than 50 substances have been identified as carcinogens. These chemicals are extremely damaging to the cardiovascular system. Specifically, these chemicals are carried in the bloodstream on low-density lipoprotein cholesterol (LDL-C), where they either damage the lining of the arteries directly or they damage the LDL-C molecule (creating oxidized LDL), which then damages the arteries. An elevated LDL-C level worsens the effect of smoking on the cardiovascular system because more cigarette toxins travel through it. Smoking contributes to elevated cholesterol presumably by damaging feedback mechanisms in the liver, which control how much cholesterol is being manufactured. Smoking also promotes platelet aggregation and elevated fibrinogen levels, two other important independent risk factors for CVD because they tend to result in the formation of blood clots. In addition, it is a well-documented fact that cigarette smoking is a contributing factor to high blood pressure.

Even passive exposure to cigarette smoke is damaging to cardiovascular health, as convincing evidence links environmental (secondhand or passive) smoke to CVD. Analysis of 10 population-based studies indicates a consistent dose-response effect related to exposure.[1] In other words, the more you are exposed to cigarette smoke the greater your risk for CVD. Evidence indicates that nonsmokers appear to be more sensitive to smoke, including its deleterious effects on the cardiovascular system. Environmental tobacco smoke actually has a higher concentration of some toxic constituents. Data after short- and long-term environmental tobacco smoke exposure show changes in the lining of the arteries and in platelet function as well as exercise capacity similar to those in active smoking. In summary, passive smoking is a relevant risk factor for CVD. In the United States it is estimated that more than 37,000 coronary heart disease (CHD) deaths each year are attributable to environmental smoke.

The good news is that the magnitude of risk reduction achieved by smoking cessation in patients with CVD is quite significant. Results from a detailed meta-analysis showed a 36% reduction in relative risk of mortality for patients with CAD who quit compared with those who continued smoking.

Elevated Blood Cholesterol Levels

Cholesterol is far from a "bad" substance—it's actually very important to our health and has many critical functions in the body. It's found in all cells of the body, where it functions as a necessary structural component of cell membranes. Cholesterol is also used by the body to make many hormones, particularly the sex hormones estrogen and testosterone, but also adrenal hormones such as cortisol and aldosterone. The body also uses cholesterol to make vitamin D.

Cholesterol is transported in the blood on carrier molecules known as lipoproteins. The major categories of lipoproteins are very-low-density lipoprotein (VLDL), low-density lipoprotein (LDL), and high-density lipoprotein (HDL). Since VLDL and LDL are responsible for transporting fats (primarily triglycerides and cholesterol) from the liver to body cells, while HDL is responsible for returning fats to the liver, elevations of either VLDL or LDL are associated with an increased risk for developing atherosclerosis (hardening of the arteries), the primary cause of heart attacks and strokes. In contrast, elevations of HDL are generally associated with a low risk of heart attacks.

It is currently recommended that the total blood cholesterol level be less than 200 mg/dl and triglyceride levels be lower than 150 mg/dl. In addition, it is recommended that the LDL cholesterol (LDL) level be less than 130 mg/dl and HDL cholesterol (HDL) greater than 35 mg/dl.

The total cholesterol to HDL and LDL:HDL ratios are referred to as cardiac risk factor ratios because they reflect whether cholesterol is being deposited into tissues or broken down and excreted. The total cholesterol to HDL ratio should be no higher than 4.2, and the LDL:HDL ratio should be no higher than 2.5. The risk for heart disease can be reduced dramatically by lowering LDL while simultaneously raising HDL levels: For every 1% drop in the LDL level, the risk for a heart attack drops by 2%. Conversely, for every 1% increase in HDL levels, the risk for a heart attack drops 3% to 4%.

Although LDL is referred to as "bad cholesterol," there are some forms that are worse than others. For example, oxidized LDL is a persistent pro-inflammatory trigger for the progression of atherosclerosis and plaque rupture. LDL molecules of higher density are associated with greater risk than larger, less dense LDL. Small, dense LDL are more likely to cause atherosclerosis than are larger and less dense LDL and are markers for CVD risk. The reason is that these smaller particles (LDL3) are more likely to be attached with sugar molecules (glycated) over the larger, more buoyant LDL. This highlights again the importance of avoiding high blood sugar levels and subsequent glycation.[2]

Another marker that deserves mention is lipoprotein (a), or Lp(a), a plasma lipoprotein whose structure and composition closely resemble that of LDL, but with an additional molecule of an adhesive protein called apolipoprotein(a). Elevated plasma levels of Lp(a) are an independent risk factor for coronary heart disease, particularly in those patients with elevated LDL levels. In fact, in one analysis a high level of Lp(a) was shown to carry with it a 10 times greater risk for heart disease than an elevated LDL level. That's because LDL on its own lacks the adhesive apolipoprotein(a). As a result, LDL does not easily stick to the walls of the artery. Actually, a high LDL level carries less risk than a normal or even low LDL with high Lp(a). Levels of Lp(a) below 20 mg/dl are associated with a low risk for heart disease; levels of 20–40 mg/dl are associated with a moderate risk; and levels above 40 mg/dl are associated with an extremely high risk for heart disease.

Elevated Triglycerides

In the past, the relation between elevations in blood triglycerides (hypertriglyceridemia) and coronary heart disease (CHD) has been uncertain. However, a large body of evidence indicates that high triglycerides are an independent risk factor for cardiovascular disease. When high triglycerides are combined with elevations in LDL, it's a recipe for an early heart attack. In one analysis, high triglycerides combined with elevated LDL and a high LDL:HDL cholesterol ratio (above 5) increased the CHD event risk approximately six-fold.

Table 7.3 -Recommended Cholesterol and Triglyceride Levels

Lipid Type	Level (mg/dl)	Result
Total cholesterol	Less than 200	Desirable
	200–239	Borderline
	240 or more	High risk
LDL cholesterol	Less than 100*	Desirable
	100–130	Borderline
	130–159	Borderline high risk
	160 or more	High risk
HDL cholesterol	Less than 35	Low (undesirable)
	35–59	Normal
	60 or more	Desirable
Triglycerides	Less than 150	Desirable
	150–199	Borderline high
	200–499	High
	500 or more	Very high

*For very-high-risk patients (those having signs and symptoms of CVD, a prior cardiovascular event, or with multiple risk factors such as diabetes, continued smoking, and high blood pressure), an LDL of less than 70 mg/dl is often recommended.

High Blood Pressure

Elevated blood pressure is often a sign of considerable atherosclerosis and a major risk factor for heart attack or stroke. In fact, the presence of hypertension is generally regarded as the most significant risk factor for stroke.

Physical Inactivity

A sedentary lifestyle is another major risk factor for CVD. *Physical activity* refers to "bodily movement produced by skeletal muscles that requires energy expenditure" and produces healthy benefits. Exercise, a type of physical activity, is defined as "a planned, structured, and repetitive bodily movement done to improve or maintain one or more components of physical fitness." Physical inactivity denotes a level of activity less than that needed to maintain good health. It applies to most Americans, as roughly 54% of adults report little or no regular physical activity, and there is also a sharp decline in regular exercise among children and adolescents.

Physical activity and regular exercise protect against the development of CVD and also favorably modifies other CVD risk factors including high blood pressure, blood lipid levels, insulin resistance, and obesity. Exercise is also important in the treatment and management of patients with CVD or increased risk including those who have hypertension, stable angina, a prior MI, peripheral vascular disease, or heart failure or are recovering from a cardiovascular event.

Other Risk Factors

In addition to the major risk factors for CVD (i.e., smoking, elevations in cholesterol, elevated blood pressure, diabetes, and physical inactivity/obesity), a number of other factors have, on occasion, been shown to be more significant than the so-called major risk factors. In fact, more than 300 different risk factors have been identified. Although there is considerable evidence that all of these risk factors and more can play a significant role in the pathogenesis of atherosclerosis, much of the current research has focused on the central role of vascular inflammation. Inflammation influences many stages in the development of atherosclerosis, from initial white blood cell recruitment to eventual rupture of the unstable atherosclerotic plaque. For example, C-reactive protein (CRP), a blood marker that reflects different degrees of inflammation, has been identified as an independent risk factor for CAD. In fact, as stated above, the CRP level has been shown to be a stronger predictor of cardiovascular events than the LDL-C level. Elevations in CRP are closely linked to insulin resistance.

It is OK to be a "Type A" Personality

"Type A" behavior is characterized by an extreme sense of time urgency, competitiveness, impatience, and aggressiveness. This behavior carries with it a twofold increase in CHD compared with non-type A behavior. Particularly damaging to the cardiovascular system is the regular expression of anger. In one study, the relationship between habitual anger coping styles, especially anger expression, and serum lipid concentrations were examined in 86 healthy subjects. Habitual anger expression was measured on four scales: aggression, controlled affect, guilt, and social inhibition. A positive correlation between serum cholesterol level and aggression was found. The higher the aggression score, the higher the cholesterol level. A negative correlation was found between the ratio of LDL-C to HDL-C and controlled affect score—the greater the ability to control anger, the lower this ratio. In other words, those who learn to control anger experience a significant reduction in the risk for heart disease, while an unfavorable lipid profile is linked with a predominantly aggressive (hostile) anger coping style.

Anger expression also plays a role in CRP levels. In one study, greater anger and severity of depressive symptoms, separately and in combination with hostility, were significantly associated with elevations in CRP in apparently healthy men and women. Here is the message I want to give: It is OK to be a type A personality, just don' let anger get the better of you. Here are ten tips to help improve coping strategies.

Table 7.4 - Ten Tips to Help Type A Personalities Improve Coping Strategies

1. **Do not starve your emotional life.** Foster meaningful relationships. Provide time to give and receive love in your life.
2. **Learn to be a good listener**. Allow the people in your life to really share their feelings and thoughts uninterruptedly. Empathize with them; put yourself in their shoes.
3. **Do not try to talk over somebody**. If you find yourself being interrupted, relax; do not try to outtalk the other person. If you are courteous and allow someone else to speak, eventually (unless he or she is extremely rude) he or she will respond likewise. If not, explain that he or she is interrupting the communication process. You can do this only if you have been a good listener.
4. **Avoid aggressive or passive behavior**. Be assertive but express your thoughts and feelings in a kind way to help improve relationships at work and at home.
5. **Avoid excessive stress in your life**. Avoid excessive work hours, poor nutrition, and inadequate rest. Get as much sleep as you can.
6. **Avoid stimulants like caffeine and nicotine**. Stimulants promote the fight-or-flight response and tend to make people more irritable in the process.

7. **Take time perform stress-reduction techniques and deep breathing exercises**.

8. **Accept gracefully those things over which you have no control**. Save your energy for those things that you can do something about.

9. **Accept yourself**. Remember that you are human and will make mistakes from which you can learn along the way.

10. **Be more patient and tolerant of other people**. Follow the golden rule, treat others the way you would like others to treat you.

Practical Steps in Tuning up the Cardiovascular System

The first step is reducing known risk factors. The second step is just committing to and following a healthier lifestyle and diet. There is significant evidence that simply adopting a healthy diet and lifestyle dramatically reduces CVD-related mortality. In a prospective trial enrolling over 20,000 men and women, it was found that the combination of four healthy behaviors (nonsmoking, being more physically active, moderate alcohol intake, and a plasma vitamin C indicative of at least 5 servings of fruit and vegetables per day) reduced total mortality fourfold compared with those who had none of these behaviors.

Of course, steps can be taken well-beyond these basics, especially strategies to improve insulin action, reduce blood cholesterol and triglyceride levels, and address other risk factors associated with atherosclerosis (e.g., antioxidant status, elevated CRP, fibrinogen levels).

Diet–General Guidelines

One of the most widely studied dietary interventions in CVD is the traditional "Mediterranean diet," which reflects food patterns typical of some Mediterranean regions in the early 1960s, such as Crete, parts of the rest of Greece, and southern Italy. Unfortunately, the modern

Mediterranean diet has deviated significantly from its healthful origin. The original Mediterranean diet had the following characteristics:

- Olive oil is the principal source of fat.
- The diet centers on an abundance of plant food (fruits; potatoes, beans, and other vegetables; breads; pasta; nuts; and seeds).
- Foods are minimally processed, and people focus on seasonally fresh and locally grown foods.
- Fresh fruit is the typical daily dessert, with sweets containing concentrated sugars or honey consumed only a few times a week at the most.
- Dairy products (principally cheese and yogurt) are consumed daily in low to moderate amounts.
- Fish is consumed regularly.
- Poultry and eggs are consumed in moderate amounts (up to four times weekly) or not at all.
- Red meat is consumed in low amounts.
- Wine is consumed in low to moderate amounts, normally with meals.

In one study, the effect of the Mediterranean diet on the lining of blood vessels and CRP was studied in patients with the metabolic syndrome. Patients in the intervention group were instructed to follow the Mediterranean diet and received detailed advice on how to increase their daily consumption of whole grains, fruits, vegetables, nuts, and olive oil; patients in the control group followed the American Heart Association (AHA) diet. After 2 years, patients following the Mediterranean diet consumed more foods rich in monounsaturated fat, polyunsaturated fat, and fiber and had a lower ratio of omega-6 to omega-3 fatty acids. Compared with patients consuming the control diet, patients consuming the intervention diet had significantly reduced serum concentrations of CRP and other inflammatory mediators; improved blood vessel function; and greater weight loss.

Although several components of the Mediterranean diet deserve special mention, it is important to stress that the total benefits reflect an interplay among many beneficial compounds rather than any single factor. That said, one of the most important aspects of the Mediterranean diet may be the combination of olive oil (a source of monounsaturated fats and antioxidants) and the intake of omega-3 fatty acids. Olive oil consists not only of monounsaturated fatty acid (oleic acid) but also of several antioxidant agents that may also account for some of its health benefits. In addition to a mild effect in lowering LDL-C and triglycerides, olive oil increases the HDL-C level and helps prevent LDL-C from being damaged by free radicals creating oxidized LDL which is even far more damaging to the arteries.

Olive Polyphenols Promote Heart Health by Affecting Gene Expression

In addition to the health effects of the mono-unsaturated fatty acid oleic acid, olives and olive oil contain compounds known as polyphenols that produce remarkable health benefits. While much of the benefits have focused on heart health, tissues throughout the body benefit from compounds from olives. For example, population-based studies have shown a higher intake of olives is associated with fewer wrinkles. Olives contain verbascoside, a polyphenol molecule that has shown exceptional protective antioxidant effects specific to the health of the skin. In detailed studies conducted by Japanese and Italian researchers, olive fruit extracts concentrated for verbacoside and other polyphenols have been shown to effectively prevent the degeneration of the skin that can lead to wrinkle formation.

Additional studies have shown extracts rich in olive polyphenols lower blood pressure blood pressure and cholesterol levels. In the largest trial to date, 232 patients with high blood pressure were given either an olive leaf extract

(500 mg twice daily) or the conventional antihypertensive drug Captopril (12.5 mg twice daily) for 8 weeks. Results showed the olive extract lower blood pressure was clinically as effectively as the drug, but without side effects.

Table 7.5–Olive Extract vs. Captopril in Patients with High Blood Pressure

Group	Beginning Blood Pressure	Blood Pressure at 8 Weeks
Olive Extract	149.3/93.9	137.8/89.1
Captopril	148.4/93.8	134.7/87.4

In addition to lowering blood pressure, olive polyphenols have been shown to lower the bad form of cholesterol (LDL cholesterol) while increasing the beneficial form (HDL cholesterol). Researchers were unsure exactly how this effect was accomplished until a recent study showed that olive polyphenols exert a very complex action on the expression of genes that made LDL and HDL cholesterol. In other words, the olive compounds blocked the expression of the DNA that would lead to the making of LDL cholesterol while simultaneously assisting the expression of DNA for making HDL cholesterol.

In addition to olive oil, the benefits of the longer-chain omega-3 fatty acids eicosapentaenoic acid (EPA), docosahexaenoic acid (DHA), and docosapentaenoic acid (DPA) for cardiovascular health has been demonstrated in more than 300 clinical trials. These fatty acids exert considerable benefits in reducing the risk for CVD. Supplementation with EPA and DHA has little effect on cholesterol levels but does lower triglyceride levels significantly, as well as producing a myriad of additional beneficial effects including reduced platelet aggregation; improved function of the lining of blood vessels and arterial flexibility; improved blood and oxygen supply to the heart; and a mild effect in lowering blood pressure.

The levels of EPA and DHA within red blood cells have been shown to be highly significant predictors of heart disease. This laboratory value has been termed the omega-3 index. An omega-3 index of 8% was associated with the greatest protection, whereas an index of 4% was associated with the least. In one analysis, the omega-3 index was shown to be the most significant predictor of CVD compared with CRP; total cholesterol, LDL-C, or HDL-C ; and homocysteine. Researchers subsequently determined that a total of a combined 1000 mg of EPA and DHA daily is required to achieve or surpass the 8% target of the omega-3 index.

The findings with the omega-3 index are not surprising, as a wealth of information has documented a clear relationship between dietary intake omega-3 fatty acids and the likelihood of developing CVD: the higher the omega-3 fatty acid intake, the lower the likelihood of CVD. It has been estimated that raising the levels of long-chain omega-3 fatty acids through diet or supplementation may reduce overall cardiovascular mortality by as much as 45%.

In general, for preventive effects against CVD, the dosage recommendation is 1,000 mg EPA+ DHA per day; for lowering triglycerides, the dosage is 3,000 mg per day. In a double-blind study, after 8 weeks of supplementation, a daily dosage of 3.4 g EPA+DHA lowered triglycerides by 27%, while a lower dosage of 0.85 g had no effect. These results clearly indicate that the effective dosage for lowering triglycerides with fish oils requires dosages of 3 g EPA+DHA per day.

Although the longer-chain omega-3 fatty acids exert more pronounced effects than alpha-linolenic acid, the shorter omega-3 fatty acid from vegetable sources (e.g., flaxseed oil, walnuts, etc.), it is important to point out that the two populations with the lowest rates of heart attack have a relatively high intake of alpha-linolenic acid: the Japanese who inhabit Kohama Island and the inhabitants of Crete. Typically, Cretans have a threefold higher serum concentration of alpha-linolenic acid than members of other European countries, owing to their frequent consumption of walnuts and the vegetable purslane. Of course another important dietary factor in both the Kohamans and Cretans is their use of oleic acid–containing oils. However, although the oleic acid content of the diet offers some degree of protection, the rates of heart attack among the Kohamans and Cretans are much lower than those in populations that consume only oleic acid sources and little alpha-linolenic acid. The intake of alpha-linolenic acid is viewed as a more significant protective factor than oleic acid.

Consider Avocado Oil in Place of Olive Oil

A few years ago while shopping at a major retail store, I spotted the availability of avocado oil at an exceptionally economical price compared to olive oil. Knowing both are excellent sources of monounsaturated fat and that the smoke point of refined avocado oil is roughly 500 degrees F versus about 400 degrees F for extra virgin olive oil, I decided to give the avocado oil a try and I am glad that I did.

Avocados are an excellent source of monounsaturated fatty acids, as well as potassium, vitamin E, B vitamins and fiber. One avocado will have the potassium content of 2-to-3 bananas (about 1,000 mg of potassium). Of course, an avocado will also have about 3 times the calories as a banana. A 3-1/2 ounce (100g) serving is about ½ of an avocado and provides 160 calories, 2.0 g protein, 14.7 g fat, 8.5 carbohydrate and 6.7 g fiber.

Avocados contain a moderate level of phytochemicals, especially polyphenols that show antioxidant activity. Avocados have the highest fruit antioxidant capacity in protecting against the formation of damaged fats (lipid peroxides) in the blood. Avocados and avocado oil promote healthy blood lipid profiles and enhance the bioavailability of fat-soluble vitamins and phytochemicals from other fruits and vegetables. For example, the consumption of avocados with salads or salsa increases the bioavailability of carotenoids multi-fold, which may add to the potential health benefits.

A total of eight clinical trials have shown consumption of avocados produce cardiovascular benefits including improvements in cholesterol levels. In subjects with high blood cholesterol levels, avocado enriched diets improved blood lipid profiles by lowering LDL-cholesterol and triglycerides and increasing HDL-cholesterol, compared to high carbohydrate diets or other diets without avocado.

Along with the benefits to cardiovascular health, several preliminary clinical studies indicate that avocados can support weight control. The calories of the avocado seem to be offset by the promotion of satiety. For example, in a randomized single blinded, crossover study of 26 healthy overweight adults when the subjects ate one-half an avocado at lunch, they reported significantly reduced hunger and desire to eat, and increased satiation as compared to the control meal.

Nuts and Seeds

Higher consumption of nuts and seeds has been shown to significantly reduce the risk of CVD in large population-based studies including the Nurses Health Study, the Iowa Health Study, and the Physicians Health Study. Researchers estimate that substituting nuts for an equivalent amount of carbohydrates in an average diet resulted in a 30% reduction in heart disease risk. Researchers calculated an even more impressive risk reduction, 45%, when fat from nuts was substituted for saturated fats (found primarily in meat and dairy products). Nuts have a cholesterol-lowering effect, which partly explains this benefit, but they are also a rich source of arginine. By increasing nitric oxide levels, arginine may help to improve blood flow, reduce blood clot formation, and improve blood fluidity (the blood becomes less viscous and therefore flows through blood vessels more easily).

Walnuts appear to be especially beneficial because they are also a rich source of both antioxidants and alpha-linolenic acid. In one study, hypercholesterolemic men and women were randomized to a cholesterol-lowering Mediterranean diet and a diet of similar energy and fat content in which walnuts replaced approximately 32% of the energy from monounsaturated fat (olive oil). Participants followed each diet for 4 weeks. Compared with the Mediterranean diet, the walnut diet improved the function of the cells that line the arteries and significantly reduced total cholesterol (-4.4%) and LDL-C (-6.4%).

Vegetables, Fruits, and Red Wine

An important contributor to the benefits noted with the Mediterranean diet is the focus on carotenoid- and flavonoid-rich fruits, vegetables, and beverages (e.g., red wine). Numerous population studies have repeatedly demonstrated that a higher intake of dietary antioxidants significantly reduces the risk of heart disease and stroke. Higher blood levels of antioxidant nutrients are also associated with lower levels of CRP. The importance of antioxidant intake in the prevention and treatment of CAD is discussed further below.

Two valuable sources of antioxidants in the Mediterranean diet are tomato products and red wine. Tomatoes are a rich source of the carotene lycopene. In large clinical studies evaluating the relationship between carotene status and heart attack (acute MI), lycopene but not beta-carotene was shown to be protective. Lycopene exerts greater antioxidant activity compared with beta-carotene in general but specifically against LDL-C oxidation.

The cardiovascular protection offered by red wine is popularly referred to as the "French paradox." Because the French consume more saturated fat than people in the United States and the United Kingdom yet have a lower incidence of heart disease, red wine consumption has been suggested to be the reason. Presumably this protection is the result of flavonoids and other polyphenols in red wine that protect against oxidative damage to LDL-C as well as helping to reduce the levels of inflammatory mediators. In fact, I don't think you need red wine at all as I believe that the major benefits of red wine consumption in protecting against CVD are due more to the effect the polyphenols have on improving the function of the cells that line the blood vessels (endothelial cells) than the effects of moderate alcohol consumption. The consumption of other polyphenols, such as those in green tea, pomegranate, and dark chocolate, like that of red wine, has also been shown in population studies to be associated with a reduced risk for CVD.

One of the most beneficial groups of plant flavonoids are the proanthocyanidins (also referred to as procyanidins or procyanidolic oligomers [PCOs]). Although PCOs exist in many plants as well as in red wine, commercially available sources of PCO include extracts from grape seeds and the bark of the maritime (Landes) pine. These flavonoids offer protection via several different mechanisms, including their antioxidant activity and effects on the cells that line blood vessels (discussed below).

The Vascular Lining - A Key Target for Nutritional Therapies

What if I told you that your body has an internal medicine chest the size of a football field that is packed full of phenomenal and powerful remedies for inflammation, poor blood flow, high blood pressure, memory loss and virtually every other condition imaginable? Would you believe it? Well, it is true. This medicine chest is the lining of cells along the interior surface of all blood vessels. The technical term for this tissue is the endothelium and the cells that form this lining are called endothelial cells. From the heart to the smallest capillary all vascular tissue has an endothelium. If all of the endothelial cells in the body were laid out flat, the endothelial surface area would be about the size of a football field. That is incredible to think about isn't it? Even more incredible is the way that nutrition and dietary supplements can impact the vascular lining. Here is a brief look at some of the important and profound functions that the endothelium is responsible for:

- Barrier function—the endothelium acts as a semi-selective barrier controlling the passage of materials and the transit of white blood cells into and out of the bloodstream. Excessive or prolonged increases in permeability of the endothelial layer are associated with inflammation and swelling.

- Inflammation—the endothelium helps to control inflammation in order to protect the deeper layers of blood vessels.

- Blood clotting (thrombosis & fibrinolysis)—the surface of the endothelium normally possesses factors that prevent the formation of blood clots. When it lacks these protective factors in can lead to the formation of blood clots that could lead to the buildup of plaque or the formation of a large clot that may break off and cause a heart attack or stroke.
- The constriction and dilation of blood vessels—hence, the endothelium plays a key role in controlling blood flow and blood pressure.
- In some organs, there are highly differentiated endothelial cells to perform specialized "filtering" functions. Examples of such unique endothelial structures include those found in the kidneys (the renal glomerulus) and those that protect the brain (the blood–brain barrier).

The loss of proper endothelial function is a hallmark for vascular diseases and the key early event in the development of atherosclerosis (hardening of the arteries). Impaired endothelial function is often seen in patients with diabetes, hypertension, high cholesterol levels, as well as in smokers.

The main causes of endothelial dysfunction are high blood sugar levels and damage caused by free radicals and pro-oxidants. One of the key consequences of this damage is a diminished ability to manufacture nitric oxide, a key chemical messenger used by the endothelial cells used to perform its duties.

The Role of Nutrition and Endothelial Function

Virtually all of the compounds that you have ever heard of that provides benefits to the vascular system, whether it is dark chocolate, pomegranate, olive oil, nuts and seeds, grape seed extract, arginine, coenzyme Q10 or fish oil, all impact endothelial function. One of the key benefits of the heart healthy Mediterranean diet is that it greatly improves endothelial function.

The amazing thing about this barrier is that it is only one cell thick. It is kind of like shingles on a roof. If this barrier is damaged, it really sets in motion all of the factors that ultimately lead to the formation of the arterial plaque that is the hallmark feature of atherosclerosis (hardening of the arteries). The endothelial cells can be damaged by free radicals and pro-oxidants as well as by immune, viral, chemical and various drugs. Therefore, it is absolutely critical to support healthy endothelial function.

One of the keys to eating a diet high in antioxidant activity is focusing on flavonoids, a type of plant pigment and a member of the larger polyphenol family. As a class of compounds, flavonoids are often called "nature's biological response modifiers" because of their anti-inflammatory, anti-allergic, antiviral and anticancer properties. Many of the super foods like cacao, acai, goji, blueberries, etc., owe their benefits to their flavonoid content. While different flavonoids have different effects in the body, the key factor may not be a high intake of any one particular flavonoid, but rather a high total flavonoid intake that also provides a high variety of flavonoids rather than any one particular flavonoid class. There are more than 8,000 different types of flavonoids out there in nature.

What the research also shows is that it does not seem to matter where the flavonoids come from, e.g., through dietary sources such as legumes, fruit, green tea, coffee, chocolate or through flavonoid-rich extracts (grape seed, ginkgo, milk thistle, pine bark, bilberry, etc.), as long as an effective dosage is being taken. The caveat is that the proanthocyanidin flavonoids must be a major part of the flavonoid intake. Good dietary sources of these compounds are found in red or black grapes (especially the seeds), apples, cacao, cocoa, dark chocolate, berries (especially blueberries, cranberries, and black currants), certain nuts (e.g., hazelnuts, pecans, and pistachios) and red wine. So, with this caveat on the importance of proanthocyanidins in mind, what is an effective dosage of flavonoids? The best evidence on determining an effective dosage of total flavonoid intake is clinical trials with either well-defined sources of flavonoids from food and beverages, or from flavonoid-rich extracts. Fortunately, there has been an explosion of good scientific studies on a wide variety of flavonoid sources. For example, there are fantastic studies with proanthocyanidin-rich extracts from grape seed, cocoa, pomegranate, and pine bark, as well as flavonoid rich extracts from citrus, soy, and green tea extract all showing significant clinical benefits including in the following health conditions:

- Asthma
- Atherosclerosis
- Attention deficit disorder
- High blood pressure
- High cholesterol levels
- Male infertility
- Mild cognitive impairment
- Menopausal symptoms
- Osteoarthritis
- Periodontal disease
- Varicose veins, venous insufficiency and capillary fragility
- Visual function, retinopathy and macular degeneration

There have also been a large number of studies with flavonoid-rich sources looking at more immediate effects, such as their effect on blood vessel function, blood flow, or antioxidant capacity. Most of the studies with the aforementioned flavonoid-rich extracts have used an average dosage of about 300 mg per day to show an effect. Longer-term studies show even more benefit. For example, one of the best examples of the practical effect seen by normalizing endothelial function is with grape seed extract (standardized to contain 95 percent procyanidolic oligomers) in people with high blood pressure. Similar studies exist with pine bark (Pycnogenol), pomegranate, hibiscus and hawthorn extracts—all natural products rich in procyanidins. And, all used a dosage close to 300 mg per day to see a clinical effect.

Endothelial Function and Erectile Dysfunction

An estimated 20 to 30 million American men suffer from erectile dysfunction (ED), a term used to signify the inability to attain or maintain erection of the penis sufficient to permit satisfactory sexual intercourse.

ED may be due to organic or psychogenic factors. In the overwhelming majority of cases the cause is organic, i.e., it is due to some physiological dysfunction. In fact, in men over the age of 50, organic causes are responsible for erectile dysfunction in over 90% of cases. The most common organic cause is atherosclerosis of the penile artery. Hence, factors that prevent atherosclerosis also prevent ED.

Often men do not really care much about their health until it affects their sex life. This study should serve as motivation to take steps to improve endothelial cell function. These cells play a role in erectile function by forming nitric oxide. Drugs like Viagra and Cialis increase nitric oxide production by these cells. Nutritional factors that improve endothelial function include the Mediterranean diet; omega-3 fatty acids; dark chocolate and other sources of flavonoids including pomegranates, green tea, red wine, grape seed extract, and legumes; and magnesium.

As far as specific nutritional recommendations for ED, the amino acids arginine and citrulline increase the formation of nitric oxide within blood vessels. Several double-blind studies have shown an ability of these amino acids to improve the hardness of an erection and satisfaction with sexual intercourse. Studies have also shown results are better if arginine or citrulline is combined with either grape seed or pine bark extract. Here are my dosage recommendations:

- L-Arginine or L-Citrulline: 1,600 to 3,200 mg daily
- Grape seed extract or pine bark extract (95% PCO content): 150 to 300 mg daily

For a Healthy Cardiovascular System Boost Magnesium and Potassium Intake

Magnesium and potassium are absolutely essential to the proper functioning of the entire cardiovascular system. Their critical roles in preventing heart disease and strokes are now widely accepted. In addition, there is a substantial body of knowledge demonstrating that magnesium or potassium supplementation or both are effective in treating a wide range of CVDs, including angina, arrhythmias, congestive heart failure, and high blood pressure. In many of these applications, magnesium or potassium supplementation or both have been used for more than 50 years.

The average intake of magnesium by healthy adults in the United States ranges from 143 to 266 mg/day. This level is well below even the recommended daily allowance (RDA) of 350 mg for men and 300 mg for women. Food choices are the main reason. Because magnesium occurs abundantly in whole foods, most nutritionists and dietitians assume that most Americans get enough magnesium in their diets. But most Americans are not eating whole, natural foods. They are consuming large quantities of processed foods. Because food processing refines a large portion of magnesium, most Americans are not getting the RDA for magnesium.

The best dietary sources of magnesium are tofu, legumes, seeds, nuts, whole grains, and green leafy vegetables. Fish, meat, milk, and most commonly eaten fruits are quite low in magnesium. Most Americans consume a low-magnesium diet because their diet is high in low-magnesium foods such as processed foods, meat, and dairy products.

People dying of heart attacks have been shown to have lower heart magnesium levels than people of the same age dying of other causes. Low magnesium levels contribute to atherosclerosis and CVD via many mechanisms including causing dysfunction of the endothelial cells resulting in an inflammatory environment. Taking a magnesium supplement insures adequate intake. I recommend magnesium bound to citrate, aspartate, or malate over the popular form of magnesium oxide. A good daily dosage is 250-300 mg daily.

Low magnesium levels can also cause high blood pressure, but even more common as a cause of high blood pressure is a diet high in sodium and low in potassium. Conversely, a diet high in potassium and low in sodium can lower blood pressure. Numerous studies have shown that sodium restriction alone does not improve blood pressure control in most people; it must be accompanied by a high potassium intake. Most Americans have a potassium-to-sodium ratio of less than 1:2, meaning they ingest more than twice as much sodium as potassium. Researchers recommend a dietary potassium-to-sodium ratio of greater than 5:1 to maintain health. The easiest way to lower sodium intake is to avoid prepared foods and table salt - use my PerfeKt Sea Salt instead. It is high in potassium, low in sodium. PerfeKt Salt is available exclusively at iHerb.com.

Using a high potassium salt to replace sodium has been shown to be a very easy and extremely effective way to lower blood pressure especially if it combined with sound nutrition. Two very large studies have shown quite clearly that a healthy diet can be effective in lowering blood pressure. These studies, the "Dietary Approaches to Stop Hypertension" (DASH) tested a diet rich in fruits, vegetables, and low-fat dairy foods, and low in saturated and total fat. The DASH diet was also low in cholesterol, high in dietary fiber, potassium, calcium, and magnesium, and moderately high in protein.

The first study showed that a diet rich in fruits, vegetables, and low-fat dairy products can reduce blood pressure in the general population and people with hypertension. The original DASH diet did not require either sodium restriction or weight loss--the two traditional dietary tools to control blood pressure--to be effective. The second study from the DASH research group found that coupling the original DASH diet with sodium restriction is more effective than either dietary manipulation alone. In the first trial, the DASH diet produced a net blood pressure reduction of 11.4 and 5.5 mmHg systolic and diastolic, respectively, in patients with hypertension. In the second trial, sodium intake was also quantified at a "higher" intake of 3,300 milligrams per day; an "intermediate" intake of 2,400 milligrams per day; and a "lower" intake of 1,500 milligrams per day. Compared to the control diet, the DASH diet was associated with a significantly lower systolic blood pressure at each sodium level. The DASH diet with the lower sodium level led to a mean systolic blood pressure that was 7.1 mmHg lower in participants without hypertension, and 11.5 mmHg lower in participants with hypertension. These results are clinically significant and indicate that a sodium intake below 1,500 mg daily can significantly and quickly lower blood pressure. And, I would definitely recommend using my PerfeKt Sea Salt to boost your potassium levels and reduce your sodium levels.

Special Foods to Lower Blood Pressure

Special foods for people with high blood pressure include beet juice; celery; garlic and onions; nuts and seeds or their oils for their essential fatty acid content; cold-water fish (salmon, mackerel, etc.) or fish oil supplements concentrated for EPA+ DHA (dosage 1,000-3,000 mg per day); green leafy vegetables as a rich source of calcium and magnesium; legumes for their fiber; and foods rich in vitamin C like broccoli and citrus fruits.

Ground flaxseeds are also helpful in high blood pressure. In a study conducted at the St. Boniface Hospital Research Centre in Winnipeg, Canada, the effects of daily ingestion of ground flaxseed on systolic (SBP) and diastolic blood pressure (DBP) in patients with peripheral artery disease was studied. While individuals with normal BP showed no effect with 6 months of flaxseed ingestion (two tablespoons daily), those patients who entered the trial with a SBP ≥ 140 mm Hg at baseline obtained an average reduction of 15 mm Hg in SBP and 7 mm Hg in DBP. In other words, this major antihypertensive effect was achieved selectively in hypertensive patients. Flaxseeds can be purchased either whole or already ground or sliced. I prefer purchasing ground/milled flaxseeds as it to enhances their digestibility and therefore their nutritional value. Most of the beneficial research have focused on the use of ground flaxseeds. Ground flaxseeds have also been shown to be helpful in improving blood lipid profiles.

What about Flaxseed Oil?

Flaxseed oil is an excellent source of both essential fatty acids: alpha linolenic (an omega-3 fatty acid) and linoleic acid (an omega-6 fatty acid). Although the body can convert alpha-linolenic acid, a short-chain omega-3 fatty acid, from flaxseed oil, it is much more efficient to get EPA and DHA from fish oils. Furthermore, there is evidence that many people, particularly many men, have a difficult time converting sufficient amounts of alpha-linolenic acid to EPA and DHA. Also, the long-chain omega-3 fatty acids, but not alpha-linolenic acid, are also transformed into prostaglandins (see above). Nonetheless, I do recommend adding flaxseed oil or flaxseeds to your diet.

First, do not cook with flaxseed oil, it is far too fragile and is easily damaged by heat and light. You can add it to foods after they have been cooked or use it as a salad dressing. Taking flaxseed oil by swigging it down or by the tablespoon is not very palatable. Use it as a salad dressing, dip your bread into it, add it to your hot or cold cereal, or spray it over your popcorn. Here is a sample salad dressing featuring flaxseed oil:

Flaxseed Oil Basic Salad Dressing.

Place all ingredients into a salad bowl and whisk together until smooth and creamy. This recipe is quick and delicious!

- 4 tablespoon organic flaxseed oil
- 1 1/2 tablespoon lemon juice
- 1 medium garlic clove, crushed
- Pinch of sea salt or salt-free seasoning
- Fresh ground pepper to taste

Jazz up this basic recipe to your own personal taste by using your favorite herbs and spices.

Celery is another particularly interesting food for lowering blood pressure. A celery seed extract standardized to contain 85% 3-n-butylphthalide (3nB) has been shown to help improve blood pressure control. 3nB is a compound that is unique to celery and is responsible for the characteristic flavor and odor of celery. It was discovered as the active component of celery in response to investigations by researchers seeking to explain some of the traditional effects of celery including lowering of blood pressure and relief of joint pain. The dosage of the extract is 75 to 150 mg twice daily. This amount would translate to about 12 ribs of celery, probably too high of amount of whole celery to eat, but easily done by juicing.

Two clinical studies have also shown grape seed extract (standardized to contain 95% procyanidolic oligomers) to normalize high blood pressure in patients with initial blood pressure in the range of 150/95 mm Hg. The dosage was 300 mg daily. This amount can be achieved through dietary means by focusing on proanthocyanidin-rich foods such as berries.

To prove the effect of dietary flavonoids producing blood pressure lowering effects, let's take a look at a study conducted at Florida State University. In the study, 48 postmenopausal women with mild hypertension were enrolled to evaluate the effects of daily blueberry consumption for 8 weeks. The women were randomly assigned to receive either 22 g freeze-dried blueberry powder or 22 g control powder daily. Approximately 22 g freeze-dried blueberry powder is equal to 1 cup fresh blueberries, an attainable dosage for people to consume on a daily basis. After 8 weeks, systolic blood pressure and diastolic blood pressure (131 mm Hg and 75 mm Hg, respectively) were significantly lower than baseline levels (138 mm Hg, 80 mm Hg), whereas there were no changes in the group receiving the control powder. Blueberry consumption was also associated with improved elasticity within the arteries.

Concise Recommendations for High Blood Pressure.

- General lifestyle, dietary, and supplement recommendations
  - Reduce excess weight

- ○ Follow a healthy lifestyle: avoid alcohol, caffeine, and smoking; exercise and use stress-reduction techniques especially deep breathing exercises
- ○ Eat a high-potassium diet rich in whole plant foods
- ○ Increase dietary consumption of celery, garlic, and onions
- ○ Reduce or eliminate the intake of animal fats while increasing the intake of olive oil and omega-3 fatty acids
- ○ Eliminate salt (sodium chloride) intake and use PerfeKt Sea Salt instead.
- ○ Supplement the diet with all of the following:
  - • High-potency multiple vitamin and mineral formula
  - • Grape seed or pine bark extract: 300 mg daily
  - • Fish oil: 1,000 to 3,000 mg of EPA+DPA+DHA daily
  - • Vitamin C: 500–1,000 mg two to three times daily
  - • Magnesium: 250 mg two to three times daily
  - • Coenzyme Q10 (CoQ10): ubiquinone form dosage is 300 mg daily; ubiquinol form dosage is 100 mg daily.
- • Additional recommendations if needed, choose one or more of the following:
  - ○ Berberine: 500 mg three times daily before meals.
  - ○ Celery Seed Extract standardized to contain 85% 3-n-butylphthalide (3nB): 75 to 150 mg twice daily.
  - ○ Hibiscus tea or extracts have demonstrated blood pressure lowering properties in clinical trials. In double-blind studies, hibiscus extract showed similar blood pressure lowering effect to popular antihypertensive drugs. But unlike the drugs, which carry a significant side effect profile, hibiscus has a 100% tolerability and safety response. Typical reductions in systolic blood pressure are 15-20 mm Hg in subjects with initial readings of 140 mm Hg. Dosage: for the tea, three 240 ml servings/day; for an extract, take enough to supply 10-20 mg anthocyanidins daily.

- ○ Olive leaf extract has been shown in clinical trials to work as effective as the conventional antihypertensive drug Captopril in lowering blood pressure, but without side effect. Dosage: 500 mg (17% to 23% oleuropein content) twice daily.

Monitor your blood pressure

You will know if these recommendations are working by monitoring your blood pressure. As a reminder, high blood pressure must not be taken lightly. By keeping your blood pressure in the normal range, you will not only lengthen your life, but you will improve the quality of your life as well.

NOTE: If you have severe hypertension you will need to work with a physician to select the most appropriate medication. If a prescription drug is necessary, ACE inhibitors alone or in combination with a diuretic appear to be the safest. If after following the above recommendations for two months and your blood pressure has not dropped below 140/105, you may also need to be on prescription medication. When satisfactory control over the high blood pressure has been achieved, work with the physician to taper off the medication.

How to Lower Cholesterols Levels

Lowering total cholesterol (TC), as well as LDL cholesterol (LDL) and triglycerides (TG), is clearly associated with reducing CVD risk. Most of the benefits noted with lowering LDL are based on a large number of randomized clinical trials involving the use of the HMG CoA (3-hydroxy-3 methylglutaryl coenzyme A) reductase inhibitors known collectively as *statin drugs*. The development of statin drugs owes their origin to red yeast *(Monascus purpureus)* fermented on rice. This traditional Chinese medicine has been used for its health-promoting effects in China for more than 2000 years. Red yeast rice is the source of a group of compounds known as *monacolins* (e.g., lovastatin, also known as monacolin K, one of the key monacolins in red yeast rice extract). The marketing of an extract of red yeast fermented on rice standardized for monacolin content as a dietary supplement in the United States caused controversy in 1997 because it contained a natural source of a prescription drug. The FDA eventually ruled that red yeast rice products could only be sold if they were free of monacolin content.

Although the data are clear that statin drugs can produce decreases in heart disease related deaths and heart attacks, the debate remains whether statin therapy reduce overall mortality in anyone other than those with serious heart disease. In people with the only risk factor being elevated LDL, statins do not appear to be effective (especially in women) and given the beneficial effects of diet therapy they certainly are not the best treatment for most people.

One interesting study compared the "Portfolio Diet" comprised of plant-based cholesterol-lowering foods to a statin. The participants were randomly assigned to undergo one of three interventions on an outpatient basis for 1 month: a diet low in saturated fat, based on milled whole-wheat cereals and low-fat dairy foods; the same diet plus lovastatin, 20 mg/day; or a diet high in plant sterols (1 g/1000 kcal), soy protein (21.4 g/1000 kcal), viscous fibers (9.8 g/1000 kcal), and almonds (14 g/1000 kcal). The control, statin, and dietary portfolio groups had mean (SE) decreases in low-density lipoprotein cholesterol of 8%, 30.9%, and 28.6%, respectively. Respective reductions in CRP were 10%, 33.3%, and 28.2%. This study and subsequent studies show that diversifying cholesterol-lowering components in the same dietary portfolio increased the effectiveness of diet as a treatment of high cholesterol levels and produced results comparable to a statin drug with effects similar to statins, but without the side effects.

Ground flaxseeds alone can be helpful in lowering cholesterol levels. Health Canada, the Canadian version of the United States FDA, allows for a therapeutic claim for ground flaxseed in its ability to lower blood cholesterol levels. Health Canada based their decision to allow the claim that ground flaxseeds lower cholesterol levels after closely examining the results from 8 clinical trials. Treatment duration ranged from 4 weeks to 12 months and the quantity of ground flaxseed consumed ranged from 30g/day to 50 g/day or roughly 4 to 6 tablespoons. The amount of drop in total cholesterol and LDL cholesterol is usually in the 5-15% range, similar to what is seen with oat bran and other high fiber foods. Modest, but still meaningful. The specific claim that Health Canada allows: Ground (whole) flaxseed helps reduce/lower cholesterol, which is a risk factor for heart disease.

While individual dietary changes may produce benefit in improving blood lipids, the best approach is to incorporate a broad-spectrum dietary approach that incorporates a wide array of dietary components shown to positively impact lipid levels. The bottom line is that it is imperative that other dietary recommendations such as reducing the dietary intake of saturated fat, trans fatty acids, and cholesterol, as well as the increasing the dietary intake of monounsaturated fats, soluble fiber, and nuts also be promoted. The Mediterranean Diet is the prototypical heart healthy diet and is appropriate as a basis for a cholesterol-lowering diet.

Despite research documenting the benefits of diet and other non-drug approaches, it is unlikely that lowering LDL with statin drugs will be supplanted as the primary therapy in lipid management and prevention of CAD anytime in the near future. In 2020, in the U.S., it is estimated that more than one of every 4 adults—over 50 million people—were taking a statin drug to lower LDL. Therefore, the focus for many will be on the support of statin therapy. For example, it appears that individuals taking statin drugs need to supplement with coenzyme Q_{10} (CoQ_{10}). HMG-CoA reductase is not only required for the synthesis of cholesterol but also CoQ_{10}. Thus, taking a statin lowers CoQ_{10} levels even at lower dosage levels. Researchers have concluded that inhibition of CoQ_{10} synthesis by statin drugs could explain the most commonly reported side effects, especially fatigue and muscle pain, as well as the more serious side effects such as rhabdomyolysis. CoQ_{10} supplementation in subjects on statin drugs has also been shown to reduce markers of oxidative damage. If you are taking a statin, please take either 300 mg of CoQ_{10} as ubiquinone or 100 mg of CoQ_{10} as ubiquinol.

Tune-Up Tip: If Cholesterol Levels are High, Rule Out Low Thyroid

People with low thyroid function have higher rates of coronary artery disease. That's because insufficient thyroid hormones can cause an increase in "bad" cholesterol and Lp(a) and a decrease in "good" cholesterol. The problem can exist even in those who do not experience symptoms of hypothyroidism. If you are trying to lower cholesterol, be sure your thyroid is functioning properly. For more information, and tips about improving thyroid function, see Chapter 5, pages 123-130.

Natural Products to Lower Dietary Cholesterol

PGX

It is well established that the soluble dietary fiber found in legumes, fruit, and vegetables is effective in lowering cholesterol levels. The greater the degree of viscosity or gel-forming nature, the greater the effect of a particular dietary fiber has on lowering cholesterol levels. New, highly viscous, soluble fiber blends are showing greater effect than previously used single fiber sources such as oat bran or psyllium seed husks. In particular, I recommend PGX for lowering cholesterol levels. I mentioned PGX in Chapter 5, it is fantastic for improving blood sugar control and insulin sensitivity. Take 2.5 to 5 grams before meals three times daily.

Niacin

Since the 1950s niacin (vitamin B_3) has been known to be effective in lowering blood cholesterol levels. In the 1970s the famed Coronary Drug Project demonstrated that niacin was the only cholesterol-lowering agent to actually reduce overall mortality. Niacin typically lowers LDL levels by 16–23% while raising HDL levels by 20–33%. These effects, especially the effect on HDL, compare quite favorably with conventional cholesterol-lowering drugs (i.e., statin drugs like Crestor, Lipitor, Zocor, etc.).

Niacin has also been shown to lower the more harmful Lp(a) lipoprotein, triglycerides, and lower markers of inflammation such as CRP and fibrinogen

Several studies have compared niacin with standard lipid-lowering drugs, including statins. These studies have shown significant advantages for niacin. While statins produce a greater LDL reduction, niacin provides better overall results as the percentage increase in protective HDL is dramatically in favor of niacin. Niacin also is very useful in patients with the more damaging small and dense form of LDL particle or lipoprotein(a). Here is a table from a study comparing niacin to Lipitor.

Table 7.6–Niacin vs. a Statin

	Atorvastatin		Niacin	
Parameter	Before	After	Before	After
Total LDL (mg/dl)	110	56	111	89
LDL peak diameter	251	256	253	263
Lipoprotein(a) (mg/dl)	45	44	37	23
HDL (mg/dl)	42	43	38	54

In addition to lowering cholesterol and triglycerides, niacin exerts additional benefits in battling atherosclerosis. Specifically, niacin produces beneficial lipid-altering effects on particle distribution in patients with coronary artery disease that are not well reflected in typical lipoprotein analysis. In addition, systemic markers of inflammation decrease in patients receiving niacin. In one study, when a modest dosage of niacin (1,000 mg daily) was added to existing therapy for 3 months in 54 subjects with stable coronary artery there was a 32% increase in large-particle HDL, an 8%

decrease in small-particle HDL, an 82% increase in large-particle LDL, and a 12% decrease in small-particle LDL. Niacin therapy also decreased lipoprotein-associated phospholipase A2 and CRP levels (20% and 15%, respectively). No significant changes from baseline were seen in any tested parameter in subjects who received placebo. These results indicate that the addition of niacin to existing medical regimens for patients with coronary artery disease and already well-controlled lipid levels favorably improves the distribution of lipoprotein particle sizes and inflammatory markers in a manner expected to improve protection against a cardiovascular event.

While niacin exerts significant benefit on its own, it does not appear to enhance the benefits of statins in well-controlled patients (LDL levels below 100 mg/dl). The AIM-HIGH study funded by the National Heart, Lung, and Blood Institute recruited 3,400 patients who were at risk for heart trouble despite the fact that their LDL was under control with the use of a statin drug (simvastatin [Zocor]) these patients were given niacin to see if there was an additive effect. The study ended 18 months early because no additional cardiovascular benefit was seen in those taking niacin.

In another trial known as the HPS2-THRIVE study, over 25,000 patients at high risk for a heart attack who were taking either simvastatin or simvastatin/ezetimibe (Vytorin) were randomized to take on top of these drugs either a placebo or Tredaptive - a drug produced by Merck containing niacin and an "anti-flushing agent" known as laropiprant. As expected, niacin caused average reductions in LDL of 10 mg/dl and triglycerides of 33 mg/dl while increasing HDL by 6 mg/dl but provided no additional benefit over the statin alone in reducing the rate of heart attacks or other vascular events.

Making matter worse, the Tredaptive group experienced a high rate serious adverse events, i.e., every 3 out of 100 niacin-treated patients suffered from increased bleeding, infections, new onset diabetes, or other serious side effect. However, since these side effects had not been seen in other niacin+statin trials, it is extremely likely the side effects were due to the anti-flushing agent. Consistent with other combination trials, the use of niacin with a statin increased the likelihood of muscle damage caused by the statin.

This trial made absolutely no sense to conduct as the average LDL in the group was 63 mg/dl—well below the recommended level of less than 100 mg/dl for this patient population. Even in high risk individuals it would be highly unlikely that further reduction of LDL would show any significant impact on reducing cardiovascular mortality.

The conventional medical community had a field day commenting on this study. There were many misleading statements being made in the press. This study does not erase the considerable scientific base of niacin as a medicine. It only casts a blow in using niacin with an anti-flushing in patients taking statin drugs who already have well-controlled LDL levels.

While niacin is definitely effective on its own and offers a viable alternative to statins, I do agree with the HPS2-THRIVE finding that niacin should not be used in high-risk patients with low LDL levels and it should definitely not be used with laropiprant.

The side effects of niacin are well known. The most common and bothersome side effect is the skin flushing that typically occurs 20 to 30 minutes after the niacin is taken. Newer timed-released preparations on the market, referred to as "intermediate-release" have solved some of the side effects of niacin and large clinical trials have shown them to be extremely well tolerated.

For best results niacin should be given at night, as most cholesterol synthesis occurs while sleeping. If pure crystalline niacin is being used, it should begin with a dose of 100 mg a day and be carefully increased over 4 to 6 weeks to the full therapeutic dose of 1.5 to 3 g daily. If a timed-released preparation (intermediate release only!) or inositol hexaniacinate is being used, a 500-mg dosage should be given at night and increased to 1500 mg after 2 weeks. If after 1 month of therapy the dosage of 1500 mg per day fails to effectively lower LDL cholesterol, the dosage should be increased to 2000 mg and if that dosage fails to lower lipids, I would recommend discontinuing it.

Fish Oils to Lower Triglyceride Levels

The benefits of the longer chain omega-3 fatty acids EPA and DHA to cardiovascular health has been demonstrated in more than 300 clinical trials. Supplementation with EPA + DHA has little effect on cholesterol levels but does lower triglyceride levels significantly, as well as produce a myriad of additional beneficial effects in protecting against CVD. In general, for preventive effects against CVD, the dosage recommendation is 1,000 mg EPA+DHA per day, but for lowering triglycerides the effective dosage is usually 3,000 EPA + DHA. The degree of reduction in triglycerides with fish oil is on par with other drug therapies (reduction of triglyceride levels 45%). Fish oils work to lower triglyceride levels via several mechanisms that basically reduce the formation of triglycerides while increasing their breakdown into energy.

Berberine

Berberine was discussed in Chapter 5 because it activates the enzyme AMPk that serves as the master switch for metabolism. It has been extensively studied in clinical trials for lowering blood sugar, lipids, and blood pressure. There have been over 30 clinical studies with berberine in these disorders. Results have showed quite convincingly that in the treatment of type 2 diabetes, berberine (500 mg two to three times daily) lowered the level of fasting blood sugar levels, after-meal blood sugar levels and glycosylated hemoglobin (HbA1c). In fact, when berberine was compared to oral hypoglycemic drugs used in type 2 diabetes like metformin, glipizide and rosiglitazone, there was no statistical significance between treatment of berberine and these drugs. In other words, the clinical results seen with berberine are on par with the drugs, but with no significant side effects.

The same sort of comparative results seen in type 2 diabetes were found in the treatment of elevated cholesterol and triglyceride levels as well as high blood pressure. In regard to its effects on blood lipids not only does it lower total and LDL cholesterol (typically 20-30%), unlike statins, berberine also lowers blood triglycerides (-20%) and raises beneficial HDL cholesterol (7-12%). Berberine has also been shown to lower apolipoprotein B by 13-15%, which is another very important risk factor to reduce heart disease. Studies also supported that berberine combined with conventional drugs in these conditions is safe and can produce better results than the drugs used alone. Side effects with berberine occurred at much lower rates and were milder than prescription drugs. The typical dosage is 500 mg two to three times a day before meals.

Berberine produces these metabolic effects on through various mechanisms. In addition to its effects on the microbiome, berberine also activates AMP-activated protein kinase (AMPk)—an enzyme involved in regulating the body's energy levels. By targeting this pathway, berberine induces the uptake of glucose into cells, where it is converted into energy. Activating AMPk is also key to berberine's function in regulating blood lipids, such as LDL cholesterol, total cholesterol and triglycerides. This enzyme acts as a master switch, regulating energy production and storage as well as lipid metabolism. It helps burn fatty acids within cells, stabilize the receptors for LDL cholesterol and inhibit the formation of lipids by the liver. Another valuable AMPk activator is PQQ. This supplement is discussed in Chapter 8 for its effects on improving memory and brain function. If you have high cholesterol levels, I would definitely recommend taking 20 mg of PQQ.

Garlic (Allium sativum) and Onion (Allium cepa)

Garlic appears to be an important protective factor against heart disease and stroke via its ability to affect the process of atherosclerosis at so many steps. A major area of focus on garlic's ability to offer significant protection against heart disease and strokes has been the evaluation of its ability to lower blood cholesterol levels, even in apparently healthy individuals. According to the results from numerous double-blind, placebo-controlled studies in patients with initial cholesterol levels greater than 200, supplementation with commercial preparations providing a daily dose of at least 10 mg alliin or a total allicin potential of 4000 mcg can lower total serum cholesterol levels by about 10% to 12%; LDL cholesterol decreases by about 15%; HDL cholesterol levels usually increase by about 10%; and triglyceride levels typically drop by 15%. However, most trials not using products that can deliver this dosage of allicin fail to produce a lipid-lowering effect.

Although the effects of supplemental garlic preparations on cholesterol levels are modest, the combination of lowering LDL and raising HDL can greatly improve the HDL-to-LDL ratio, a significant goal in the prevention of heart disease and strokes. Garlic preparations have also demonstrated blood pressure–lowering effects, inhibition of platelet aggregation, reduction of plasma viscosity, promotion of fibrinolysis, prevention of LDL oxidation, and an ability to exert positive effects on endothelial function, vascular reactivity, and peripheral blood flow.

Pantethine

Pantethine is the stable form of pantetheine, the active form of vitamin B_5 or pantothenic acid. Pantothenic acid is the most important component of coenzyme A (CoA). This enzyme is involved in the transport of fats to and from cells, as well as to the energy-producing compartments within the cell. Without coenzyme A, the cell's fats cannot be metabolized to energy.

Pantethine has significant lipid-lowering activity while pantothenic acid has little (if any) effect in lowering cholesterol and triglyceride levels due to pantethine ability to be converted to cysteamine. Pantethine administration (standard dose 900 mg/day) has been shown to significantly reduce serum triglyceride (32%), total cholesterol (19%), and LDL cholesterol (21%) levels while increasing HDL cholesterol (23%) levels. It appears to be especially useful in diabetics.

The lipid-lowering effects of pantethine are most impressive when its toxicity (virtually none) is compared with conventional lipid-lowering drugs. Its mechanism of action is due to inhibited cholesterol synthesis and acceleration of the use of fat as an energy source.

Bergamot

Bergamot is a bitter, yellowish-orange citrus fruit native to southern Italy. It is cultivated mainly for an essential oil from the colored peel that is used to scent foods, cosmetic products, and perfumes. It is also what gives Earl Grey tea its distinctive taste.

Bergamot has also historically been used to improve cardiovascular function. Multiple clinical trials have now shown evidence that bergamot can reduce total cholesterol and LDL cholesterol. Like berberine, flavonoids and other polyphenols from the bergamot enhance AMPk activity. They also exert antioxidant and anti-inflammatory effects. The typical dosage of bergamot polyphenol fraction extract is 1,000-1,500 mg per day.

Table 7.7 - Comparative effects on blood lipids of several natural compounds in patients with high cholesterol and triglyceride levels*s

	Niacin	Berber-ine	Garlic	Pantethine	Bergamot
Total cholesterol (% decrease)	-18%	-24%	-10%	-19%	-24%
LDL cholesterol (% decrease)	-23%	-30%	-15%	-21%	-28%
HDL cholesterol (% increase)	+32%	+20%	+31%	+23%	+26%
Triglycerides (% decrease)	-26%	-20%	-13%	-35%	-25%

*Typically, lipid lowering agents will show a greater percentage reduction when cholesterol or triglyceride levels are high. These effects noted in this table are not entirely accurate as results are showed in a range of elevated levels in the studies included in this illustration.

Guidelines on What Cholesterol-lowering Natural Product to Use

Here are some general guidelines for choosing the best product for you.

- PGX should be used if you also are overweight or have diabetes or insulin resistance. Can be used with other agents including statins.
- Niacin should be used if you have high LDL cholesterol, low HDL levels, and high triglycerides (with fish oils as well). S
- Berberine should be used if you are also overweight, have diabetes or insulin resistance, or high blood pressure.
- Garlic should be used if your LDL is only slightly elevated and you have low HDL levels.
- Pantethine should be used if you primarily have high triglyceride levels, but also high LDL and low HDL levels.
- Bergamot should be used if you do not want to take niacin and have high LDL cholesterol, low HDL levels, and high triglycerides (with fish oils as well).

Eat Walnuts for Heart Health and More

Walnuts are one of the most nutritious foods on the planet. They provide an excellent source of essential fatty acids and other beneficial oils, protein (twenty percent by weight), vitamin E, calcium, iron, and zinc. Walnuts are often regarded as a "brain food." This belief probably originally stems from the wrinkled, brain-like appearance of the nutmeat and its shell, but it also is true because of the brain-nourishing substances the nuts contain. Based upon recent research, walnuts should also be considered "heart food." In addition to population-based studies showing walnut consumption offers significant protection against heart disease, there are two clinical studies that have shown moderate walnut consumption significantly lowers LDL by twelve to sixteen percent and reduces the ratio of LDL to HDL cholesterol.

Walnuts are best purchased as whole, uncracked nuts. Whole walnuts stored in a cool, dry environment can be stored up to one year. Walnuts can be eaten alone as a snack food or used in recipes. Here is one of my favorite recipes:

Dr. Murray's Greens and Walnuts
One of my all-time favorite dishes—simple but absolutely delicious and good for your heart too.

2 large bunches greens (such as spinach, kale, mustard greens, chard, etc.), washed, trimmed and coarsely chopped
2 tablespoons olive oil
1 cup diced green onion (optional)
1 or 2 cloves of garlic (thinly sliced)
1 cup coarsely chopped walnuts
1 teaspoon balsamic vinegar
Lemon wedges

Heat 2 tablespoons of olive oil and 1 teaspoon of balsamic vinegar in large skillet or wok over medium-high heat. Add greens, onions, garlic, and walnuts, and sauté until softened. Serve with lemon wedges. Makes 6 servings.

Case History: Grizzly Bear to Teddy Bear

Jerry was a 52-year old retired United States Postal Service employee. In the eleven years, since he'd turned forty-one, Jerry had undergone seven different heart surgeries—three coronary artery bypass operations and four angioplasties. Despite all of these procedures and all of the drugs he was taking, Jerry had tremendous angina—upon exertion.

A fascinating feature in Jerry's case is that he had no risk factors identifiable by conventional testing. His cholesterol levels were perfect, his blood pressure was actually low, he did not smoke, he was not overweight. For years, his doctors had been at a loss to explain why he had such severe heart disease.

It didn't take long for me to figure it out. Jerry seemed like a very affable, mild-mannered guy. But when I asked him how he would evaluate his ability to control his temper I could see that he often "went postal." He told me that he was a real hothead and that his temper was a major problem in his life. I once made the mistake of asking him to give me some examples of what makes him mad. His face turned red, the veins in his neck and forehead popped out, and his voice became quite loud as he told me a few things that really ticked him off. Shortly into this tirade he stopped for a second or two to pop a nitroglycerin pill.

At that point, I seized the opportunity to help him make the connection between his inability to control his anger and his heart disease. He was quite resistant at first, because he just wanted me to prescribe some natural medicines. I suggested the following regimen that I have used successfully in congestive heart failure, angina, and arrythmias:

- High-potency multiple vitamin and mineral formula
- Coenzyme Q10: 300 mg per day
- Magnesium (citrate): 250 mg three times daily
- Hawthorn extract (1.8% vitexin-4'-rhamnoside): 250 mg three times daily

At first, Jerry was completely uninterested in taking a look at his emotional life. In fact, it was not until the next visit one month later that he really opened up and became receptive to my ideas. At our follow-up visit I told Jerry that I wanted him to read a book by my friend Stephen Sinatra, MD: *Heartbreak & Heart Disease* (Keats, 1996). It is an excellent account of the role emotions play in heart disease. I also referred Jerry to a psychotherapist for biofeedback training and to a yoga instructor so that he could start taking yoga classes.

Over the course of next year and a half, Jerry progressively got better. He went from popping nitroglycerin tablets practically every time he got up out of his chair to walking nearly four miles per day and was completely free of his angina medications. Even more impressive than his incredible improvements in his physical health were his changes in his emotional health and personality. What impressed me most, however, were the changes in Jerry's relationships with his wife and kids.

So, what led to the improvement? Was it the natural medicines I prescribed Jerry, or the changes he made in his emotional responses? No doubt the supplements improved his physical well-being. But I am convinced that the most important factor for Jerry's remarkable case was the emotional change.

Cerebral Vascular Insufficiency

While severe disruption of blood and oxygen supply results in a stroke, minor reductions in blood and oxygen supply to the brain—cerebral vascular insufficiency is characterized by one or more of the following symptoms short-term memory loss; dizziness; headache; ringing in the ears; depression; blurred vision. It is extremely common among the elderly in the United States due to the build-up of atherosclerotic plaque in the carotid arteries—the main arteries that supply blood to the brain located on each side of the neck running parallel to the jugular vein. Prevention of strokes and cerebral vascular insufficiency involve the same guidelines as preventing a heart attack since both are caused by atherosclerosis.

Anyone who experiences signs and symptoms of cerebral vascular insufficiency should consult a physician immediately for proper evaluation. In the past evaluation of blood flow to the brain involved invasive techniques, but it now involves the use of non-invasive ultrasound techniques. These techniques determine the rate of blood flow and the degree of blockage by using sound waves. Symptoms of cerebral vascular insufficiency may indicate the occurrence of "mini-strokes" known as transient ischemic attacks (TIAs).

For people with cerebral vascular insufficiency, instead of grape seed or pine bark extract for the source of flavonoids, I recommend Ginkgo biloba extract (GBE). The quality of research on GBE in cerebral vascular insufficiency is exemplary. In numerous well-designed studies, GBE has produced significant regression of all the major symptoms of cerebral vascular insufficiency without significant side effect. GBE has also been shown to promote a speedier and more complete recovery from a stroke. Typical dosage recommendation of GBE is 240-320 mg per day.

Varicose Veins

One of the most common cardiovascular disorders, especially in women, is varicose veins—twisted and engorged superficial veins of the legs. Blood in veins is on its way back to the heart; it is blue because it lacks oxygen. Normally, valves in the veins prevent blood from falling back down the leg. In some people, though, the valves become weak or "leaky." The blood collects in the veins, causing them to swell. The problem is more of a cosmetic concern than a medical one, but the legs may feel heavy, tight, and tired.

A more serious form of varicose vein involves obstruction and valve defects of veins that lie deeper in the leg. This can lead to thrombophlebitis (vein inflammation), pulmonary embolism (blood clot in the lungs), heart attack, or stroke. Varicose veins affect nearly one out of two middle-aged adults. Women are four times as likely to have them as men.

It is possible to relieve varicose veins through lifestyle methods including exercise and through dietary strategies such as the use of supplements and botanical medicines. The main goal is to strengthen the wall of the vein, improve circulation, and provide your body with nutrients that prevent formation of blood clots. While small "spider veins" may resolve entirely, well-formed large varicose veins should not be expected to magically go away. In these cases, elastic compression stockings are occasionally beneficial, but they are a nuisance to put on and take off.

Fortunately, many of my patients with varicose veins have found that by using botanical medicines they do not have to put up with the hassles of wearing those compression stockings. The most effective botanical medicine is an extract of horse chestnut (*Aesculus hippocastanum*) concentrated for the compound escin. Good clinical studies have found that horse chestnut seed extract is as effective as using support stockings. Escin reduces the permeability of the veins, which helps prevent swelling and inflammation. It also improves the ability of the vein to contract. There are other useful herbs. Gotu kola (*Centella asiatica*) contains compounds that enhance the connective tissue structure of the veins to give them additional support and improve blood flow. Butcher's broom (*Ruscus aculeatus*) contains ruscogenins, which prevent inflammation and promote vein constriction. For simplicity, I am going to recommend that you give Vein Sense from Natural Factors a try. It contains fantastic natural support to vein structures. In addition to the herbal extracts, it contains a special form of the flavonoid diosmin. It is produced through a process known as micronization that involves a high-technology grinding process with a jet of air at supersonic velocities in order to reduce the particle size far smaller than possible otherwise. As a result there is better and faster absorption, which produces greater clinical efficacy. Micronized diosmin at a dosage of 500 to 1,000 mg per day has shown considerable benefits in improving blood flow in varicose veins and promoting the healing of venous leg ulcers and hemorrhoids.

There is one other consideration in varicose veins. Many people with varicose veins have a decreased ability to break down fibrin, the protein involved in blood clots. Fibrin is deposited in the tissue near varicose veins, causing skin to become hard and lumpy. Inability to break down fibrin (fibrinolysis) increases the risk of blood clots and other serious heart conditions. See the discussion above on natural ways to increased fibrinolytic activity.

Longevity Matrix Lifestyle Tune-Up #7–Develop Positive Relationships

Positive human relationships sustain us and nourish us — body and soul. They are absolutely as critical to heart health. In fact, data from large, well-controlled population studies have shown that loneliness, isolation, unfulfilling jobs and relationships, and a "broken heart" were as important a risk factor for heart disease and premature death as smoking, high blood pressure, high blood cholesterol, obesity, and physical inactivity. In contrast, having positive relationships and support structure is linked to better health and lower absenteeism, lower incidence of cancer and heart disease, and reduced hospital stays. In one study cited by Dr. Ken Pelletier, of the University of California, San Francisco, School of Medicine, and author of Sound Mind, Sound Body (Simon & Shuster, 1994), researchers divided 1,337 medical students into two groups: one made up of students who were not close to their parents and were dissatisfied with their personal relationships, and one that had better relationships with their parents and others. The first group was found to have a three to four times higher risk of cancer later in life than the students with better relationships.

The bottom line here is that good scientific research is telling us something that most of us already know. We all need relationships and the love and acceptance that they should bring to us. In fact, the desire to be loved and appreciated is one of the main drivers of human behavior. Unfortunately, many of us do not always act in manner that allows us to achieve something that is so vital to our existence.

What is the biggest roadblock to positive human relationships? In my opinion it is poor listening skills. The quality of any relationship ultimately comes down to the quality of its communication. Poor listening skills lead to poor communication. When we are truly listening, we are telling the person that he or she is important to us and that we respect him or her. Here are seven tips to being a good listener:

- Be empathetic. When we put ourselves in the other person's shoes it is amazing how it opens up the lines of communication. If you first seek to understand, you will find yourself being better understood.

- Be an active listener. This means that you must act really interested in what the other person is communicating. Listen to what they are saying instead of thinking about your response. Ask questions to gain more information or clarify what they are telling you. Good questions open lines of communication.

- Be a reflective listener. Restate or reflect back to the other person your interpretation of what they are telling you. This simple technique shows the other person that you are both listening and understanding what they are saying. Restating what you think is being said may cause some short-term conflict in some situations, but it is certainly worth the risk.

- Do not interrupt. Wait to speak until the person or people you want to communicate with are listening. If they are not ready to listen, no matter how well you communicate your message will not be heard.

- Don't try to talk over somebody. If you find yourself being interrupted, relax, don't try and out talk the other person. If you are courteous and allow them to speak, eventually (unless they are extremely rude) they will respond likewise. If they don't, point out to them that they are interrupting the communication process. You can only do this if you have been a good listener. Double-standards in relationships seldom work.

- Help the other person become an active listener. This can be done by asking them if they understood what you were communicating. Ask them to tell you what is was that they heard. If they don't seem to be understanding what it is you are saying, keep after it until they do.

- Don't be afraid of long silences. Human communication involves much more than human words. A great deal can be communicated during silences, unfortunately in many situations silence can make us feel uncomfortable. Relax. Some people need silence to collect their thoughts and feel safe in communicating. The important thing to remember during silences is that you must remain an active listener.

With good communication in our relationships, it usually translates to greater intimacy. Words are not enough, however, in our most intimate relationships. What I mean is that it is not enough to simply feel love in your friendships and intimate relationships, we must express these feelings. We must demonstrate to our loved ones just how important they are to us. We must continually find ways to communicate our deepest feelings through our actions. Have you ever heard the expression "words are cheap?" I would not go that far, but what I think this expression symbolizes is that we must show our loved ones just how much we love and appreciate them.

One of the key principles of life is that whatever you sow, so shall you reap, but multiplied a hundred times. When you plant a tomato seed, you get a bush of tomatoes, a tomato plant that has dozens of tomatoes on it each of which has dozens of seeds. The law of nature always gives back more than it receives. And really, it is the same for human beings. We all need and want to be loved and appreciated, but in order to receive these gifts we must first give them. The more you give, the more you receive.

If you truly are not a "people person," here is the next best thing - get a pet. A relationship with a pet can be almost as positive as human relationship. Studies have shown that owning or caring for a pet can relieve loneliness, depression, and anxiety, and even promote a quicker recovery from illness.

CHAPTER 8:

Breaking Free from Stress and Depression

All of us know stress. In fact, most of us have accepted the fact that everyday stress is part of modern living. Job pressures; family arguments; financial pressures; and running late are just a few of the "stressors" most of us are faced with on a daily basis. Although we most often think one of these examples of something that causes us to feel "stressed out," technically speaking a stressor may be almost any disturbance—heat or cold, environmental toxins, toxins produced by microorganisms, physical trauma, and strong emotional reaction—that can trigger a number of biological changes to produce what is commonly known as the "stress response."

Fortunately for us, control mechanisms in the body are geared toward counteracting the effects of stress. Most often the stress response is so mild they go entirely unnoticed. However, if stress is extreme, unusual, or long lasting, these control mechanisms can be overwhelming and quite harmful. In fact, I have seen many people age rapidly, sometimes literally overnight, due to the effects of stress. It is absolutely critical to develop a stress management strategy and utilize natural approaches to reduce stress and its effects as part of the longevity matrix.

Recognizing Stress

Have you ever been suddenly frightened? That is the extreme end of the stress response. What you were feeling is adrenaline surging through your body. Adrenaline is released from your adrenal glands, a pair of glands that lie on top of each kidney. Adrenaline was designed to give the body that extra energy boost to escape from danger. Unfortunately, it can also make us feel stress, anxiety, and nervousness.

In modern life many people experience stress but may not be able to tell you exactly what it is that is causing them to feel stressed out. What these people may notice are the side effects of stress such as insomnia, depression, fatigue, headache, upset stomach, digestive disturbances, and irritability.

Understanding Stress

Before discussing methods on how to deal effectively stress, it is important to understand the stress response. Ultimately, the success of any stress management program is dependent on its ability to improve an individual's immediate and long-term response to stress.

The stress response is actually part of a larger response known as the "general adaptation syndrome." To fully understand how to combat stress, it is important that we take a closer look at the general adaptation syndrome. The general adaptation syndrome is broken down into three phases: alarm, resistance, and exhaustion. These phases are largely controlled and regulated by the adrenal glands and our nervous system.

The General Adaptation Syndrome

The initial response to stress is the alarm reaction that is often referred to as the "fight or flight response." The fight or flight response is triggered by reactions in the brain which ultimately cause pituitary gland, the master gland of the entire hormonal system of the body that is located at the center of the base of the brain, to release a hormone called adrenocorticotropic hormone (ACTH) which causes the adrenals to secrete adrenaline and other stress-related hormones like cortisol.

The fight or flight response is designed to counteract danger by mobilizing the body's resources for immediate physical activity. As a result, the heart rate and force of contraction of the heart increases to provide blood to areas necessary for response to the stressful situation. Blood is shunted away from the skin and internal organs, except the heart and lung, while at the same time the amount of blood supplying needed oxygen and glucose to the muscles and brain is increased. The rate of breathing increases to supply necessary oxygen to the heart, brain, and exercising muscle. Sweat production increases to eliminate toxic compounds produced by the body and to lower body temperature. Production of digestive secretions is severely reduced since digestive activity is not critical for counteracting stress. And, blood sugar levels are increased dramatically as the liver dumps stored glucose into the blood stream.

While the alarm phase is usually short-lived, the next phase - the resistance reaction - allows the body to continue fighting a stressor long after the effects of the fight or flight response has worn off. Other hormones, such as cortisol and other corticosteroids secreted by the adrenal cortex, are largely responsible for the resistance reaction. For example, these hormones stimulate the conversion of protein to energy so that the body has a large supply of energy long after glucose stores are depleted as well as promote the retention of sodium to keep blood pressure elevated.

As well as providing the necessary energy and circulatory changes required to deal effectively with stress, the resistance reaction provides those changes required for meeting emotional crisis, performing strenuous tasks and fighting infection. However, while the effects of adrenal hormones are quite necessary when the body is faced with danger, prolongation of the resistance reaction or continued stress increases the risk of significant disease (including diabetes, high blood pressure, and cancer) and results in the final stage of the general adaptation syndrome, i.e., exhaustion.

Prolonged stress places a tremendous load on many organ systems, especially the heart, blood vessels, adrenals, and immune system. Exhaustion may manifest by a total collapse of a body function or a collapse of specific organs.

Table 8.1 - Conditions Strongly Linked to Stress

- Angina
- Asthma
- Autoimmune disease
- Cancer
- Cardiovascular disease
- Common cold
- Diabetes (adult onset - Type II)
- Depression
- Headaches
- Hypertension
- Immune suppression
- Irritable bowel syndrome
- Menstrual irregularities
- Premenstrual tension syndrome
- Rheumatoid arthritis
- Ulcerative colitis
- Ulcers

Stress: A Healthy View

The "godfather" of modern stress research was Hans Selye, M.D. Having spent most of his life studying stress this brilliant man probably had the best perspective on the role of stress in our lives. According to Dr. Selye, stress should not be viewed as a negative factor. It is not the stressor that determines the response; instead it is the individual's internal reaction that triggers the stress response. This internal reaction is highly individualized. What one person may experience as significant stress; the next person may view it entirely different. Dr. Selye perhaps summarized his view best in a passage in his book "The Stress of Life" (McGraw Hill, New York, NY, 1978):

"No one can live without experiencing some degree of stress all the time. You may think that only serious disease or intensive physical or mental injury can cause stress. This is false. Crossing a busy intersection, exposure to a draft, or even sheer joy are enough to activate the body's stress mechanisms to some extent. Stress is not even necessarily bad for you; it is also the spice of life, for any emotion, any activity causes stress. But, of course, your system must be prepared to take it. The same stress which makes one person sick can be an invigorating experience for another."

The key statement Selye made is "your system must be prepared to take it." It is my goal to help prepare and bolster your stress-fighting system, boost your mood, and help you get a good night's sleep.

What is the difference between stress and anxiety?

When we experience stress, it is often accompanied with feelings of anxiety. Technically, anxiety is defined as "an unpleasant emotional state ranging from mild unease to intense fear." Anxiety differs from fear, in that while fear is a rational response to a real danger, anxiety usually lacks a clear or realistic cause. Experiencing some anxiety is normal and, in fact, healthy, but higher levels of anxiety are not only uncomfortable, they are linked to all of the issues with long-term stress.

Anxiety is often accompanied by a variety of symptoms. The most common symptoms relate to the chest such as heart palpitations (awareness of a more forceful or faster heartbeat), throbbing or stabbing pains, a feeling of tightness and inability to take in enough air, and a tendency to sigh or hyperventilate. Tension in the muscles of the back and neck often leads to headaches, back pains, and muscle spasms. Other symptoms can include excessive sweating, dryness of mouth, dizziness, digestive disturbances, and the constant need to urinate or have a bowel movement.

Severe anxiety will often produce what are known as "panic attacks" - intense feelings of fear. Panic attacks may occur independent from anxiety but are most often associated with generalized anxiety or agoraphobia. Agoraphobia is defined as an intense fear of being alone or being in public places. As a result, most people with agoraphobia become housebound. How common are panic attacks? Very. Its estimated that about 15% of the United States population experience a panic attack in their lifetimes, and 3% report regular panic attacks.

Stress Assessment

One useful tool to assess the role that stress may play in a person's life is the "social readjustment rating scale" developed by Holmes and Rahe. The scale was originally designed to predict the risk of a serious disease due to stress. Various life-changing events are numerically rated according to their potential to cause disease. The standard interpretation of the social readjustment rating scale is that a total of 200 or more units in one year is considered to be predictive of a high likelihood of experiencing a serious disease. However, rather than using the scale solely to predict the likelihood of serious disease, I recommend it as simply a tool to determine your level of stressor exposure, because everyone reacts differently to stressful events. If you score is greater than 200, however, I strongly encourage you to be very aggressive in your stress management.

Table 8.2 - The Social Readjustment Rating Scale

Rank	Life event	Mean value
1	Death of spouse	100
2	Divorce	73

3	Marital separation	65
4	Jail term	63
5	Death of a close family member	63
6	Personal injury or illness	53
7	Marriage	50
8	Fired at work	47
9	Marital reconciliation	45
10	Retirement	45
11	Change in health of family member	44
12	Pregnancy	40
13	Sex difficulties	39
14	Gain of a new family member	39
15	Business adjustment	39
16	Change in financial state	38
17	Death of a close friend	37
18	Change to different line of work	36
19	Change in number of arguments with spouse	35
20	Large mortgage	31
21	Foreclosure of mortgage or loan	30
22	Change in responsibilities at work	29
23	Son or daughter leaving home	29
24	Trouble with in-laws	29
25	Outstanding personal achievement	28
26	Spouse begins or stops work	26
27	Beginning or end of school	26
28	Change in living conditions	25
29	Revision of personal habits	24
30	Trouble with boss	23
31	Change in work hours or conditions	20
32	Change in residence	20
33	Change in schools	20
34	Change in recreation	19

35	Change in church activities	19
36	Change in social activities	18
37	Small mortgage	17
38	Change in sleeping habits	16
39	Change in number of family get-togethers	15
40	Change in eating habits	15
41	Vacation	13
42	Christmas	12
43	Minor violations of the law	11

Dealing with Stress

Throughout our lives, each of us develops our own ways of coping with stress. Some of those strategies are healthier than others. For example, one person might relieve stress by taking long, relaxing walks or watching funny movies. Another might drink alcohol or use drugs. If your coping strategy appears on the following list, you will definitely need to develop better methods for managing stress.

- Dependence on chemicals
- Drugs (legal and illegal)
- Alcohol
- Tobacco
- Overeating
- Watching too much television
- Emotional outbursts
- Feelings of helplessness
- Overspending
- Excessive or reckless behavior (promiscuous sex, thrill-seeking, etc.)

Chemical Dependencies

The United States appears to be a nation of addicts. The level of addiction ranges from the responsible person who "can't get started in the morning" without a cup of coffee to the strung-out crack addict. Check out these sobering statistics:

- Americans consume 450 million cups of coffee each day.
- At least 20 million Americans drink six or more cups of coffee each day.
- Of American adults, 30% smoke at least half a pack of cigarettes each day.
- At least 10% of the population is addicted to alcohol.
- Approximately one-third of the adult population consumes more than four drinks daily.
- Every year Americans swallow more than 10 billion tranquilizers like Valium, Xanax, Ambien, and Lunesta.
- Cocaine addiction afflicts at least 2.2 million persons.

In many instances, people claim that they smoke, drink alcohol, or take drugs because it calms them. In reality, these substances actually complicate matters. The relaxation or chemical high these drugs are short-lived and ultimately lead to adding even more stress to the system. Individuals suffering from stress, anxiety, depression, insomnia, or other psychological conditions must absolutely stop drinking coffee and other sources of caffeine; and alcohol. They also need to quit smoking and using other recreational drugs. In short, these people must choose health.

Is There a Built in Need to Get High?

There appears to be an inherent need for humans to get high. Does this need to be the chemical high that most Americans seek? No. Think back to some fantastic moments in your life. Most of us have experienced an extreme natural high at least once in our lives. What was the moment in your life that seemed almost magical? Was it the first time your wife or lover said they loved you? How about the birth of your first child? Or, how about when you accomplished one of your dreams? Didn't these moments seem almost unreal? Did you feel as if you were naturally high?

All the drugs that act on the brain do so by mimicking or enhancing the activity of natural compounds already present in the brain. Within you lies all the chemicals required for every emotion you can possibly experience. The key is not to take drugs to try and duplicate these feelings, but rather learn how to create the feelings inside of you so that you can conjure them up whenever you want. Your mind is such a powerful tool in determining how you feel. You can use your mind to create powerful positive emotions that can give you a natural high that can help you cope with stress.

Here is how you can do it. First recreate a powerful positive experience in your life. Do your best to relive those feelings to the fullest. Turn up the dial of intensity as high as you possibly can. Put this book down and do it now.

How do you feel now? It is within you to experience more of the feelings that you really want to have in life. It is easy for us to be overcome by incredible feelings of love, appreciation, and energy when we recall powerful positive events in our life. In particular, I believe that we are wired to experience and express gratitude in our lives. By regularly recalling positive feelings and moments on a regular basis conditions your mind to continue to experience these emotions which will allow you to be in a more resourceful state of mind in dealing with the stress of life.

All of this may sound a bit funny to you but believe me it does work. In an effort to provide some guidance in helping you develop a mental attitude that can help deal with stress I offer seven key steps below.

Seven Steps to a Stress Busting Attitude

Step 1. Prime Yourself for Success. The first step is to employ the priming exercise I detail in Chapter 1.

Step 2. Become an Optimist. We are, by nature, optimists. Optimism is a vital component of good health and an ally in the healing process. Focus on the positives even in challenging situations. Look for the gift.

Step 3. Become Aware of Your Self-Talk. There is a constant dialog taking place in our heads. Our self-talk makes an impression onto our subconscious mind. In order to develop or maintain a positive mental attitude you must guard against negative self-talk. Become aware of your self-talk and then consciously work to imprint positive self-talk on the subconscious mind. Two powerful tools in creating positive self-talk are questions and affirmations ("I am" statements).

Step 4. Ask Better Questions. The quality of your life is equal to the quality of the questions you habitually ask yourself. Whatever question you ask your brain—you will get an answer. Let's look at the following example: An individual is met with a particular challenge or problem. He or she can ask a number of questions when in this situation. Questions many people may ask in this circumstance include: "Why does this always happen to me?" Or, "Why am I always so stupid?" Do they get answers to these questions? Do the answers build self-esteem? Does the problem keep reappearing? What would be a higher quality question? How about, "This is a very interesting situation, what do I need to learn from this situation so that it never happens again?" Or, how about "What can I do to make this situation better?"

In another example, let's look at an individual who suffers from depression. What are some questions they might ask themselves that may not be helping their situation? How about—Why am I <u>always</u> so depressed? Why do things <u>always</u> seem to go wrong for me? Why am I so unhappy?

What are some better questions they may want to ask themselves? How about - What do I need to do to gain more enjoyment and happiness in my life? What do I need to commit to doing in order to have more happiness and energy in my life? After they have answered these questions, I will have my depressed patients ask themselves this one—If I had happiness and high energy levels right now, what would it feel like?—You will be amazed at how powerful questions can be in your life. When the mind is searching for answers to these questions, it is reprogramming your subconscious into believing you have an abundance of energy. Unless there is a physiological reason for the chronic fatigue (e.g., anemia, hypothyroidism, etc.), it won't take long before your subconscious believes. Regardless of the situation, asking better questions is bound to improve your attitude. If you want to have a better life, simply ask better questions. It sounds simple, because it is. If you want more energy, excitement, and/or happiness in your life, simply ask yourself the following questions on a consistent basis.

- What am I most happy about in my life right now?
  - Why does that make me happy?
  - How does that make me feel?
- What am I most excited about in my life right now?
  - Why does that make me excited?
  - How does that make me feel?
- What am I most grateful about in my life right now?
  - Why does that make me grateful?
  - How does that make me feel?
- What am I enjoying most about in my life right now?
  - What about that do I enjoy?
  - How does that make me feel?
- What am I committed to in my life right now?
  - Why am I committed to that?
  - How does that make me feel?
- Who do I love? (Starting close and moving out)
  - Who loves me?

Step 5. Employ Positive Affirmations. An affirmation is a statement with some emotional intensity behind it. Positive affirmations can make imprints on the subconscious mind to create a healthy, positive self-image. In addition, affirmations can actually fuel the changes you desire. You may want to have the following affirmation in plain sight to recite them over the course of the day:

- I am blessed with an abundance of energy!
- I am thankful to God for all of my good fortune!

- I am blessed to have had so many wonderful moments in my life!
- I am aware that love, joy, peace, and happiness flow through me with every heartbeat.

Here are some very simple guidelines for creating your own affirmations. Have fun with it! Positive affirmations can make you feel really good if you follow these guidelines.

- Always phrase an affirmation in the present tense. Imagine that it has already come to pass.
- Always phrase the affirmation as a positive statement. Do not use the words not or never.
- Do your best to totally associate to the positive feelings that are generated by the affirmation.
- Keep the affirmation short and simple, but full of feeling. Be creative.
- Imagine yourself really experiencing what you are affirming.
- Make the affirmation personal to you and full of meaning.
  - Using these above guidelines and examples, write down five affirmations that apply to you. State these affirmations aloud while you are taking your shower, driving, or when you are praying.

Step 6. Practice Positive Visualizations. Positive visualization or imagery is another powerful tool in creating health, happiness, or success. Many believe that we have to be able to see our lives the way we want it to be before it happens. You can use visualization in all areas of your life, but especially in your health. In fact, some of the most promising research on the power of visualization involves enhancing the immune system in the treatment of cancer. Be creative and have fun with positive visualizations. They are powerful and inspirational. In fact, the famous author Anatole France said something about dreams and life that we think really hits home - "existence would be intolerable if we were never to dream."

Step 7. Laugh Long and Often. Humor may be the most powerful stress buster around. By laughing frequently and taking a lighter view of life, you will also find that life is much more enjoyable and fun. I covered some tips on how to increase laughter in your life at the end of Chapter 6. Go back and refresh your memory if you need to. I want you to laugh hard and often.

Calming the Mind and Body

Another important step in fighting stress is learning to calm the mind and body. For me that is priming and doing deep breathing exercises. For me, it produces physiologic response known as a *relaxation response*—a response that is exactly opposite to the stress response that reflects activation of the parasympathetic nervous system. Although an individual may relax by simply sleeping, watching television, or reading a book, relaxation techniques are designed specifically to produce the relaxation response.

Relaxation response was a term coined by Harvard professor and cardiologist Herbert Benson in the early 1970s to describe a physiologic response that he found in people who meditate that is just the opposite of the stress response. With the stress response (Table 8.3), the sympathetic nervous system dominates. It is designed to protect us against immediate danger. With the relaxation response (Table 8.4), the parasympathetic nervous system dominates. The parasympathetic nervous system controls bodily functions such as digestion, breathing, and heart rate during periods of rest, relaxation, visualization, meditation, and sleep. Although the sympathetic nervous system is designed to protect against immediate danger, the parasympathetic system is designed for repair, maintenance, and restoration of the body.

The relaxation response can be achieved through a variety of techniques. It doesn't matter which technique you choose, because all techniques have the same physiologic effect—a state of deep relaxation. The most popular techniques are meditation, prayer, progressive relaxation, self-hypnosis, and biofeedback. To produce the desired long-term health benefits, the patient should use the relaxation technique for at least5 to 10 minutes each day.

Table 8.3 - The Stress Response

- The heart rate and force of contraction of the heart increase to provide blood to areas necessary for response to the stressful situation.
- Blood is shunted away from the skin and internal organs, except the heart and lung, while at the amount of blood supplying required oxygen and glucose to the muscles and brain is increased.
- The rate of breathing rises to supply necessary oxygen to the heart, brain, and exercising muscle.
- Sweat production increases to eliminate toxic compounds produced by the body and to lower body temperature.
- Production of digestive secretions is severely reduced because digestive activity is not critical to counteracting stress.
- Blood sugar levels are raised dramatically as the liver dumps stored glucose into the blood stream.

Table 8.4 - The Relaxation Response

- The heart rate is reduced and the heart beats more effectively. Blood pressure is reduced.
- Blood is shunted towards internal organs, especially those organs involved in digestion.
- The rate of breathing decreases as oxygen demand is reduced during periods of rest.
- Sweat production diminishes, because a person who is calm and relaxed does not experience nervous perspiration.
- Production of digestive secretions is increased, greatly improving digestion.
- Blood sugar levels are maintained in the normal physiologic range.

Getting a Good Night's Sleep

My first big step helping people deal with stress, anxiety, depression, or low energy levels is almost always to try to improve their sleep quality. It's a great quick fix to feeling better. Think of a time in your life where you did not sleep well for a few days. Were you more easily stressed? Maybe you were irritable or easily angered. For sure your energy levels were down and likely your mood was as well. Now, quickly think of a time in your life where you slept fantastic and woke up with an abundance of energy. Undoubtedly the world looked brighter and you dealt with people in a friendlier manner and probably felt stress free. I realize that if you are reading this book that it has probably been a while since you regularly felt this way, but I hope you get my point. Everything is better after a good night's sleep.

Human sleep is perhaps one of the least understood body processes, but its value to human health and proper functioning is without question. Sleep is absolutely essential to both the body and mind. Impaired sleep, altered sleep patterns, and sleep deprivation impair mental and physical function. Many health conditions, particularly depression, chronic fatigue syndrome, and fibromyalgia, are either entirely or partially related to sleep deprivation or disturbed sleep.

Sleep Deprivation in the United States

Over the course of a year, over one-half of the U.S. population will have difficulty falling asleep. About 33% of the population experiences insomnia on a regular basis with 17% of the population claiming that insomnia is a major problem in their lives. Many use over-the-counter sedative medications to combat insomnia, while others seek stronger prescription medications from their physicians. Each year up to 12.5% of adults in the U.S. receive prescriptions for drugs to help them go to sleep.

The Problem with Sleeping Pills

Most sleeping pills are technically "sedative hypnotics." This specific class of drugs is also widely used to treat anxiety and stress. Examples include:

- alprazolam (Alprazolam, Xanax)
- chlordiazepoxide (Librium)
- diazepam (Valium)
- eszopiclone (Lunesta)
- flurazepam (Dalmane)
- quazepam (Doral)
- ramelteon (Rozerem)
- temazepam (Restoril)
- triazolam (Halcion)
- zaleplon (Sonata)
- zolpidem tartrate (Ambien)

All of these drugs are associated with significant risks. Problems with these drugs include the fact that most are highly addictive and very poor candidates for long-term use. Common side effects include dizziness, drowsiness, and impaired coordination, it is important not to drive or engage in any potentially dangerous activities while on these drugs. Alcohol should never be consumed with these drugs as it could be fatal.

The most serious side effects of the conventional anti-anxiety drugs relate to their effects on memory and behavior. Because these drugs act in a powerful manner on brain chemistry, significant changes in brain function and behavior can occur. Severe memory impairment and amnesia of events while on the drug, nervousness, confusion, hallucinations, bizarre behavior, and extreme irritability and aggressiveness may result. They have also been shown to increase feelings of depression, including suicidal thinking.

The Dark Side of Sleeping Pills

Daniel F. Kripke, M.D., Professor of Psychiatry Emeritus at the University of California of San Diego worked for over 30 years assessing the risk of sleeping pills. His findings are stunning. The most shocking of his findings was that people who take sleeping pills die sooner than people who do not use sleeping pills. Dr. Kripke examined data from a very large study known as the Cancer Prevention Study I (CPSI). In this study, American Cancer Society volunteers gave questionnaires to over 1 million Americans and then determining six years later whether the participants had survived. Dr. Kripke and his colleagues found that 50% more of those who said that they "often" took sleeping pills had died, compared to participants of the same age, sex, and reported health status who "never" took sleeping pills.

To re-examine these risks, the American Cancer Society agreed to ask new questions about sleeping pills to participants in a new study, called The Cancer Prevention Study II or CPSII. In 1982, American Cancer Society volunteers gave health questionnaires to 1.1 million new participants. The survival of these people was ascertained in 1988.

In the CPSII, it was again found that people who said that they used sleeping pills had significantly higher mortality. Those who reported taking sleeping pills 30 or more times per month had 25% more mortality than those who said that they took no sleeping pills. Those that took sleeping pills just a few times per month showed a 10-15% increased mortality, compared to those who took no sleeping pills. Sleeping pills appeared unsafe in any amount.

Deaths from common causes such as heart disease, cancer, and stroke were all increased among sleeping pill users. In addition, though the risk was small, daily use of sleeping pills increased the suicide risk by 7 times in men and two times in women.

As of 2020, over 20 population studies have found that use of sleeping pills showed increased mortality risk. Three of these studies specifically found that use of sleeping pills predicted increased risk of death from cancer. There is preliminary data that sleeping pills can increase the risk of certain cancers. But, the strongest explanation for the increased risk of mortality with sleeping pill use is that it is associated with an increased frequency of depression. Considerable evidence shows that depression is also associated with an increased risk for an early death.

So, what does all of this data really mean? First, it may mean that the use of sleeping pills is just an indicator of stress, anxiety, insomnia, and depression. In other words, maybe these people were taking sleeping pills because they were really stressed out and/or depressed it was actually the stress or depression that did them in. Or, it could be that the drugs produce complications. For example, it is possible that these drugs interfere with normal sleep repair mechanisms as well as promote depression.

Although all of the benefits of sleep are still a mystery, one of the ways in which sleep recharges the energy within our cells is by removing harmful chemicals from the body (particularly the brain). Sleep functions to enhance antioxidant mechanisms in order to reduce the damage from highly reactive compounds known as free radicals that can damage our cellular components including our DNA.

Do Sleeping Pills Impair Sleep Quality?

Another explanation for the potential negative effects of sleeping pills on longevity is that they actually interfere with normal sleep patterns. From observation of eye movement and brain wave tracings (electroencephalographic [EEG] recordings), sleep is divided into two distinct types, REM (rapid eye movement) sleep and non-REM sleep. During REM sleep the eyes move rapidly and dreaming takes place. When people are awakened during non-REM sleep, they report that they were thinking about everyday matters but rarely report dreams.

Non-REM sleep is divided into stages 1 through 4 according to level of brain wave activity and ease of arousal. As sleep progresses there is a deepening of sleep and slower brain wave activity until REM sleep, when suddenly the brain becomes much more active. In adults, the first REM sleep cycle is usually triggered 90 minutes after going to sleep and lasts about 5 to 10 minutes. After the flurry of activity, brain wave patterns return to those of non-REM sleep for another 90-minute sleep cycle.

Each night most adults experience five or more sleep cycles. REM sleep periods grow progressively longer as sleep continues; the last sleep cycle may produce a REM sleep period that can last about an hour. Non-REM sleep lasts approximately 50% of this 90-minute sleep cycle in infants and about 80% in adults. As people age, in addition to less REM sleep, they tend to awaken at the transition from non-REM to REM sleep.

Disturbance of the normal rhythm of sleep as well as impairing the ability to reach the deeper stages (3 and 4) of non-REM sleep have long been known to be a problem with many sedative hypnotic drugs. It's the main reason why these drugs will often produce a morning "hangover" feeling. In contrast, natural sleep enhancers (e.g., melatonin, 5-HTP, L-theanine, etc.) appear to actually increase the time spent in the deeper levels of non-REM sleep allowing for the brain and body to get fully recharged. When I talk about sleep quality, what I am really referring to is spending sufficient time in those deeper levels of sleep. While sleeping pills increase sleeping time, they do not improve sleep quality. And, based upon the population-based studies do not appear to improve our health, but actually rob it.

Given the problems with these drugs, every effort should be made to avoid their use. Certainly they are not suitable for long term use for insomnia.

Improving Sleep Quality Naturally

Like other health conditions, the most effective ways to improve sleep quality is based upon identifying and addressing factors that impair sleep. For example, let's take a look at the most common form of insomnia— sleep maintenance insomnia. In this form, people are able to get to sleep, but awaken 3, 4 or 5 hours later and have a really tough time getting back to sleep. What I have found is that most people with sleep maintenance insomnia suffer from faulty blood sugar control. Basically, these people are on what I refer to as the "blood sugar rollercoaster." New techniques in blood sugar monitoring have shown quite clearly that nighttime fluctuations in blood sugar levels are the major cause of sleep maintenance insomnia. The recommendations given in Chapter 5 and below to improve blood sugar control are critical in helping many people with sleep maintenance insomnia get the good night's sleep they need and desire.

Other common causes of insomnia are stress, depression, anxiety, sensitivity to caffeine, and certain medications—there are well over 300 drugs that can interfere with normal sleep. Elimination of the cause is by far the best treatment.

One of the first steps to improve sleep quality in many people is eliminating caffeine. The average American consumes 150-225 mg of caffeine daily, or roughly the amount of caffeine in one to two cups of coffee. Although most people can handle this amount, there is a huge—15-fold—variation in the rate at which people detoxify stimulants such as caffeine. Due to the genetic variation in the liver enzyme that breaks down caffeine it means that some people can eliminate caffeine while others have a form that works so slowly it make take them as much as 12 to 24 hours to fully eliminate the caffeine from a single cup of coffee. Anyone who has trouble sleeping should simply try caffeine avoidance for seven to ten days. This avoidance has to be strict, so all sources, not just coffee, but tea, chocolate, drugs with caffeine, energy drinks, etc. must be avoided.

Alcohol must also be eliminated in people with regular insomnia. Alcohol causes the release of adrenaline and disrupts the production of serotonin (an important brain chemical that initiates sleep). Although not considered a stimulant, sugar and refined carbohydrates can interfere with sleep. Eating a diet high in sugar and refined carbohydrates and eating irregularly, can cause a reaction in the body that triggers the fight or flight response, causing wakefulness.

Seven Additional Tips for a Good Night's Sleep

1. **Make your bedroom primarily a place for sleeping**. It is not a good idea to use your bed for paying bills, doing

work, watching TV, etc. Help your body recognize that this is a place for rest or intimacy. Make sure your room is well ventilated and the temperature consistent. And try to keep it quiet. You could use a fan or a "white noise" machine to help block outside noises.

2. **Incorporate bedtime rituals**. Listening to soft music or sipping a cup of herbal tea cues your body that it's time to slow down and begin to prepare for sleep. Try to go to bed and wake up at the same time every day, even on the weekends. Keeping a regular schedule will help your body expect sleep at the same time each day. Don't oversleep to make up for a poor night's sleep—doing that for even a couple of days can reset your body clock and make it hard for you to get to sleep at night.

3. **Relax for a while before going to bed**. Spending quiet time can make falling asleep easier. This may include meditation, relaxation and/or breathing exercises, or taking a warm bath. Try listening to recorded relaxation or guided imagery programs.

4. **Get out of bed if unable to sleep**. Don't lie in bed awake. Go into another room and do something relaxing until you feel sleepy. Worrying about falling asleep actually keeps many people awake.

5. **Don't do anything stimulating**. Don't read anything job related or watch a stimulating TV program (commercials and news shows tend to be alerting). Don't expose yourself to bright light. The light gives cues to your brain that it is time to wake up.

6. **Perform progressive relaxation**. This technique is based on a very simple procedure of comparing tension against relaxation, see page 296 on how to do it.

7. **Consider changing your bedtime**. If you are experiencing sleeplessness or insomnia consistently, think about going to

bed later so that the time you spend in bed is spent sleeping. If you are only getting five hours of sleep at night, figure out what time you need to get up and subtract five hours (for example, if you want to get up at 6:00 am, go to bed at 1:00 am). This may seem counterproductive and, at first, you may be depriving yourself of some sleep, but it can help train your body to sleep consistently while in bed. When you are spending all of your time in bed sleeping, you can gradually sleep more.

Melatonin

Melatonin is by far the most popular natural sleep aid. Melatonin has been shown to be very effective in helping induce and maintain sleep in both children and adults and in both people with normal sleep patterns and those with insomnia. However, the sleep-promoting effects of melatonin are most apparent if melatonin levels are low. In other words, using melatonin is not like taking a sleeping pill. It has a sedative effect only when melatonin levels are low. When melatonin is taken just before going to bed in normal subjects or in patients with insomnia who have normal melatonin levels, it produces no sedative effect. This is because just before going to bed, people normally have a rise in melatonin secretion. Melatonin supplementation appears to be most effective in treating insomnia in the elderly, in whom low melatonin levels are quite common.

A dose of 3 mg at bedtime is more than enough, because doses as low as 0.1 and 0.3 mg have been shown to produce a sedative effect when melatonin levels are low. Although melatonin appears to have no serious side effects at recommended doses, melatonin supplementation could conceivably disrupt the normal circadian rhythm. In one study, a dosage of 8 mg/day for only 4 days resulted in significant alterations in hormone secretions.

5-HTP (5-Hydroxytryptophan)

5-HTP is converted in the brain to serotonin - an important initiator of sleep. It is one step closer to serotonin than l-tryptophan and has shown more consistent results in promoting and maintaining sleep, even though used at lower dosages. One of the key benefits of 5-HTP is its ability to increase REM sleep (typically by about 25%) while increasing deep sleep stages 3 and 4 without lengthening total sleep time. The sleep stages that are reduced to compensate for the increases are non-REM stages 1 and 2—the least important stages. The dosage recommendation to take advantage of the sleep-promoting effects of 5-HTP is 50 to 150 mg 30 to 45 minutes before retiring. Start with the lower dose for at least 3 days before increasing it.

L-Theanine

L-theanine is a unique amino acid found almost exclusively in tea (*Camellia sinensis*). Clinical studies have demonstrated that L-theanine reduces stress, improves the quality of sleep, diminishes the symptoms of the premenstrual syndrome, heightens mental acuity and reduces negative side effects of caffeine. At typical dosages, e.g., 100-200 mg L-theanine does not act as a sedative, but it does significantly improve sleep quality. It is an excellent support agent to melatonin and 5-HTP. As described above, these ingredients exert synergistic effects to promote restful sleep. NOTE: At higher single dosages, e.g., 600 mg L-theanine does exert sedative action.

Valerian

In terms of herbal medicine, there is no question that valerian (*Valeriana officinalis*) is the most popular remedy for insomnia. Recent scientific studies have substantiated valerian's ability to improve sleep quality and relieve insomnia. In a large double-blind study involving 128 subjects it was shown that an aqueous extract of valerian root improved the subjective ratings for sleep quality and sleep latency (the time required to get to sleep) but left no "hangover" the next morning.

In a follow-up study, valerian extract was shown to significantly reduce sleep latency and improve sleep quality in sufferers of insomnia under laboratory conditions and was suggested to be as effective in reducing sleep latency as small doses of benzodiazepines. The difference, however, arises in the fact that these drugs also result in increased morning sleepiness. Valerian on the other hand, actually reduces morning sleepiness.

As a mild sedative, valerian may be taken at the following dose thirty to forty-five minutes before retiring:

- Dried root (or as tea) - 1-2 grams
- Tincture (1:5) - 4-6 ml (1-1.5 tsp.)
- Fluid extract (1:1)- 1-2 ml (0.5-1 tsp.)
- Valerian extract (0.8% valeric acid) - 150-300 mg

If morning sleepiness does occur, reduce dosage. If dosage was not effective be sure to eliminate those factors that disrupt sleep such as caffeine and alcohol before increasing dosage.

The Effects of Sleep Loss on Cortisol Levels

Our society seems to attach high value to sleeping as little as possible and to extending the waking period. Also wreaking havoc on sleep cycles is shift work at 24-hour, around-the-clock, operations—including hospitals. Sleep deprivation is a major problem in America.

Researchers are attempting to discover a physiological marker of sleep loss and stress. One of the best appears to be measuring cortisol levels at various times during the day. One recent study showed that even partial sleep loss of only 4 hours resulted in loss of cortisol regulation by the body.

Chronic sleep loss may set the stage for poor stress response and symptoms of cortisol excess, including depression, fatigue, and loss of blood sugar control. A vicious cycle ensues, high cortisol levels mean that your body converts less tryptophan into serotonin. Since serotonin is an important initiator of sleep and is also converted to melatonin, insomnia and poor sleep quality are generally associated with elevated cortisol levels. Low serotonin levels can also lead to craving of carbohydrates, depression, migraine headaches and other problems. The amino acid 5-hydroxytryptophan (5-HTP) can be quite helpful to break the vicious cycle of high cortisol levels.

Resetting the Biological Clock

While low nighttime melatonin can lead to insomnia, higher daytime levels can lead to excessive daytime sleepiness. Several studies have shown that vitamin B_{12} in the form of methylcobalamin (dosage 1.5 to 3 mg upon awakening) is an effective treatment to improve sleep in shift workers as well as in people with excessive daytime sleepiness, restless nights, and frequent nighttime awakenings. The subjects taking methylcobalamin experienced improved sleep quality, increased daytime alertness and concentration, and in some cases, they also reported improved mood. Much of the benefit appears to be a result of methylcobalamin's ability to cause a significant decrease in daytime melatonin levels while increasing nighttime levels.

To reset the biological clock I recommend 3 mg of melatonin at night and 3 mg of methylcobalamin in the morning for one month.

Tuning-Up the Adrenal Glands

The first step in improving adrenal health is stabilizing blood sugar levels and improving the sensitivity of the cells throughout the body to insulin. I really do believe that insulin resistance is the biggest underlying threat to the health of most Americans. This statement may sound strong, but it is 100% accurate. Insulin resistance is the key underlying factor that leads to weight gain, the inability to lose weight, increased risk for heart disease, and the development of type 2 diabetes. It also leads to blood sugar volatility or as I refer to it as "the blood sugar roller coaster." And, that roller coaster leads to repeated stimulation of the adrenal glands to secrete adrenalin and cortisol—mirroring the effects of the fight or flight response. Elevated cortisol levels are not only associated with increased feelings of stress, but also loss of appetite control, cravings for sugar, and weight gain.

Table 8.5 - Are You Riding the Blood Sugar Roller Coaster?

Do any of the following apply to you?

- My waist circumference is larger than my hips.
- It is difficult for me to lose weight.
- I crave sweets.
- I feel much better after I eat.
- I am very irritable if I miss a meal.
- I often cry for no reason.
- Sometimes I feel a bit spacey and disconnected.
- I have elevated blood sugar or triglyceride levels.
- I get anxious for no apparent reason.
- I wake up often during the night.
- I feel hungry all of the time.
- I often get very sleepy in the afternoon.

The Negative Effects of Excess Cortisol

To fully appreciate the effect of excessive cortisol secretion on our physiology, let's take a look at the well-known side effects of a drug form of cortisol, prednisone. Used primarily in allergic and inflammatory conditions like asthma and rheumatoid arthritis, prednisone is by far the most often prescribed oral corticosteroid. It blocks many key steps in the allergic and inflammatory response, including the production and secretion of compounds that promote inflammation by white blood cells. This disruption of the normal defense functions of the white blood cells is great at stopping the inflammatory response, but it essentially cripples the immune system. Long term use of prednisone also causes abdominal obesity, puffiness of the face ("moon face"), and accumulation of fat in the upper back ("buffalo hump").

Common side effects of long-term prednisone use at higher dosage levels include: depression, insomnia, mood swings, personality changes, and even psychotic behavior; high blood pressure; diabetes; peptic ulcers; acne; excessive facial hair in women; muscle cramps and weakness; thinning and weakening of the skin; osteoporosis; and susceptibility to the formation of blood clots. Unfortunately, every single one of prednisone's side effects, both short and long term, can occur in our bodies due to excessive cortisol secretion.

Cortisol excess is almost always associated with weight gain. Not only does cortisol signal the brain to eat more, it increases the amount of visceral (abdominal) fat.

Table 8.6 - Conditions Linked to Elevated Cortisol Levels

- Atherosclerosis
- Chronic fatigue syndrome
- Cushing's syndrome
- Depression
- Fibromyalgia
- High blood pressure
- Hypoglycemia
- Hypothyroidism
- Immune system depression
- Insomnia
- Menstrual abnormalities
- Obesity
- Osteoporosis
- Rapid aging
- Stress

Cortisol, Mood, and Sleep

Many of the detrimental effects of cortisol on appetite, mood, and sleep are the result of lowering brain serotonin levels. Serotonin is an important brain chemical that promotes a sense of relaxation and positive mood (happiness). When your brain is low in serotonin, carbohydrate cravings result. What the brain is trying to accomplish by signaling a carbohydrate craving is increasing the manufacture of serotonin from the amino acid tryptophan. Tryptophan has a difficult time getting into the brain because it competes with other amino acids for transport across the blood brain barrier. After a high-carbohydrate meal, there are fewer molecules of amino acids that compete with tryptophan circulating in the bloodstream thanks to our friend insulin. While insulin's primary job is to remove sugar from the blood and help it pass into the cells, it also promotes the absorption of certain amino acids into muscle tissue. As a result, there are fewer amino acids to compete with tryptophan for transport through the blood-brain barrier. Therefore, as long as either a person has insulin resistance or high cortisol levels it will lead to low brain serotonin levels. That may result in strong carbohydrate cravings, depression, or insomnia.

Stabilizing blood sugar levels is the key to stabilizing cortisol levels. Stabilizing blood sugar levels requires eating a low glycemic diet and using the unique dietary fiber PGX (see Chapter 5, pages 131-144).

Potassium to Nourish the Adrenals

Another important dietary recommendation for adrenal health is to restore your potassium-sodium balance. Most Americans consume half as much potassium (which scientists abbreviate K) as they do sodium (abbreviated Na), leading to a K:Na ratio of 1:2. Ideally, however, we should get at least *five times* as much potassium as sodium (a ratio of 5:1). In other words, most people today are getting only one-tenth of the potassium they need.

Reduce sodium in your diet by avoiding the intake of salt. Eat at least five servings of fruit and vegetables per day, because most of these foods have a K:Na of at least 100:1 (see Table 8.7). As you probably know, bananas are the princes of potassium because they have over 400 times as much of this nutrient as they do sodium. Another key recommendation is to use my PerfeKt Sea Salt (see above).

Table 8.7 - Potassium:Sodium Ratio in Fruits and Vegetables

Fruit	K:Na Ratio
Apples	90:1
Asparagus	165:1
Bananas	440:1
Carrots	136:1
Potatoes	110:1
Oranges	260:1
Strawberries	125:1

Key Nutrients to Support the Adrenals

Other nutrients especially important in supporting adrenal function are vitamin C, vitamin B6, zinc, magnesium, and pantothenic acid. All of these nutrients play a critical role in the health of the adrenal gland as well as the manufacture of adrenal hormones. There is evidence that indicates that during times of stress, the levels of these nutrients in the adrenals can plummet.

For example, it is well known that during times of chemical, emotional, psychological, or physiological stress, the urinary excretion of vitamin C is increased signifying an increased need for vitamin C during these times. Examples of chemical stressors include cigarette smoke, pollutants, and allergens. Extra vitamin C in the form of supplementation along with an increased intake of vitamin C-rich foods is often recommended to keep the immune system working properly during times of stress.

Equally important during high periods of stress or in individuals needing adrenal support is pantothenic acid (B vitamin). Pantothenic acid deficiency results in adrenal atrophy characterized by fatigue, headache, sleep disturbances, nausea, and abdominal discomfort. Pantothenic acid is found in whole-grains, legumes, cauliflower, broccoli, salmon, liver, sweet potatoes, and tomatoes. In addition, it is a good idea to take at least an additional 100 mg of pantothenic acid daily. The other key nutrients—

vitamin B6, zinc, and magnesium—should be taken at levels at least equal to the recommended dietary intake (RDI).

DHEA

In the 1990s, there was a lot of interest in the use of DHEA as a strategy for tuning up the metabolism and supporting adrenal function. Its popularity has waned and that is too bad because it can be very effective in promoting health and vitality. After age 25 or so your DHEA levels decline significantly. DHEA supplements boosts energy and well-being, increases sexual appetite and performance, and offset age-related changes in sexuality and mental function. In short, many people regard DHEA is a kind of hormonal fountain of youth.

I believe that DHEA may offer significant benefits to certain people, but only when used appropriately. The only time I recommend use of DHEA by people under forty years of age is if the patient is a woman with an autoimmune disease such as lupus, rheumatoid arthritis, or multiple sclerosis. If you fall into this category, have your doctor evaluate your DHEA levels. The dosage of DHEA I suggest for patients with these autoimmune diseases is 50 to 100 mg daily. The most common side effect from this regimen is acne.

I do not recommend use of DHEA by other women who have not gone through menopause, because many women naturally experience an increase of DHEA as they approach the "change of life." Too much DHEA can cause masculinizing side effects, such as growth of facial hair as well as menstrual abnormalities. There simply is no reason to take DHEA for most premenopausal women. For women after menopause, I usually recommend conservative doses no higher than 5 to 15 mg daily. However, for older women with lupus, higher dosages may be helpful. In a series of clinical studies conducted at Stanford University in women with lupus dosages were as high as 200 mg daily. Again, if you have an autoimmune disease like lupus, I suggest talking to your doctor about DHEA.

Most men who ask me about DHEA complain about low energy and low sex drive. They are hoping for treatment that will increase their sense of well-being and help them feel younger. Before suggesting the use of DHEA, I measure the blood levels of DHEA and testosterone. If these are abnormally low, I recommend that men between the ages of forty and fifty take a dose of DHEA between 15 and 25 mg per day. Older men usually need somewhat higher doses of 25 to 50 mg per day. People over age 70 may need even higher doses to compensate for the continuing decline of their own natural supply of DHEA.

If you are taking DHEA and you are not under the care of a physician, I strongly urge you to get one the test kits available to consumers that measure the level of DHEA in saliva. Just make sure the lab is certified as Clinical Laboratory Improvement Amendments (CLIA). You can use the results to make sure that you are not taking too much.

DHEA for Age-related Mental Decline and Depression

Typically, as people age there is a significant drop in the production of DHEA. Preliminary studies in animals and later in humans indicate that taking supplemental DHEA appears to offset some of the effects of aging including age-related decline in mental function and depression. For example, in a study conducted at the Department of Psychiatry at the University of California School of Medicine, San Francisco, it was shown that elderly patients with major depression and low DHEA levels respond quite well to DHEA supplementation. The dosage used in the study ranged from 30 to 90 mg per day. Improvements in mood and mental function were directly related to increases in the blood levels of DHEA and DHEA-sulfate.

Table 8.8- DHEA Supplementation in the Elderly

Benefits:

DHEA has been shown in double-blind clinical trials to:
- Improve mood and cognition; relieve depression
- Promote increased sense of well-being
- Improve erectile dysfunction
- Improve blood sugar control in diabetics

- Boost immune function
- Higher DHEA levels are also associated with a lower risk for many chronic disease including heart disease

Risks:

Theoretically may increase the risk for breast and prostate cancer

Natural Products for Stress, Anxiety, and Depression

Before discussing natural products to use for stress and anxiety, it is first important to mention that often people suffering from these conditions also suffer from depression and vice versa. This often reflects low levels of brain serotonin, an important neurotransmitter—a chemical messenger responsible for transmitting information from one nerve cell to another. Serotonin has been referred to as the brain's own mood elevating and tranquilizing drug. There is a lot of support for this sentiment. Because the manufacture of serotonin in the brain is dependent upon how much tryptophan is delivered to the brain, in experimental studies researchers can feed human volunteers or animals diets absent in tryptophan and note the effects of such a diet. The results from these sorts of studies have contributed greatly in our understanding on just how vital proper levels of serotonin are to a positive human experience.

Table 8.9 - The Effects of Different Levels of Serotonin

Optimal Level of Serotonin	Low Level of Serotonin
Hopeful, optimistic	Depressed
Calm	Anxious
"Good-natured"	Irritable
Patient	Impatient
Reflective and thoughtful	Impulsive
Loving and caring	Abusive
Able to concentrate	Short attention span
Creative, focused	Blocked, scattered

Able to think things through	"Flies off the handle"
Responsive	Reactive
Does not overeat carbohydrates	Craves sweets and high carbohy- drate foods
Sleeps well with good dream recall	Insomnia and poor dream recall

The lower the level of serotonin, the more severe the consequences. For example, low levels of serotonin are linked to depression with the lowest levels being observed in people who have committed or attempted suicide.

Anti-depressant drugs

In the treatment of depression conventional medicine primarily focuses on increasing the effects of serotonin. Once serotonin is manufactured in the brain it is stored in nerve cells waiting for release. Once released, the serotonin carries a chemical message by binding to receptor sites on the neighboring nerve cell. Almost as soon as the serotonin is released enzymes are at work that will either breakdown the serotonin or work to uptake the serotonin back into the brain cells. Either event results in stopping the serotonin effect. It is at this point that various drugs typically work to either inhibit the reuptake of serotonin or prevent its breakdown. Most popular drugs are referred to as SSRIs—short for selective serotonin reuptake inhibitor. As a result of inhibiting serotonin reuptake, there is more serotonin hanging around capable of binding to receptor sites and transmitting the serotonin effect.

Table 8.10–Examples of SSRIs

- citalopram (Celexa, Cipramil, Cipram, Dalsan, Recital, Emocal, Sepram, Seropram, Citox, Cital)
- dapoxetine (Priligy)
- escitalopram (Lexapro, Cipralex, Seroplex, Esertia)
- fluoxetine (Prozac, Fontex, Seromex, Seronil, Sarafem, Ladose, Motivest, Flutop)

- fluvoxamine (Luvox, Fevarin, Faverin, Dumyrox, Favoxil, Movox)
- paroxetine (Paxil, Seroxat, Sereupin, Aropax, Deroxat, Divarius, Rexetin, Xetanor, Paroxat, Loxamine, Deparoc)
- sertraline (Zoloft, Lustral, Serlain, Asentra)
- vilazodone (Viibryd)

The effectiveness of antidepressant drugs has been the subject of several reviews. The results indicate that they have not been shown to work any better than placebo in cases of mild to moderate depression, the most common reason for prescription medication, and claims that antidepressants are more effective in more severe conditions have little evidence to support them. In fact, the research indicates that SSRIs and other antidepressant drugs might actually increase the likelihood of suicides in adults and children.

An additional alarming finding is that 25% of patients taking antidepressants do not even have depression or a diagnosable psychiatric problem. So, the bottom line is millions of people are using antidepressants for a problem they do not have, and for the people who have a diagnosable condition, these medications do not work in most cases anyway and may cause significant side effects. As one group of researchers concluded "Given doubt about their benefits and concern about their risks, current recommendations for prescribing antidepressants should be reconsidered." This statement is a clear mandate to consider natural medicine to deal with the causes of these mood disorders.

While antidepressant drugs are only marginally successful in alleviating depression at best, they do produce many side effects. Approximately 20% of patients experience nausea; 20% headaches; 15% anxiety and nervousness; 14% insomnia; 12% drowsiness; 12% diarrhea; 9.5% dry mouth; 9% loss of appetite; 8% sweating and tremor; and 3% rash. SSRIs also definitely inhibit sexual function. In studies where sexual side effects were thoroughly evaluated, 43% of men and women taking SSRIs reported loss of libido or diminished sexual response. There is also a significant risk for weight gain and the development of type 2 diabetes.

SSRIs, Weight Gain, and Diabetes

A little-known side effect of SSRIs is weight gain. Statistics show that once weight gain begins while taking these medications it usually does not stop. These drugs induce weight gain because they alter an area of the brain that regulates both serotonin levels and the utilization of glucose. While the human brain will usually make up 2% of our overall body mass, it is so metabolically active that it uses up to 50% of glucose in the body for energy. Evidently the SSRIs disrupt the utilization of glucose in the brain in such a way that the brain senses that it is low in glucose. That sets in motion very powerful signals to eat. And, typically if a person has had sugar or other food cravings they will be dramatically enhanced by the drug. Other changes produced by the drug will lead to insulin resistance, setting the stage for inevitable weight gain and, perhaps, even type 2 diabetes. Studies have shown that individuals predisposed to diabetes are two to three times more likely to become diabetic if they use an antidepressant medication.

Alternatives to SSRIs

There are effective alternatives to antidepressant drugs. For example, there are a number of lifestyle and dietary factors that lead to reduced serotonin levels. Chief among these factors are cigarette smoking, alcohol abuse, a high sugar intake, too much protein, blood sugar disturbances (hypoglycemia and diabetes), and various nutrient deficiencies. All of these factors have one thing in common—they lower serotonin levels by impairing the conversion of tryptophan to serotonin. A health-promoting lifestyle and diet go a long way in restoring optimal serotonin levels and relieving depression. But, in the interim, natural agents like 5-HTP, S-adenosylmethionine (SAMe), or lavender extract can provide the necessary boost in mood to help make important changes in diet and lifestyle easier to accomplish. Both natural agents are discussed below and a program for weaning off SSRIs is given in the Final Comments section in this chapter.

Table 8.11 - Non-drug Approaches to Depression

- Psychological therapy has been shown to be as effective as antidepressant drugs in treating moderate depression.
- Organic factors which are known to contribute to low serotonin levels, i.e., nutrient deficiency or excess, drugs (prescription, illicit, alcohol, caffeine, nicotine, etc.), hypoglycemia, consumption, hormonal derangement, allergy, and environmental factors.
- Depression is often a first or early manifestation of low thyroid function. Thyroid hormone appears to be necessary in the conversion of tryptophan to serotonin.
- Elimination of sugar and caffeine has been shown to produce significant benefits in clinical trials in patients with depression. This effect is due to improving the conversion of tryptophan to serotonin as well as other mechanisms.
- Increased participation in exercise, sports, and physical activities is strongly associated with decreased symptoms of anxiety, depression, and malaise indicating an association with higher serotonin levels.
- Low levels of magnesium, B6, and vitamin D3 are among the nutritional causes of depression. Correcting these nutrient deficiencies can result in significant improvement in mood.
- An insufficiency of the long chain omega-3 fatty acids eicosapentaenoic acid (EPA) and docosahexaenoic acid (DHA) has been linked to depression. Recommended dosage is 1,000 to 2,000 mg EPA+DHA for clinical benefits to be noted.

5- Hydroxytryptophan (5-HTP)

5-HTP is the direct building block for serotonin. It exerts significant advantage over L-tryptophan, which has to be converted to 5-HTP before being converted to serotonin. While only 3% of an oral dose of L-tryptophan is converted to serotonin, more than 70% of an oral dose of 5-HTP is converted to serotonin. In addition to increasing serotonin levels, 5-HTP causes an increase in endorphin levels. Numerous double-blind studies have shown that 5-HTP has "equipotency" with SSRIs and tricyclic antidepressants in terms of effectiveness and is less expensive, better tolerated, and associated with fewer and much milder side effects.

In many studies in depression researchers use a rating scale called the Hamilton Depression Scale (HDS). The HDS score is determined by having the test subject complete a series of questions in which he or she rates the severity of symptoms on a numerical basis, as follows:

- 0—not present
- 1—present but mild
- 2—moderate
- 3—severe
- 4—very severe

Symptoms assessed by the HDS include depression, feelings of guilt, insomnia, gastrointestinal symptoms and other bodily symptoms of depression (e.g., headaches, muscle aches, heart palpitations), and anxiety. The HDS is popular in research because it provides a good assessment of the overall symptoms of depression. Table 8.12 shows the results of a study comparing 5-HTP to tryptophan and a placebo.

Table 8.12–Hamilton Depression Scale from a comparative study of 5-HTP, Tryptophan, and Placebo

Result	5-HTP	Tryptophan	Placebo
Beginning of the study	26	25	23
End of the study (30 days)	9	15	19

In one study, 5-HTP was compared in the study with the SSRI fluvoxamine (Luvox). Fluvoxamine is used primarily in the United States as a treatment for obsessive compulsive disorder (OCD), an anxiety disorder characterized by obsessions and compulsions affecting an estimated 5 million Americans. Fluvoxamine exerts antidepressant activity comparable to (if not better than) other SSRIs like Prozac, Zoloft, and Paxil. In the study, subjects received either 5-HTP (100 mg) or fluvoxamine (50 mg) three times daily for 6 weeks. The assessment methods used to judge effectiveness included the HSD, self-assessment depression scale (SADS), and physician's assessment (Clinical Global Impression). The percentage decrease in depression was slightly better in the 5-HTP group (60.7% vs. 56.1%). 5-HTP was quicker acting than the fluvoxamine, and a higher percentage of patients responded to 5-HTP than to fluvoxamine.

Table 8.13 - Improvement in Specific Depression Symptoms

Symptom	5-HTP	Fluvoxamine
Depressed mood	67.5%	61.8%
Anxiety	58.2%	48.3%
Physical symptoms	47.6%	37.8%
Insomnia	61.7%	55.9%

The advantages of 5-HTP over fluvoxamine were really evident when looking at the subcategories of the HDS: depressed mood, anxiety, physical symptoms, and insomnia. For depressed mood, 5-HTP produced a 65.7% reduction in severity compared with 61.8% for fluvoxamine; for anxiety, 5-HTP produced a 58.2% reduction in severity compared with 48.3% for fluvoxamine; for physical symptoms, 5-HTP produced a 47.6% decrease in severity compared with 37.8% for fluvoxamine; and for insomnia, 5-HTP produced a 61.7% decrease in severity compared with a 55.9% decrease for fluvoxamine. However, perhaps more important than simply relieving insomnia is 5-HTP's ability to improve the quality of sleep. By contrast, antidepressant drugs greatly disrupt sleep processes. On the SADS, 5-HTP produced a 53.3% drop in SADS values compared with a drop of 47.6% for the fluvoxamine group. A drop greater than

50% is an excellent result. In fact, a 50% drop is the best SSRIs generally produce.

5-HTP is equal to or better than standard antidepressant drugs, and the side effects are much less severe. In the study comparing 5-HTP with fluvoxamine, this is how the physicians described the differences among the two groups: Whereas the two treatment groups did not differ significantly in the number of patients sustaining adverse events, the interaction between the degree of severity and the type of medication was highly significant: fluvoxamine predominantly produced moderate to severe side effects; 5-HTP produced primarily mild forms of adverse effects. Fourteen (38.9%) of the patients receiving 5-HTP reported side effects compared with 18 patients (54.5%) in the fluvoxamine group. The most common side effects with 5-HTP were nausea, heartburn, and gastrointestinal problems (flatulence, feelings of fullness, and rumbling sensations). These side effects were rated as being very mild to mild. In contrast, most of the side effects experienced in the fluvoxamine group were of moderate to severe intensity. The only subject to drop out of the 5-HTP group did so after 35 days (5 weeks), while four subjects in the fluvoxamine group dropped out after only 2 weeks. The longer that 5-HTP is used (e.g., after 4 to 6 weeks of use), the less the problem with mild nausea.

5-HTP has been shown to have "equipotency" with SSRIs and tricyclic antidepressants in terms of effectiveness but offers several advantages in that it is better tolerated and associated with fewer and much milder side effects. In addition, many people prefer to use a natural substance like 5-HTP over synthetic drugs.

S-Adenosylmethionine (SAMe)

Another alternative to SSRIs is SAMe - a compound that we naturally produce that is involved in the manufacture of important brain chemicals including neurotransmitters and phospholipids like phosphatidylcholine and phosphatidylserine. Normally, the brain manufactures all the SAMe it needs from the amino acid methionine. However, SAMe synthesis is impaired in depressed patients. Supplementing the diet with SAMe in depressed patients results in increased levels of serotonin, dopamine, and phosphatidylserine, and improved binding of neurotransmitters to receptor sites, resulting in increased serotonin and dopamine activity and improved brain cell membrane fluidity, and thus significant clinical improvement.

The results of a number of clinical studies suggest that SAMe is one of the most effective natural antidepressants. Unfortunately, its use is still limited due to its higher price. Many clinical trials used injectable SAMe. However, more recent studies using oral preparations have demonstrated that SAMe is just as effective orally as it is when given intravenously. SAMe is better tolerated and has a quicker onset of antidepressant action than typical antidepressant drugs. Overall in the double-blind studies comparing SAMe to antidepressant drugs, 76% of the SAMe group showed significant improvements in mood compared to only 61% in the drug group.

No significant side effects have been reported with oral SAMe. The typical dosage for SAMe is 200 mg twice daily. If after two weeks no significant improvement is noted the dosage can be increased as high as 400 mg four times daily.

Individuals with bipolar (manic) depression should not take SAMe. Because of SAMe's antidepressant activity, these individuals are susceptible to experiencing hypomania or mania. This effect is exclusive to some individuals with bipolar depression.

Caffeine in depression and anxiety

The importance of eliminating caffeine was stressed in Chapter 3 in regard to improving sleep quality. It also seems important in people prone to feeling depressed or anxious. Several studies have looked at caffeine intake and depression. For example, one study found that, among healthy college students, moderate and high coffee drinkers scored higher on a depression scale than did low users. Interestingly, the moderate and high coffee drinkers also tended to have significantly lower academic performance. Several other studies have shown that depressed patients tend to consume fairly high amounts of caffeine (e.g., >700 mg/day). In addition, caffeine intake has been positively correlated with the degree of mental illness in psychiatric patients.

The combination of caffeine and refined sugar seems to be even worse than either substance consumed alone. Several studies have found an association between this combination and depression. In one of the most interesting studies, 21 women and 2 men responded to an advertisement requesting volunteers "who feel depressed and don't know why, often feel tired even though they sleep a lot, are very moody, and generally seem to feel bad most of the time." After baseline psychological testing, the subjects were placed on a caffeine- and sucrose-free diet for 1 week. The subjects who reported substantial improvement were then challenged in a double-blind fashion. The subjects took either a capsule containing caffeine and a Kool-Aid drink sweetened with sugar or a capsule containing cellulose and a Kool-Aid drink sweetened with NutraSweet. Each challenge lasted up to 6 days. About 50% of test subjects became depressed during the test period with caffeine and sucrose.

Another study using a similar format as the Kool-Aid study described earlier found that 7 of 16 depressed patients were depressed with the caffeine and sucrose challenge but symptom free during the caffeine- and sucrose-free diet and cellulose and NutraSweet test period.

The average American consumes 150 to 225 mg of caffeine daily, or roughly the amount of caffeine in one to two cups of coffee. Although most people appear to tolerate this amount, some people are more sensitive to the effects of caffeine than others. Even small amounts of caffeine, as found in decaffeinated coffee, are enough to affect some people adversely. The bottom line appears to be that anyone with depression or any psychological disorder should avoid caffeine completely.

L-theanine

L-theanine has been approved for use in Japan as an aid to conquer stress and promote relaxation. It is a very is a popular ingredient in functional foods and beverages as well as dietary supplements designed to produce mental and physical relaxation, without inducing drowsiness. L-theanine is fast-acting. Generally, the effects are felt within the first 30 minutes, and have been shown to last up to 8 to 12 hours.

Based on the results of clinical studies, it has been established that L-theanine is effective in the range of 50 - 200 mg. If you have higher levels of stress take at least 100 to 200 mg one to three times daily. Although L-theanine is completely safe and without any known adverse drug interaction, as a general guideline it is recommended to take no more than 600 mg within a 6-hour period and no more than 1,200 mg within a 24-hour period.

PharmaGABA

GABA (gamma-aminobutyric acid) is a natural calming agent in the brain. In fact, it is one of the brain's most important regulators of proper function and neurotransmitter. It appears that many people with anxiety, insomnia, epilepsy, and other brain disorders do not manufacture sufficient levels of GABA. Many popular drugs such as Valium, Neurontin, baclofen, and Valproate act by increasing the effects of GABA within the brain.

PharmaGABA is a special form of GABA naturally manufactured from *Lactobacillus hilgardii*—the bacteria used to ferment vegetables in the preparation of the traditional Korean dish known as kimchi. PharmaGABA has been shown to produce relaxation as evidenced by changes in brain wave patterns, diameter of the pupil, and heart rate as well as reduce markers of stress including salivary cortisol levels. These effects are thought to be the result of activation of the parasympathetic nervous system rather than the PharmaGABA crossing the blood-brain barrier. Remember that activation of the parasympathetic nervous system produces the relaxation response.

Unlike chemically produced, synthetic GABA, PharmaGABA appears to be able to increase brain alpha waves and lowers beta waves. PharmaGABA is more powerful in this action compared to L-theanine, hence, its effects are a bit more noticeable.

Clinical studies with PharmaGABA have yielded some very interesting results. For example, one study had subjects who were afraid of heights transverse a long walking suspension bridge that spanned a 150-foot canyon. Halfway across the bridge a saliva sample was obtained, and blood pressure was determined. What the researchers were looking for in the saliva was the level of secretory IgA—an important antibody in saliva that helps fight infection. Typically, during times of stress saliva levels drop, sometimes quite precipitously. This event happened when the subjects were given a placebo, but when they were given PharmaGABA the secretory IgA levels in the saliva were maintained halfway across the bridge and actually increased upon completion of the crossing.

The typical dosage for PharmaGABA is 100 to 200 mg up to three times daily. Though no side effects have been reported, as a general guideline it is recommended to take no more than 1,000 mg within a 4-hour period and no more than 3,000 mg within a 24-hour period.

Herbal Adaptogens to Support the Adrenals and Stress Response

Chinese ginseng *(Panax ginseng)* and Siberian ginseng *(Eleutherococcus senticosus)*, rhodiola *(Rhodiola rosacea)*, and ashwaganda *(Withania somnifera)* all exert beneficial effects on adrenal function and enhance resistance to stress and are often referred to as "adaptogens." These plants have historically been used to:

• Restore vitality in debilitated and feeble individuals

- Increase feelings of energy
- Improve mental and physical performance
- Prevent the negative effects of stress and enhance the body's response to stress

In addition, I have found the water-soluble extract of lavender to be another important consideration in helping people with stress and anxiety. It works primarily to improve mood and promote a greater sense of serenity.

Ginseng

Both Siberian and Chinese ginseng have been shown to enhance the ability to cope with various stressors, both physical and mental. Presumably this anti-stress action is mediated by mechanisms that control the adrenal glands. Ginseng delays the onset and reduces the severity of the alarm phase response of the general adaptation syndrome.

People taking either of the ginsengs typically report an increased sense of wellbeing. Clinical studies have confirmed that both Siberian and Chinese ginsengs significantly reduce feelings of stress and anxiety. For example, in one double-blind clinical study, nurses who had switched from day to night duty rated themselves for competence, mood, and general well-being, and were given a test for mental and physical performance along with blood cell counts and blood chemistry evaluation. The group who were given *P. ginseng* demonstrated higher scores in competence, mood parameters, and mental and physical performance compared with those receiving placebos. The nurses taking the ginseng felt more alert, yet more tranquil, and were able to perform better than the nurses who were not taking the ginseng.

In addition to these human studies, several animal studies have shown the ginsengs to exert significant anti-anxiety effects. In several of these studies, the stress-relieving effects were comparable to those of diazepam (Valium); however, diazepam causes behavior changes, sedative effects, and impaired motor activity, but ginseng has none of these negative effects.

On the basis of the clinical and animal studies, ginseng appears to offer significant benefit to people suffering from stress and anxiety. *P. ginseng* is generally regarded as being more potent than Siberian ginseng. *P. ginseng* is probably better for the person who has experienced a great deal of stress, is recovering from a longstanding illness, or has taken corticosteroids such as prednisone for a long time. For the person who is under mild to moderate stress and is experiencing less obvious impairment of adrenal function, Siberian ginseng may be the better choice. Dosages are as follows:

Panax ginseng (Chinese or Korean ginseng):
- High-quality crude ginseng root: 1.5 to 2 g one to three times daily
- Fluid extract (:containing a minimum of 10.5 mg/mL ginsenosides with Rg1:Rb1 greater than or equal to 0.5 by HPLC): 2 to 4 ml (1/2 to 1 tsp) one to three times daily
- Dried powdered extract standardized to contain 5% ginsenosides with a Rb1/Rg1 ratio of 2:1: 250 to 500 mg one to three times daily

Siberian ginseng (Eleutherococcus senticosus):
- Dried root: 2 to 4 g one to three times daily
- Fluid extract (1:1): 2 to 4 mL (1/2 to 1 tsp) 2 to 4 g one to three times daily
- Solid (dry powdered) extract (20:1 or standardized to contain more than 1% eleutheroside E): 100 to 200 mg 2 to 4 g one to three times daily

Rhodiola rosea

Rhodiola rosea (artic root), a popular plant in traditional medical systems in Eastern Europe and Asia, is another useful botanical medicine to support stress management. Modern research has confirmed the adaptogenic actions of *R. rosea* are different from those of Chinese and Siberian ginsengs, which act primarily on the hypothalamus-pituitary-adrenal axis. In contrast, *R. rosea* seems to exert its adaptogenic effects by working on neurotransmitters and endorphins. *R. rosea* appears to offer an advantage over other adaptogens in circumstances of acute stress because it produces a greater feeling of relaxation and anti-anxiety effects. A single dose of Rhodiola extract prior to acute stressful events has been shown to prevent stress-induced disruptions in function and performance, but like the ginsengs, *R. rosea* has also shown positive results with long-term use. In one randomized, placebo-controlled trial of 60 patients with stress-related fatigue, Rhodiola was found to have an anti-fatigue effect that increased mental performance, particularly the ability to concentrate, as well as decreased the cortisol response to awakening stress.

On the basis of results of clinical trials with a standardized *R. rosea* extract, the therapeutic dose varies according to the rosavin content. For a dosage target of 3.6 to 7.2 mg of rosavin, the daily dose would be 360 to 600 mg for an extract standardized for 1% rosavin; 180 to 300 mg for 2% rosavin; and 100 to 200 mg for 3.6% rosavin. When *R. rosea* is used as an adaptogen, long-term administration is normally begun several weeks before a period of expected increased physiologic, chemical, or biologic strain and continued throughout the duration of the challenging event or activity. When *R. rosea* is used as a single dose for acute stress (e.g., for an examination or athletic competition), the suggested dose is three times the dose used for long-term supplementation. No side effects have been reported in the clinical trials, but at higher dosages, some individuals might experience greater irritability and insomnia.

Withania somnifera (Ashwagandha)

Two proprietary extract of roots and leaves from *Withania somnifera* known as KSM-66 and Sensoril and KSM-66 have shown impressive clinical results in dealing with stress. These extracts with the body's natural biological systems to help restore balance to the body and normalize body functions. They help to increase the body's resistance to stress and reduce physiological responses to stress events. Ashwagandha's comprehensive mechanism of action, by balancing and harmonizing body systems, delivers a variety of benefits to maintaining good health. Among other things, KSM-66 and Sensoril:

- Helps counteract the negative effects of stress.

- Increases resistance to fatigue.
- Helps promote mental clarity and concentration.
- Supports healthy weight management by inhibiting stress responses that can lead to overeating.
- Helps increase resistance to stress and tension.
- Helps protect against the effects of aging by protecting against free radical damage to cells.

The typical dosage for Sensoril is 125 mg once or twice daily while the dosage of KSM-66 is typically 300 mg once or twice daily.

Effective Stress Management with Natural Products: Putting it All Together

The use of natural medicines as part of stress management program can be utilized according to one's need to provide a more personalized program. Here is how I generally determine when people require additional support.

Level 1 Support

In addition to following the appropriate lifestyle and dietary approaches to stress reduction as well as regular utilization of techniques to calm the mind and body, Level 1 Support simply involves using natural products on an as needed basis such as following those recommendations for getting a good night's sleep (e.g., 5-HTP, L-theanine, and/or melatonin), for stabilizing blood sugar levels (PGX), or taking L-theanine or PharmaGABA when experiencing situational stress.

Level 2 Support

Level 2 Support involves all of the above and using either L-theanine or PharmaGABA on an ongoing basis if there are more pervasive feelings of stress or nervousness. If the primary issue is more depression than anxiety, choose either 5-HTP (especially if weight loss is desired) or SAMe (better choice if the liver needs support).

Level 3 Support

Level 3 Support involves using the above plus one of the adrenal adaptogens at the dosages recommended above.

Level 4 Support

For people who are starting to experience or are experiencing significant signs of adrenal fatigue and generalized exhaustion, Level 4 Support is recommended. This level involves using all of the above plus a combination of at least two of the herbal adaptogens.

Recommendations if You are on a Prescription Drug for Anxiety, Insomnia, or Depression

If you are taking any prescription drug for stress, anxiety, depression, or insomnia and wish to discontinue, you need to work with your physician. In general, discontinuing any drug for these conditions has to be done gradually—especially with the benzodiazepines. The same is true for SSRIs. Stopping an SSRI too quickly is associated with symptoms such as dizziness, loss of coordination, fatigue, tingling, burning, blurred vision, insomnia, and vivid dreams. Less often, there may be nausea or diarrhea, flu-like symptoms, irritability, anxiety, and crying spells.

To help support weaning off of SSRIs, 5-HTP and/or SAMe can be used. A concern when mixing antidepressant drugs with 5-HTP is producing what is referred to as the "serotonin syndrome" - characterized by confusion, fever, shivering, sweating, diarrhea, and muscle spasms. Although it is theoretically possible that combining 5-HTP with standard antidepressant drugs could produce this syndrome, to my knowledge no one has actually experienced this syndrome with the simultaneous use of 5-HTP with an SSRI. Nonetheless, my recommendation is that when using 5-HTP in combination with standard antidepressant drugs that you be closely monitored by your doctor for any symptoms suggestive of the serotonin syndrome. If these symptoms appear, elimination of one of the SSRI entirely may be indicated. There is no concern with using SAMe and SSRIs simultaneously.

To taper off the SSRI, work with your physician to reduce the dosage of the SSRI by 50% and take 50 mg of 5-HTP three times daily and/or 200 mg SAMe daily. After two weeks reduce the dosage of the SSRI by ½ again. Stay on this dosage for a month before finally discontinuing the SSRI. If needed the dosage of 5-HTP can be increased to 100 mg three times daily and the dosage of SAMe can be as high as 400 mg four times daily.

Case Study: Getting the Stress Out

Patty, thirty-nine-year-old woman, was a website manager for an Internet company. She complained of stress, anxiety, and insomnia. When she did sleep, she didn't dream.

In taking her medical history, I identified many possible contributing factors. First was diet, which did not support health at all. Like many people living in Seattle, Patty had a great affection for Starbuck's coffee. She was regularly drinking four tall lattes a day and at least two cans of Diet Pepsi a day (another major source of caffeine). Instead of breakfast she opted for a double latte. Her first "food" of the day was usually a candy bar from the vending machine during her first coffee break. Lunch was usually her only significant meal. For dinner, she usually had a bowl of popcorn washed down with (you probably guessed it) a Diet Pepsi.

To make matters even worse, stress was a major factor in Patty's life. She was going through a divorce, changing jobs, and looking for new apartment. She told me she felt like she was "going nuts." She had tried benzodiazepines (Valium-like drugs) as well as Ambien, an insomnia drug, but did not like the way they made her feel. She also reacted quite poorly to the antidepressant Prozac. "I just can't take it anymore," she said, I was her "last resort."

After taking her medical history, I asked Patty what changes in her diet and lifestyle did she think she needed to make to support her body and mind. In my experience, most patients pretty much know what they to do to improve their health. Patty was no different. She admitted she needed to eat more nutritiously, cut down on the caffeine intake, and start exercising more regularly.

I told Patty that maybe the anxiety she was feeling arose from excitement over the endless possibilities that were now available to her (plus, of course, her excess caffeine intake). If we took away the caffeine, perhaps everything else would fall into place. We spent most of the hour-long office visit discussing what an exciting time it was in her life. If you think about the physical feeling of excitement is very close to the feelings of anxiety (Imagine a roller-coaster ride!). Perhaps the biggest difference is the label we put on it. I asked Patty such questions as, "What are the things in life that you are most excited about?" "Why does this make you feel excited?" It was amazing to watch the transformation occurring before me. Her anxiety and fear were replaced with excitement and hope. I could tell that Patty was going to be O.K., but we needed to improve her physiology so that her natural, positive mental attitude could shine. Here was her prescription:

- Switch to decaffeinated coffees.
- Quit eating those candy bars and drinking those diet soft drinks!
- Eat breakfast, even if it was simply a piece of fruit like an apple or banana on her drive to work.
- Consume a salad (no dressing) at lunch. Continue with her other healthy lunch choices.
- Don't fill up on popcorn at dinner. Plan ahead and plan meals at least a day in advance.
- Join a health club.
- Take the following supplements:
  - A high-potency multiple vitamin and mineral formula): 1 tablet three times daily.

- Kava: 200 mg of an extract standardized to contain 30% kavalactones three times daily.
- 5-HTP: 100 mg at bedtime.

A repeat office visit four weeks later was phenomenal. Her whole life had been transformed. Patty told me that the first week was hard as she did experience some caffeine withdrawal (she took acetaminophen to help with headaches). But after that first week she noticed that her energy levels were higher. She felt "the weight of the world" was finally off her shoulders. Coincidentally, she had found a great place to live, her divorce had been finalized, she had several men pursuing her at the health club she joined, she was sleeping normally again, and she was dreaming again for the first time in years. We eventually weaned her off the kava, but she continued to use the 5-HTP because she liked the way it helped her get a good night's sleep as well as dream.

Longevity Matrix Lifestyle Tune-Up #8—Become a "Good Finder"

In order for a person to be really happy with themselves and life, I believe that they must become what motivation expert Zig Ziglar refers to as a "good finder" - someone who looks for the good in other people or situations.

A classic experiment illustrates just how powerful an effect looking for the good can have on others. The study conducted at Harvard University by Dr. Robert Rosenthal involved three groups of students and three groups of rats. He informed the first group of students, "You're in luck. You are going to be working with genius rats. These rats have been bred for intelligence and are extremely bright. They will perform the tests like running through a maze with great ease."

The second group was told, "Your rats are just average. They are not too bright, not too dumb, just a bunch of average rats. Don't expect too much from them, because they are just average." The third group was told, "Your rats are really dumb. If they find the end of the maze, it will be purely by accident."

For the next six weeks, the students conducted experiments with the rats involving having individual rats run through a maze. Their performance was timed. Not surprisingly, the genius rats behaved like geniuses and had the lowest times. The average rats were average, and the dumb rats were really dumb.

O.K., so what is so amazing about this study? Well, it turns out that all of the rats were from the same litter. There were no genius, average, or dumb rats. The only difference between them was the direct result of the difference in attitude and expectations of the students conducting the experiments.

Does the same thing happen with humans? Most definitely. Studies conducted with teachers and children produced the same kind of results as the studies with the rats. Remarkable as it may seem, it has been shown many times in controlled experiments that parents, teachers, managers, and others will get exactly what they expect. A name has been given to this phenomenon; it is called the "Pygmalion Effect."

According to Greek mythology, Pygmalion was a sculptor and King of Cyprus who fell in love with one of his creations. The ivory statue came to life after Pygmalion's repeated prayers to the Goddess of Love, Venus. Pygmalion's vision was so powerful and his faith so strong, his vision became his reality. The myth exemplifies the truth that what we see reflected in many objects, situations, or persons is what we put there with our own expectations. We create images of how things should be, and if these images are believed, they become self-fulfilling prophecies.

If we expect only the worst from people, that is exactly what we see. If we can focus our attention on the positives, if we can look for the good in people and situations, that becomes our reality. In addition, if we are constantly criticizing and looking for the negatives in people, especially our loved ones, this attitude is reflected. We too are harshly judged and criticized.

To be happy and have positive relationships, you absolutely must become a good finder. You must look for the good in people. You must expect the best from people. And, you must reinforce the good that you see. You must also demonstrate your love and appreciation.

It is not enough to simply feel love in our friendships and intimate relationships, we must express these feelings. We must demonstrate to our loved ones just how important they are to us. We must continually find ways to communicate our deepest feelings through our actions whether they are verbal, written, through touch, or by our behavior. We all need to see, hear, and physically feel loved and appreciated. I strongly urge you to seek out ways to continually tell those around you how much you love and appreciate them. It creates a powerful feedback cycle that raises your own feelings of self-worth.

CHAPTER 9:

Boosting and Protecting
Your Brain

A strong argument could be made that the human brain is the most astonishing structure in the known universe. Merely to look at it, you wouldn't know the brain held such power. The human brain is about the size of medium-sized cantaloupe. It's full of folds and fissures, like a walnut. And, it has the consistency of cold oatmeal. Yet this mass of densely packed, interwoven nerve cells, weighing only about three and half pounds, has thousands of times more calculating power than the largest computer ever built. It regulates every function within your body. It processes and coordinates signals from thousands of nerves to help you perceive, make sense of, and respond to the world around you. It stores your memories so efficiently that you can instantly recall the lyrics and melody of a song you may not have heard for thirty years. And, that brain power should definitely last and NOT be affected by aging

Let me be very clear here. Memory loss and decreased brain power is NOT inevitable as we age. Steps can be taken to not only stop memory loss and mental decline, but also reverse it. Brain cells are the most complex, long living and nutritionally demanding cells in the body. Scientific studies have shown that intelligence, memory, behavior and concentration are all influenced by the quality of brain nutrition. Young or old, our nutritional status plays a vital role in determining how well our brain functions. Trying to sidestep this fundamental fact by trying to address brain health solely through prescription drugs or even dietary supplements and herbal products aids is foolish, yet it is the dominant model. Especially in conventional medicine whether a person is showing memory loss, depression, ADHD, or other brain issue the only solution being offered is a prescription. The reality is that this approach is very limited and far from ideal.

The Role of Dietary Fat and the Growth of the Human Brain

A larger, more metabolically active brain is one of the key differences between humans and other primates. It has been theorized by some evolutionists that a shift in dietary intake of fats was the likely stimulus for the brain growth in ancient humans. The shift itself was likely the result of limited food availability forcing early humans to collect shellfish and hunt grazing mammals such as antelope and gazelle in addition to their gathering plant foods. Archeological data supports this association— brains of humans started to grow and become more developed at about the same time as evidence shows an increase of shellfish consumption and the presence of animal bones being butchered with stone tools at early villages. Data also shows that the early humans who lived near water sources and ate seafood experienced the biggest brain change. An increased intake of the omega-3 fatty acid docosahexaenoic acid (DHA) found primarily in fish and seafood, but also wild game, was perhaps the largest dietary contributor to brain growth.

The thought is that a higher DHA intake led to bigger brains in humans. And, with a bigger brain, early humans were able to engage in more complex social behavior, which led to improved foraging and hunting tactics, which in turn led to even higher quality food intake fostering additional brain evolution. In contrast, inland pre-historic man did not have sufficient access to DHA, and the Neanderthals chose to focus on low DHA content meat from larger animals. As a result, both got stuck with limited brain capacity and died off.

The importance of DHA to brain function relates to its role in the composition of brain cell membranes and as result it influences:

- The fluidity of brain cell membranes.
- Neurotransmitter synthesis.
- Neurotransmitter binding.
- Signal transmission.
- The activity of key enzymes that break down neurotransmitters like serotonin, epinephrine, dopamine, and norepinephrine.

While improved dietary quality alone cannot fully explain why human brains grew, it definitely appears to have played a critical role. Our brain is largely composed of fats. Specifically, 2/3 of the dry weight of the brain is from fats. Traditionally fish has been described as "brain food"—a claim that was dismissed as an 'old wives tale' for many years but recent research into the links between fish and brain function suggest that this old wives' tale may have more than a small grain of truth behind it. It is now known that a large part of the brain is made up of omega-3 fatty acids. In fact, as much as 60% of the fats in the brain are omega-3 fatty acids with DHA ideally being the main type. And, since fish, especially cold-water, more fatty fish are the best source of preformed DHA it truly is a good brain food.

A higher intake of DHA during pregnancy and early childhood was especially important to human evolution. DHA is critical for healthy brain development both in the womb and in early childhood. About 75% of brain cells are in place before birth and the other 25% are in place by the age of 1 year—making DHA an essential nutrient both for pregnant mothers and young children. DHA is so important for early brain development that it is now automatically added to baby milk formula and pregnant women should also strive to get sufficient levels by regularly eating fish or taking fish oil supplements.

Proper brain and nerve function also require the monounsaturated fat oleic acid, the main component of olive oil as well as the chief oil in almonds, pecans, macadamias, peanuts, and avocados. Myelin, the protective sheath that covers communicating neurons, is composed of 30% protein and 70% fat with the key fat being oleic acid. Again, the key point is the right fat has beautiful effects in your brain.

Eating the Right Type of Fats Can Make You Smarter

The next time someone calls you a fathead, take it as a compliment. Your brain is basically a vat of fat. The type of fat that you regularly consume plays a major role in how well your brain functions. Like other cells in your body, nerve cells are enveloped by membranes composed chiefly of essential fatty acids in the form of compounds known as phospholipids. These phospholipids play a major role in determining the integrity and fluidity of cell membranes. What determines the type of phospholipid in the cell membrane is the type of fat consumed. A brain cell that is packed full of phospholipids composed of saturated fat and omega-6 fatty acids differs considerably in structure and function from a brain cell packed full of essential fatty acids. A diet composed mostly of saturated fat, animal fatty acids, cholesterol, and omega-6 fatty acids produces cell membranes that are much less fluid in nature than the membranes of people who eat optimum levels of omega-3 fatty acids.

In fact, a deficiency of omega-3 fatty acids in cellular membranes makes it virtually impossible for the cell membrane to perform its vital functions. Without a healthy membrane, cells lose their ability to hold water, vital nutrients, and electrolytes. They also lose their ability to communicate with other cells and be controlled by regulating hormones. They simply do not function properly. An alteration in cell membrane function is the central factor in the development of cell injury and death.

How this all relates to impaired mental function (cognition) was illustrated in a study published in the American Journal of Epidemiology. The study indicated that the intake of linoleic acid (an omega-6 fatty acid) was positively associated with impaired cognition. The major dietary sources of linoleic acid were butter, vegetable oils (corn, safflower, sunflower, and soy), and cheese. In contrast, fish consumption (a good source of omega-3 fatty acids) was associated with improved mental function. The more fish consumed, the higher the mental function test scores. And, in a Scottish study looking at fish and brain function, researchers found that people who ate oil-rich fish like salmon, trout, mackerel or herring had an IQ level that was 13% higher than people who never ate fish. The study also found that people who ate fish were less likely to show early signs of Alzheimer's disease. I am happy to see that my grandmother was right—fish really is a "brain food"!

EPA and DHA Levels are Dangerously Low in Vegans and Vegetarians

As humans, we all have some basic and essential nutritional needs whether we choose to be omnivores, vegetarians, or vegans. Is one of these diets healthier than the next? Only within their contexts if they can provide adequate levels of essential and/or health promoting compounds.

When talking about the many health benefits of the long-chain omega-3 fatty acids from fish oils in my lectures, one of the regular questions I am asked: "is there a vegetarian answer to providing EPA and DHA?" Until recently the answer has been no, but now there are marine algae sources that are being used to provide these valuable omega-3 fatty acids. Based upon a new analysis of the fatty acid profiles in vegetarians and vegans it seems essential that supplementation with these marine algae sources.

The main omega-3 fatty acid in the vegetarian diet is alpha-linolenic acid (ALA), which is derived from foods such as flaxseed and walnuts, as well as their oils. While some ALA is converted to EPA, it is a rather inefficient conversion and supplementation with ALA from flaxseed oil has little effect on raising DHA levels. Not surprisingly, several studies have demonstrated that vegetarians and vegans have much lower blood levels of DHA and EPA, when compared to those who eat fish or take fish oil supplements.

Based upon a considerable body of evidence, the health benefits of EPA+DHA appear when the concentration within red blood cells achieves a value greater than 8%. Levels under 4% are considered high risk for over 60 different health conditions. Previous studies have shown vegans and vegetarians, as well as omnivores who do not eat fish or take fish oil supplements, are typically below 4% EPA+DHA in their blood.

Several studies have shown that vegetarians and vegans have much lower blood levels of EPA and DHA compared to those who eat fish. A study was conducted to better define the level of these omega-3 fatty acids in vegans and to determine the effects of a vegan omega-3 supplement on blood measurements from marine algae providing 254 mg EPA+DHA a day for 4 months.

A total of 165 vegans participated in the study for blood measurement. A subset of 46 subjects with a baseline omega-3 index of <4% were given a vegetarian omega-3 supplement for 4 months and then retested. The average level of EPA+DHA in the blood of the 165 vegans was 3.7% with roughly 2 out of 3 vegans having levels below 4% and 1 out of 3 even lower at less than 3%. These results clearly show that a substantial number of vegan subjects have low omega-3 status.

In the subset that received the marine microalgae derived EPA+DHA supplement, blood levels increased from 3.1% to 4.8%. These results indicate that while there was a very good response to the relatively low dose of EPA+DHA given higher dosages are required to achieve the target of 8% in these individuals. The likely dosage is at least 1,000 mg EPA+DHA daily.

What About Meat Sources of DHA?

One dietary fad right now that has been getting a lot of attention is the "paleo diet." There are several different versions out there and there is much that I agree on with the principles of eating more whole foods and avoiding processed foods. One of the offshoots of the paleo diet movement is that it has increased the awareness of how much our food supply has changed over the years.

There is a very big difference in the meat that our ancestors consumed compared to the meat we find in the supermarkets today. For example, domesticated animals like beef have a much higher fat level than wild counterparts (25-30% or higher fat content in domesticated animals compared to a fat content of lower than 4% for free-living animals or wild game). The type of fat is also considerably different. Domestic beef fed primarily corn and soy contains primarily saturated fats, omega-6 fatty acids, and virtually undetectable amounts of omega-3 fatty acids. In contrast, the fat of wild animals or grass fed beef contains very good amounts of beneficial omega-3 fatty acids (approximately 4%) including DHA and a much lower omega-6 to omega-3 ratio (>20:1 in grain fed beef and about 2-3:1 in grass fed beef).

Grass-fed beef also contains ten times as much conjugated linoleic acid (CLA) as grain-fed animals. CLA is a slightly altered form of the essential fatty acid linoleic acid. It occurs naturally in meat and dairy products. CLA was discovered in 1978 when researchers at the University of Wisconsin were looking for cancer-causing compounds that result from cooking. Instead, they found CLA, which appears to be an anticancer compound. Preliminary studies show that CLA might help some people lose weight as well as reduce the risk of heart disease and cancer. Bottom line is if you are going to eat beef make sure it is grass fed. As for chicken and eggs, make sure the chickens are free range fed.

Brain Assessment

Circle the number that best describes the intensity of your symptoms on the following scale:

0 = I do not experience this symptom

1 = Mild

2 = Moderate

3 = Severe

Score 0 for each No answer and 10 for each Yes.

1.	Often forgetful	0	1	2	3
2.	Forget people's names especially when recently introduced	0	1	2	3
3.	Lose track of time	0	1	2	3
4.	Ringing in the ears	0	1	2	3
5.	Feel dizzy at times	0	1	2	3
6.	Difficulty focusing	0	1	2	3
7.	Sense of smell is not as strong	0	1	2	3
8.	Exhaustion from slightest effort	0	1	2	3
9.	Loss of grip strength	0	1	2	3
10.	Feel mentally tired	0	1	2	3
11.	Feel nervous for no reason	0	1	2	3
12.	Can't get enough sleep	0	1	2	3

TOTAL _____

Scoring

- 12 or more: High Priority
- 5-12: Moderate Priority
- 1-4: Low Priority

Interpreting Your Score

These questions are designed to alert you to possible problems with the way your brain. Your brain is an energy hog, demanding a disproportionate amount of blood sugar to function. Your brain accounts for only about two percent of your body weight, but it consumes twenty percent of your body's energy and oxygen. If not enough blood reaches the brain, or if the blood contains inadequate supplies of glucose or oxygen, you may experience such symptoms as poor memory, lightheadedness or dizziness.

In some ways, the connections between brain cells are like very delicate wires that conduct electrical signals. At maturity, the brain contains perhaps ten billion neurons (or a hundred billion; no one seems quite sure). Given all these neurons, each with many branches, your brain has an estimated 100 trillion (with a "T") connections. If the brain cells do not receive adequate nutrients, the signals can slow to a crawl. If brain energy levels are particularly low, the signal cannot travel to its destination. That can lead to poor memory and cognition.

Blood Flow and Cardiovascular Health are Critical to Brain Health

There is a very strong link between cardiovascular health and brain health. Not surprisingly, many of the same dietary, lifestyle, and supplement strategies to support heart health have the additional benefit (either directly or indirectly) of supporting brain health as well.

Cerebral vascular insufficiency—decreased blood supply to the brain—is extremely common among the elderly in developed countries due to the high prevalence of atherosclerosis (hardening of the arteries). The artery affected in most cases is the carotid artery. A pair of carotid arteries—one on each side of the neck running parallel to the jugular vein—are the main arteries that supply blood to the brain.

Symptoms of cerebral vascular insufficiency (CVI) are caused by a reduced blood flow and oxygen supply to the brain. Severe disruption of blood and oxygen supply results in a stroke. The official definition of a *stroke* is "loss of nerve function for at least twenty-four hours due to lack of oxygen." Some strokes are quite mild; others can leave a person paralyzed, in a coma, or unable to talk, depending on which part of the brain is affected. Smaller "mini-strokes," or *transient ischemic attacks* (TIAs), may result in loss of nerve function for an hour or more, but less than twenty-four hours. TIAs may produce transient symptoms of CVI: dizziness, ringing in the ears, blurred vision, confusion, and so on. Repeated TIAs are serious as they can over time result in substantial, progressive damage to brain function. What makes this so insidious is that the lack of a sudden event can mask the problem, so it is not recognized until too late.

Ginkgo biloba Extract (GBE) has been the subject of over forty double-blind studies in the treatment of CVI. In these well-designed studies, GBE has produced a statistically significant regression of the major symptoms of CVI as well as impaired mental performance. These symptoms included short-term memory loss, vertigo, headache, ringing in the ears, lack of vigilance, and depression. The significant regression of these symptoms by GBE suggests that vascular insufficiency, not a true degenerative process, may be the major cause of these so-called age-related cerebral disorders.9

In a comprehensive review, an analysis was made of the quality of research in over forty clinical studies of GBE in the treatment of cerebral insufficiency. The results of the analysis indicate that GBE is effective in reducing all symptoms of cerebral insufficiency, including impaired mental function (senility). The typical dosage of the 24% ginkgoflavonglycoside extract is 240 to 320 mg per day.

Mild Cognitive Impairment

Mild cognitive impairment (MCI) is a recently recognized distinct medical condition that reflects an intermediate stage between the expected cognitive decline of normal aging and the more serious decline of dementia. People with mild cognitive impairment can have problems with memory, language, thinking and judgment, but generally not to a degree to cause significant problems in their day-to-day life and usual activities.

Mild cognitive impairment may increase the risk of later progressing to Alzheimer's disease or other dementia, but not everyone with MCI progresses to dementia.

Because MCI is a newly recognized and affects up to 42% of seniors, the drug companies have been very busy trying to seize market share. Drugs known as cognitive enhancers used to treat Alzheimer's disease are becoming popular prescriptions for MCI, but the research does NOT show these drugs to provide any benefit despite their popularity and have the potential to cause significant side effects. One drug, tacrine (Cognex) has already been removed from the market.

Drugs Don't Work to Boost Brain Function in MCI

The Drug Efficacy and Safety Network of the Canadian Institute of Health Research evaluated the safety and efficacy of various drugs referred to as "cognitive enhancers" (donepezil [Aricept], rivastigmine [Exelon], galantamine [Razadyne], or memantine [Nemenda]) on mild cognitive impairment. Their results showed these drugs did NOT improve cognition or function among patients with mild cognitive impairment and were associated with a greater risk of side effects especially nausea, diarrhea and vomiting than placebo. Researchers concluded "Our findings do not support the use of cognitive enhancers for mild cognitive impairment." Wow, they found these drugs are not effective at all and lead to significant side effects.

Boosting Brain Function with Nutrition

A key goal to boosting brain function is not only to improve blood flow, but to bath the brain in "super nutrition." Numerous studies have shown that brain function is directly related to nutritional status and not just the type of fats in the diet (see above). Higher nutritional status produces higher mental function. Given the frequency of nutrient deficiency in the elderly population, it is likely that many cases of impaired mental function may have a nutritional cause. What this may mean is that many people basically locked in nursing homes may not need to be there at all.

Let's take a look at a study conducted at Oxford's Department of Clinical Neurosciences that highlights the impact of supplemental B vitamins. By the way, it does not get more authoritative than Oxford. The study involved 156 elderly patients who had mild cognitive impairment and a high risk of dementia and Alzheimer's disease. The patients were divided into two groups: one group took a daily supplement with 800 micrograms of folic acid, 20 milligrams of vitamin B6, and 500 micrograms of vitamin B12; the other group took a placebo supplement. Those levels of folic acid, B6, and B12 are what you might typically find in a high potency multiple vitamin and mineral formula.

Before the trial and during the testing period, the researchers utilized magnetic resonance imaging (MRI) to measure the patients' atrophy levels of grey matter in their brains. Atrophying (shrinking) grey matter is a sign of the progression of Alzheimer's disease and other forms of dementia.

Upon completion of the two-year study, researchers found that those given the B vitamin supplement had about seven times less grey matter shrinkage than did the placebo group.

The researchers also found that those whose grey matter shrunk fastest had higher levels of homocysteine, and those with higher homocysteine levels initially received the greatest benefit from the B vitamin supplements. Homocysteine is a metabolite of the amino acid methionine that will be increased if B12, B6, or folic acid levels are low. Homocysteine can lead to oxidative damage and is linked to atherosclerosis and Alzheimer's disease.

In their conclusion the Oxford researchers stated: "Our results show that B-vitamin supplementation can slow the atrophy of specific brain regions that are a key component of the Alzheimer disease process and that are associated with cognitive decline."

Another study conducted at Oxford University found that having higher levels of omega-3 fatty acids in the brain boosted the benefits of B vitamins in improving cognitive function. More than 250 people with MCI were given a set of tests to measure their cognition and had a blood test to determine the levels of the omega-3 fatty acids EPA and DHA in their blood. The participants were split into two randomly selected groups, who received either a B-vitamin supplement or a placebo pill over two years. Their cognitive performance was also measured, and the results compared with the baseline results from the start of the study.

What the researchers found was that for people with low levels of EPA+DHA, the B vitamin supplement had little to no effect. But for those with high baseline EPA+DHA levels, the B vitamins were very effective in preventing cognitive decline compared to the placebo. These results are game changing because they show a clear interaction and that B vitamins only slow the rate of brain atrophy in MCI in those with a good level of EPA+DHA.

Of course, higher intakes of these omega-3 fatty acids are associated with better mood and mental function scores on their own. For example, a study conducted in Sweden found that people with the highest blood levels of DHA had a 47% lower risk of developing dementia and a 39% lower risk of developing Alzheimer's compared to people with the lowest levels of DHA. This study suggests that simply eating fish 2-3 times a week or taking a fish oil providing at least 1,000 mg of EPA+DHA daily may help reduce the risk of developing Alzheimer's or dementia by nearly 40%. In other words out of ten people who develop Alzheimer's disease that do not eat or supplement with EPA+DHA supplementation, four people would not have developed the condition if they simply would have consumed higher intakes of omega-3 fatty acids.

Bottom line is that in taking a high potency multiple vitamin and mineral formula that supplies sufficient B vitamins along with taking 1,000 to 2,000 mg of EPA+DHA from a quality fish oil can dramatically reduce the risk of mental decline with aging, dementia, and Alzheimer's disease.

Boost Choline Levels

The nutrient choline is critical to proper brain function as it plays a role in the formation of the key brain chemical of memory, acetylcholine, and the composition of an important fatty substance in the brain, phosphatidylcholine. Two highly bioavailable forms of choline have shown effects in boosting brain function as well as in aiding recovery from traumatic brain injuries or a stroke: citicoline (CDP-choline) and glycerophosphocholine (GPC). Both are phenomenally efficient in boosting brain choline levels helping to produce acetylcholine as well as activating neuron-to-neuron signaling used in learning, memory storage and recall. These dietary supplements are supported by more than 100 published clinical papers. For example, in one study investigating CDP-choline's effect on attention and mental performance in middle-aged women found that after 28 days, subjects taking 500 mg/d of CDP-choline demonstrated significant improvement in cognitive performance measures as compared to placebo, with the most marked improvement shown in attentional performance. Another study in an elderly population also found improvements in mental performance and memory. Subjects were evaluated on free recall, word recall, immediate recall and delayed recall, with the CDP-choline group showing marked improvement over placebo. The authors suggested the results may be due to CDP-choline's effect on neuron regeneration and circulation within the brain. Similar effects have been noted with GPC.

You don't need to take both, take either CDP-choline 1,000 to 2,000 mg daily or GPC 600 to 1,200 mg daily. There are no known side effects of interactions.

For Brain Health, Fall in Love with Dark Chocolate and Raw Cacao

Chocolate has been referred to as nature's best medicine. I am not going to go that far as I believe raw cacao is much better, but I will say that including chocolate in your diet has many health benefits including phenomenal effects on your vascular and brain health. At the center of these health benefits are the flavonoids of chocolate. The key flavonoids are flavanols similar to those found in green tea as well as proanthocyanidins (also called procyanidins) similar to those found in grape seed extracts, berries, and pine bark extract. The darker the chocolate, the richer the concentration of these key compounds.

Chocolate flavonoids improve both blood flow and brain health. Harvard researchers back in 2013 investigated the relationship between chocolate consumption and brain health. They conducted a study in a group of 60 older people (aged 72.9 ± 5.4 years) without dementia. The participants drank two cups of hot cocoa per day for 30 days and did not consume any other chocolate during the study. One group consumed a high flavanol hot cocoa providing 609 mg cocoa flavanols and the other group consumed a low flavanol version providing 13 mg.

At the beginning of the study and then again after 30 days the participants were given tests of memory and thinking skills, as well as had ultrasounds tests to measure the amount of blood flow to the brain during the tests.

What these researchers and others are showing is that as different areas of the brain need more energy to complete their tasks, they also need greater blood flow. This relationship, called neurovascular coupling, plays an important role developing dementia and/or Alzheimer's disease.

Of the 60 participants, 18 had impaired blood flow at the start of the study. Those people had an 8.3-percent improvement in the blood flow to the working areas of the brain by the end of the study, while there was no improvement for those who started out with regular blood flow.

The people with impaired blood flow also improved their times on a test of working memory, with scores dropping from 167 seconds at the beginning of the study to 116 seconds at the end. There was no change in times for people with regular blood flow. A total of 24 of the participants also had MRI scans of the brain to look for tiny areas of brain damage. The scans found that people with impaired blood flow were also more likely to have these areas of brain damage.

Interestingly, there was no clear difference between the two study groups. In other words, both the high and low flavanol content hot cocoa was shown to produce benefits. This outcome is quite interesting and suggests that flavanol molecules are not the only beneficial compounds in chocolate and hot cocoa. Other beneficial compounds that could have contributed to the effects noted include theobromine (a caffeine-like compound) and arginine– an amino acid that is required in the production of nitric oxide. Nitric oxide helps regulate blood flow, inflammation, and blood pressure.

In a smaller study conducted at Columbia University 37 healthy men and women aged 50 to 69 received either high-dose flavanol cocoa (900 mg per day) or low-dose flavanol cocoa (10 mg per day) for three months. Brain imaging and memory tests were administered to each participant before and after the study. The brain imaging measured blood volume in the dentate gyrus, a measure of metabolism, and the memory test involved a 20-minute pattern-recognition exercise designed to evaluate a type of memory controlled by the dentate gyrus. Results showed that the participants in the high-dose group had improvements in their dentate gyrus area of the brain and their memory skills improved to a level comparable to people who were 20 to 30 years younger, whereas minimal improvement was seen in participants in the low-dose group.

There are several ways that I get my chocolate fix. In order to provide the most healthful choices of chocolate products, let me offer some suggestions. First, for the biggest flavonoid bang for your caloric buck, always choose high-quality dark chocolate. Make sure the cocoa content is at least 72% in order to qualify it as a high-quality dark chocolate and choose organic, fair trade sources. Most experts agree that the recommended daily "dose" of chocolate is approximately 1 to 2 ounces of dark chocolate. So, don't go above this intake level. To help meter your chocolate intake, you may want to consider buying your dark chocolate bars in small serving size such as 0.35 oz bites. Several brands, including major brands like Ghirardelli and Lindt, as well as health food store brands like Endangered Species offer very dark chocolate bites (e.g., >85% cocoa) in these bite size forms. These are good to have on hand as an after meal treat.

Another way that I get my cacao fix is a special brew that I have almost every day that I create with organic raw cacao powder. There are several brands of raw cacao powder that I alternate. I also add 1 packet of Cocovia providing 375 mg of cocoa flavanols. This product was developed Mars Chocolate. I start the process by heating either almond or coconut milk, then pour it into a big mug. I then add two to three tablespoons of the cacao powder, one tablespoon of my Dr. Murray's AllSweet Plus Sweetener, which features allulose (you can also use xylitol or erythritol). Often, I will enhance the flavor of my special brew by:

- Adding 1 tablespoon of coconut oil
- Adding ½ to 1 tsp of cinnamon.
- Adding ¼ to ½ tsp of nutmeg
- Adding two drops of vanilla extract.
- Adding two drops of peppermint oil.

Other Special Foods to Boost Brain Function

In addition to fish, omega-3 fatty acids, dark chocolate, and raw cacao, there are many other foods to boost brain function. For example, research from Rush University Medical Center in Chicago found that eating just one serving of leafy green vegetables a day takes a decade off an aging brain. Two servings produced even greater effects. The study involved the 960 participants of the Memory and Aging Project, ages 58-99 years, who completed a food frequency questionnaire and had ≥2 cognitive assessments over a mean 4.7 years. Higher consumption of green leafy vegetables was associated with brain function that was the equivalent of being 11 years younger in age. The conclusion was very clear, consumption of approximately 1 serving per day of green leafy vegetables and foods rich in phylloquinone, lutein, nitrate, folate, α-tocopherol, and kaempferol help to slow cognitive decline with aging.

Another food that is particularly helpful in boosting brain power are blueberries or blueberry extracts. In animal studies researchers have found that blueberries help protect the brain from oxidative stress and memory loss. When older rats were given the human equivalent of 1 cup of blueberries a day, they demonstrated significant improvements in both learning capacity and motor skills, making them mentally equivalent to much younger rats. When the rats' brains were examined, the brain cells of the rats given blueberries were found to communicate more effectively than those of the other older rats that were not given blueberries. An alternative to eating more blueberries is taking a flavonoid-rich extract like grape seed or pine bark extract (100 to 300 mg daily).

Even something as simple as celery consumption may offer benefit in improving brain function. Celery and celery seed extracts contains a unique compound, 3-n-butylphthalide (3nB), that is both responsible for the characteristic odor of celery and its health benefits. In human and animal studies, 3nB treatment significantly improved learning deficits, as well as long-term spatial memory. Currently 3nB, as a purified compound, is being investigated as a treatment of CMI as well as traumatic brain injury and Alzheimer's disease. In fact, researchers have concluded "3nB shows promising preclinical potential as a multi-target drug for the prevention and/or treatment of Alzheimer's disease." If you want to take a celery extract, take enough to provide a dosage of 150 mg of 3nB daily.

Mitochondrial Enhancers to Boost Brain Function

There is growing research documenting the role of mitochondrial dysfunction in aging, including MCI. It makes sense. The brain accounts for only about two percent of our body weight, but it consumes more than twenty percent of the body's energy and oxygen. The brain requires exceptional mitochondrial energy production in order for it to function optimally. Enhancing mitochondrial function requires a 7-step process:

- Provide all essential nutrients
- Utilize mitochondrial enhancers
  - Cofactors in energy metabolism (B vitamins are particularly important)
  - Coenzyme Q10, Alpha Lipoic Acid, Carnitine, Ribose
  - Pyrroloquinoline quinone (PQQ)
  - Polyphenols and other phytochemicals
- Provide antioxidants to protect mitochondria from damage
- Improve insulin sensitivity
- Enhance detoxification processes
- Activate AMP-activated protein kinase (AMPk)
- Reduce damaging factors

- ○ Environmental toxins
- ○ Drugs (Rx, OTC, and illicit)

In regard to mitochondrial enhancers, two supplements that have been shown to work together very well in boosting memory and cognition - coenzyme Q10 (CoQ10) and pyrroloquinoline quinone (PQQ). CoQ10 is very well known, but PQQ is just beginning to get popular. PQQ is a powerful antioxidant that specifically protects against mitochondrial damage. It also promotes the spontaneous generation of new mitochondria within aging cells, a process known as mitochondrial biogenesis. This effect is why PQQ is so exciting as an anti-aging strategy.

While PQQ is effective on its own, when it is combined with coenzyme Q10 even better results have been noted. This synergistic effect was first seen in animal studies and further demonstrated in human double-blind, placebo-controlled clinical trials. In one study of 71 middle-aged and elderly people aged between 40-70, supplementation with 20 mg per day of PQQ resulted in improvements on tests of higher cognitive function compared to the placebo group, but in the group receiving 20 mg of PQQ along with 300 mg of CoQ10 the results were even more dramatic. PQQ and CoQ10 are both involved in mitochondrial energy production, so these results are not that surprising.

Herbal Approaches to Boosting Brain Power

Ginkgo biloba extract (GBE) is probably the best-known herbal approach to boosting brain power. Originally thought to be a potential preventor of Alzheimer's disease, at this time it appears that at best GBE only helps in mild cognitive impairment, probably mainly through improving blood flow to the brain. A better choice in most people with MCI is Huperzine A (Hup A), a naturally occurring alkaloid compound found in Chinese club moss (*Huperzia serrata*) that exerts a multitude of pharmacological actions that produce clinically meaningful effects in poor memory and cognition. Hup A is discussed in more detail below. For MCI, I recommend a dosage of 200 mcg twice daily.

Another popular herbal brain booster is the extract of *Bacopa monniera*. This plant has been used in the Ayurvedic system of medicine for centuries. Traditionally, it was used as a brain tonic to enhance memory development, learning, and concentration, and to provide relief to patients with anxiety. Emerging clinical evidence is validating its benefit to people with mild cognitive impairment. In one double-blind, placebo-controlled, 46 healthy volunteers (ages 18-60) were randomly and evenly divided into treatment and placebo groups. The study used a bacopa extract (300 mg daily) containing 55-percent combined bacosides. At the end of the 12-week study, results indicated a significant improvement in verbal learning, memory, and speed of early information processing in the bacopa group compared to placebo.

Curcumin, the yellow pigment of turmeric, is showing incredible promise as a brain protector including an ability to prevent and possibly reverse Alzheimer's disease (AD). Residents of rural India, who eat large amounts of turmeric, have been shown to have the lowest incidence of Alzheimer's disease in the world: 4.4 times lower than that of Americans. In addition, researchers have also demonstrated that curcumin is able to prevent the development of Alzheimer's brain lesions in mice specifically bred to develop AD and may actually reverse the tangled mess of damaged brain cells that characterize the disease. Of course, turmeric (the main component of curries) can be liberally consumed in the diet, but taking a curcumin extract may prove to be very important in the battle against age-related memory loss as well as more serious conditions like AD. In a study conducted at UCLA, 40 adults between the ages of 50 and 90 years who had MCI were randomly assigned to receive either a placebo or Theracurmin, a highly bioavailable form of curcumin, at a dosage of 90 milligrams of curcumin twice daily for 18 months.

All 40 subjects received standardized cognitive assessments at the start of the study and at six-month intervals and after 18 months. Thirty of the volunteers underwent positron emission tomography, or PET scans, to determine the levels of characteristic lesions of Alzheimer's disease in their brains at the start of the study and after 18 months.

The people who took curcumin experienced significant improvements in their memory and attention abilities, while the subjects who received placebo did not. In memory tests, the people taking curcumin improved by 28 percent over the 18 months. Those taking curcumin also had mild improvements in mood, and their brain PET scans showed significantly less damage in the amygdala and hypothalamus - regions of the brain that control several memory and emotional functions that are typically damaged in Alzheimer's disease.

Quick Tips for Using Turmeric

In addition to taking curcumin as a supplement, I do recommend liber use of turmeric (and ginger) as a spice. Turmeric is available as a ground powder, but like ginger is also available as the fresh rhizome. Fresh turmeric should be free of dark spots and be crisp and kept in the refrigerator where it will keep for 1 month.

Since turmeric's deep yellow and orange color can easily stain, avoid getting it on clothing. To avoid a permanent stain, quickly wash any affected area with soap and plenty of water. Depending upon how much you plan on handling it, it might be a good idea to wear latex gloves when preparing foods with turmeric.

- Like ginger, fresh turmeric can be juiced and consumed as a shot or as a component of fresh fruit and vegetable juices.
- Turmeric a heavily relied on spice in the cuisines of Southeast Asia, India, and Mexico as it is a primary ingredient in curry powders.
- To make your own curry powder combine in a grinder 1 tablespoon cumin, 1 tablespoon mustard seed, 1/2 tablespoon coriander, 1 teaspoon each fenugreek, fennel, ginger, and turmeric. Store this powder combination in a cool, dark, dry place for up to 6 months.

- Turmeric is a great spice to complement recipes that feature legumes, particularly lentils.
- Give salad dressings an orange-yellow hue by adding some turmeric powder to them.

Putting it All Together for Boosting Brain Function

Hey, if you are showing signs of MCI, you must act now and be very aggressive in your diet, lifestyle, and supplement strategy. Remember, blood flow is a big factor in brain function, so make sure you are doing all you can in that area as well. Here are the supplements that I recommended above all in one place:

- Foundation Supplements:
    - High potency multiple vitamin and mineral formula
    - Take extra key anti-aging nutrients:
        - Vitamin C: 500 to 1,000 mg daily
        - Vitamin D3: 2,000-4,000 IU daily
    - Fish oil supplement: 2,000 to 3,000 mg of EPA+DHA+DPA daily.
    - Grape seed extract (>95% procyanidolic oligomers): 150 to 300 mg daily
- Phosphatidylserine 300 mg daily
- Boost choline by taking either:
    - CDP-choline 1,000 to 2,000 mg daily or GPC 600 to 1,200 mg daily
- One or two tablespoons of raw cacao daily or a high flavanol containing cocoa or cacao product. I take Cocovia. Try to get 900 mg of flavanols daily.
- PQQ 20 mg and CoQ10 300 mg daily
- Huperzine A 200 mcg twice daily
- Theracurmin 60 to 90 mg twice daily.

Heavy Metal Analysis

Numerous studies have demonstrated a relationship between high levels of various other heavy metals such lead, mercury, and cadmium with Alzheimer's disease, poor mental function, various psychological diseases (especially depression), and childhood learning disabilities including attention deficit disorder (ADD). Heavy metal toxicity can masquerade as serious diseases such as amyotrophic lateral sclerosis (Lou Gehrig's disease) and multiple sclerosis. If you are suffering from any of these conditions, or if you are employed in a profession with extremely high exposure to heavy metals (battery makers, gasoline station attendants, printers, roofers, solders, and dentists), please get a hair mineral analysis or more sophisticated assessments now available to rule out heavy metal toxicity.

Preventing Dementia and Alzheimer's Disease

Of all the many problems that afflict us as we age, the thought of losing our memory and mental function is perhaps the most frightening. Most of us have seen a family member or friend deal with Alzheimer's disease (AD), a degenerative brain disorder associated with progressive deterioration of memory and cognition. In the United States, Alzheimer's affects 1.6% of the population before the age of 74 years, with the rate increasing to 19% in the 75–84 years group and to 42% in the greater than 84 years group. These numbers are striking when compared to data from the 1960s when only 2% of people over the age of 85 years had AD. The tremendous increase in AD in people over 85 years of age is often referred to as the "Alzheimer's epidemic."

AD is the result of damage to many aspects of brain structure and function that affect memory and cognition. The distinct brain lesions of AD are the result of deposits of a substance known as beta-amyloid. Amyloid is a general term for protein fragments that the body produces normally. Beta-amyloid is a fragment snipped from an amyloid precursor protein (APP). In a healthy brain, these fragments are broken down and eliminated by immune cells in the brain. In Alzheimer's disease beta-amyloid protein fragments accumulate to form hard plaques between brain cells, blocking the transmission of messages and leading to the death of brain cells and lesions known as "neurofibrillary tangles," and ultimately, dementia. Tau is the major constituent of neurofibrillary tangles and is produced when beta-amyloid levels become toxic.

How Diet Affects Epigenetic Factors in Alzheimer's Disease

Genetic factors play a major role, but diet is the major factor contributing to the epidemic of AD. There are 2 distinct types of AD—early-onset (EOAD) and late-onset (LOAD). EOAD occurs in people 30-60 years of age. It is rare, representing less than 5% of all people who have AD and is has a very strong genetic component (see below "Should You Get Your Genes Tested for Alzheimer's Risk?). Most cases of AD are the late-onset form, which develops after 60 years of age. LOAD also has a strong genetic link, but diet, environmental, and lifestyle factors greatly influence a person's risk for developing the disease.

The tremendous increase in LOAD parallels the rise in type 2 diabetes; a condition that is primarily the result of dietary and lifestyle factors that lead to a dampening of the effects of the hormone insulin. When cells throughout the body become resistant to insulin, glucose (blood sugar) cannot enter the cells. As a result, it can oxidize and damage cell structures or it can also act like superglue in attaching to protein structures on cells in a way that leads to damage and loss of proper cellular function.

LOAD is so closely linked to insulin resistance some researchers have referred to it as diabetes of the brain and even "type 3 diabetes." Individuals with type 2 diabetes have a 1.5 to 4-fold risk for LOAD as well as dementia caused by damage to the blood vessels of the brain. Insulin resistance in the brain is associated with poor uptake of glucose by brain cells leading to oxidative damage and localized inflammation that leads to beta-amyloid formation. Hence measures to improve blood sugar control and improve insulin sensitivity appear to be important steps in the prevention of LOAD.

In regard to the genetics of LOAD, the breakdown of the process to clear beta-amyloid from the brain first involves amyloid binding to apolipoprotein E (ApoE); if beta-amyloid is unbound to ApoE or "free," it begins to build up and form toxic clusters. There are three forms of ApoE coded for by the APOE gene:

- ApoE2, which is associated with decreased risk of LOAD.
- ApoE3, which is the most common form and is not known to affect LOAD risk.
- ApoE4, which is associated with an up to 12 times increased risk for LOAD.

So, a person's risk for LOAD for many years was likely simply the result of their genetic expression of ApoE. If that had ApoE4, they were at risk, otherwise they were not. But, with the huge increase in LOAD occurrence it is clear that other factors are now the biggest contributors in determining the clearance of beta-amyloid from the brain.

Results from a recent study provide some valuable insight on how diet can moderate factors involved in clearing beta-amyloid. The study involved 27 cognitively normal participants and 20 with mild cognitive impairment suggestive of LOAD. These participants were randomly assigned to 1 of 2 diets that were identical in terms of total calories:

- High fat, high carbohydrate diet: This diet provided 45% energy from total fat (25% from saturated fat), 35% to 40% from carbohydrates, and 15% to 20% from protein. A typical meal for these participants might include cheeseburgers, soda, and fries. The diet also had a very high glycemic index meaning that it contained a lot of foods that quickly raised blood sugar levels like soft drinks, breads, cereals, and pasta.
- Low fat, low glycemic diet: Participants in this group ate food with a very low glycemic index and low in fat. This diet consisted of 25% energy from fat (less than 7% from saturated fat), 55% to

60% from carbohydrates, and 15% to 20% from protein. A typical meal in this group was fish, brown rice, and steamed vegetables.

Since the spinal fluid bathes the human central nervous system including the brain, a spinal tap was performed at the beginning and at the end of the study to determine the levels of free beta-amyloid and beta-amyloid bound to the forms of ApoE. At the beginning of the study, the researchers found that those with mild cognitive impairment had a greater fraction of their beta-amyloid in the free state than the participants with normal mental function. Those carrying the genetic risk factor ApoE4 had an even higher level of free beta-amyloid.

At the end of the study, in those with ApoE2 and ApoE3 it was shown that the high fat, high glycemic diet further increased free beta-amyloid levels, while the low fat, low glycemic diet produced significant decreases in free beta-amyloid levels in these groups. But the different diets had little impact on free beta-amyloid in those subjects with ApoE4.

The study also showed that the changes in beta-amyloid were inversely correlated with cerebrospinal fluid insulin. In other words, lower insulin levels were associated with higher levels of free beta-amyloid. Insulin is critical for proper brain function for many reasons. When insulin resistance occurs as in obesity and type 2 diabetes, higher levels of insulin in the blood result in impaired transport of insulin into the brain. So, low levels of insulin in the cerebrospinal fluid reflect systemic insulin resistance.

In the normal brain, insulin plays an important role in maintaining synapses and memory. So, with the lower brain insulin noted in this study and others, it seems appropriate that LOAD is often referred to as "type 3 diabetes."

What all of these results mean is that in individuals with a low risk for LOAD because of their ApoE type, a high fat, high glycemic diet produces the same sort of changes in beta-amyloid seen in those with ApoE4 genetic predisposition to LOAD. In other words, dietary habits can nullify the protection that a person's genetic code can provide. On the flip side, the dietary changes used in this study were not enough to reduce the genetic predisposition towards LOAD in high-risk subjects. Does that mean the disease is inevitable? Hardly, it just means that additional dietary and supplement strategies are necessary in order to address this predisposition.

Should You Get Your Genes Tested for Alzheimer's Risk?

The conventional medicine answer to this question is no. A lot of reasons are given to argue against genetic testing, but perhaps the real reason is that there is no drug that can offer protection against either EOAD or LOAD. But there are steps you can take with diet, lifestyle, and supplements that can definitely reduce your risk even if you have a genetic predisposition. So, in my opinion, I think that there are clearly some indications where genetic testing makes a lot of sense. Specifically, if you have a family history of AD, either EOAD or LOAD, my advice is to get tested as early as possible. Note, EOAD testing involves markers other than ApoE4 such as amyloid precursor protein, presenilin 1, and presenilin 2 (PSEN2)

Testing for risk for LOAD always includes ApoE4, but there are now additional markers being tested for as well. In European countries ApoE4 gene testing is offered as a direct-to-consumer test. At one time, consumers in the United States were able to use laboratories like 23andMe to determine their ApoE status and other genetic markers linked to AD, but currently the FDA is blocking this service. So, for now, if you live in the U.S., you will need to find a physician that will order these tests for you.

In interpreting the results, the big caveat is that your genes do not fully determine your health destiny. What genetic testing offers is identification of risk. Just because you may be positive for a marker like ApoE4, it does not mean that you are destined to get LOAD. It provides great information for taking even more aggressive steps with diet, lifestyle, and supplementation in order to significantly reduce the risk. My feeling is that genetic testing coupled with a personalized nutritional prescription is the future of medicine.

Dietary Factors that Prevent Beta-Amyloid Accumulation

There are a number of dietary approaches that can prevent beta-amyloid formation or accumulation, and/or promote its clearance even in subjects with ApoE4. Many of these protective dietary factors for LOAD are shared with heart disease prevention. For example, following the Mediterranean Diet is associated not only with a reduced risk for heart disease, but also with a significantly reduced risk of LOAD.

These benefits are the result of the ability of the Mediterranean Diet to improve blood supply to the brain, reduce inflammation, improve insulin sensitivity, and reduce beta-amyloid formation. The key dietary factors in the Mediterranean Diet that reduce LOAD risk are thought to be the higher fish consumption (and omega-3 fatty acids), monounsaturated fatty acids (primarily from olive oil), light to moderate alcohol use (primarily red wine), and increased non-starchy vegetable and fruit consumption.

As previously stated, there is tremendous synergy among all the components of the diet rather than one specific factor responsible for all of the benefits. Nonetheless, several individual factors within the Mediterranean Diet have been shown to work directly on reducing beta-amyloid formation or deposition. For example, polyphenols found in grapes, grape seed extract, and red wine have been shown to prevent beta-amyloid formation and promote its clearance. Even something as simple as drinking coffee or regularly consuming apples or celery may offer significant protection against LOAD.

Many large population-based studies indicate moderate coffee consumption (approximately 3 cups of caffeinated coffee per day) reduces the risk for LOAD. The reduction in risk is significant. For example, one study found that moderate coffee consumption during middle adulthood produced a 65% decrease in the risk of LOAD. Animal studies have shown that both caffeine as well as coffee's polyphenol components like chlorogenic acid can prevent beta-amyloid formation and its damaging effects on brain cells. Similar studies exist for green tea. So, if you can tolerate caffeine, either source can be very good for your brain health.

In regard to apples, can an apple a day fight LOAD? It does not even have to be that frequent. According to research conducted by Dr. Thomas Shea, Director of the Center for Cellular Neurobiology & Neurodegeneration Research at the University of Massachusetts, consuming at least 3 apples per week could reduce risk of LOAD by as much as 75%. His studies show that the antioxidant compounds in apples protect the brain from inflammation and damage. They also prevent the accumulation of beta-amyloid.

Dr. Shea and his colleagues conducted a clinical trial in which 21 institutionalized individuals with moderate-to-severe LOAD consumed two 4-oz glasses of apple juice daily for 1 month. Participants demonstrated no change in mental function in this short trial, but the caregivers reported an approximate 27% improvement in behavioral and psychotic symptoms with the largest changes in anxiety, agitation, and delusion. These results suggest that apple juice may be a useful in helping prevent the decline in mood that accompanies progression of LOAD. However, I hope in the next study they use fresh, raw apple juice vs. pasteurized apple juice. The active compounds are much higher in the fresh apple juice and as a result will certainly produce better results.

In regard to celery (discussed above) and its key component 3nB, in an animal model of LOAD, 3nB treatment also significantly reduced total cerebral beta-amyloid plaque deposition and lowered brain beta-amyloid levels. It also significantly improved learning deficits, as well as long-term spatial memory. In China, synthetic 3nB is being developed as a drug to not only prevent LOAD, but also to prevent stroke; improve blood flow to the brain; protect the brain and enhance energy production within the brain; and improve mild impairment of cognitive function.

Huperzine A in Alzheimer's Disease

Huperzine A inhibits the breakdown of the neurotransmitter acetylcholine (ACH) by reversibly blocking the enzyme acetylcholinesterase. A deficiency of action of ACH is one of the hallmark features of Alzheimer's disease (AD) as well as poor memory and concentration. By preventing the breakdown of ACH, Hup A can enhance its action and produce clinically meaningful effects in AD.

ACH plays a central role in memory, especially the encoding of new memories, in certain key areas of the brain. AD is characterized by damage to these same key areas (e.g., entorhinal cortex and hippocampus) and displaying primary neurotransmitter deficit of acetylcholine function. Not surprisingly, acetylcholinesterase (AChE) inhibitors have emerged as the dominant treatment target. However, the currently available arsenal of these drugs have shortcomings including poor tolerability and lack of action on key brain AChE receptors. These drugs include donepezil (Aricept), rivastigmine (Exelon), and galantamine (Razadyne). Tacrine (Cognex), the first AchE inhibitor approved for AD was also on this list, but lack of effect and poor tolerability led to its removal from the market. Side effects included nausea, vomiting, dizziness, diarrhea, seizures, and syncope. Also, four times a day dosing regimen was required, and patients required periodic blood monitoring due to liver toxicity.

If these drugs have shown limited effects and poor tolerability in AD, how is Hup A different? First, Hup A is a highly selective, reversible, and potent AchE inhibitor. Hup A is 8- and 2-fold more potent than donepezil and rivastigmine, respectively, in increasing brain acetylcholine levels, with a longer-lasting effect. Hup A also has a higher oral bioavailability compared to conventional drug AChE inhibitors. It is also able to cross the blood-brain-barrier more efficiently. Hup A exerts a number of other actions that are important to its overall effects besides inhibiting the breakdown of acetylcholine including:

- Reduces beta-amyloid toxicity
- Prevents brain cell damage against neurotoxins
- Enhancing the activities of the brain's antioxidant enzymes

- Increases nerve growth factor production
- Promotes the generation new brain cells in the key areas affected by AD

Hup A is the drug of choice in China for the treatment of AD and memory disorders since the early 1990s and has been used with no serious adverse effects. In addition to the considerable clinical data produced from studies conducted in China, detailed clinical trials have been conducted with Hup A in AD in over 30 sites in the US and Europe. A detailed meta-analysis of 20 randomized clinical trials with 1823 participants concluded that "Huperzine A appears to have beneficial effects on improvement of cognitive function, daily living activity, and global clinical assessment in participants with Alzheimer's disease." The dosage in these trials was typically 200 mcg twice daily. However, this dosage level may not be sufficient. For example, a trial using a lower dose of 200 mcg twice daily showed no improvement on the Alzheimer's Disease Assessment Scale-cognitive subscale (ADAS-cog) scores, but a different trial using a higher dose of 400 mcg twice daily showed statistically significant improvement in the ADAS-cog scores compared to placebo. Therefore, it appears that in AD, a dosage of 400 mcg twice daily is required. This dosage does carry with it a higher rate of minor gastrointestinal side effects (nausea, vomiting and diarrhea) in about 10-20% of users. That said, Huperzine A has demonstrated an excellent safety profile in all clinical trials.

There are a few important distinctions that must be made. First, all of the clinical research and safety studies have been performed using the purified compound. This compound is substantially different from crude *Huperzia serrata* extracts, whether standardized or not for Hup A. The isolated Huperzine A is a pure compound, clinically shown to be the dietary supplement gold-standard for improvement of memory and cognition. In contrast, when it comes to crude *Huperzia serrata* extracts, there is no research and the composition of these extracts contains compounds with strong sedative and anti-cholinergic properties that exert effects on memory and cognition that are opposite to Hup A. In 1998, the head of the Drug Discovery Program at Georgetown University Medical Center published the following statement: "... the use of the product [*Huperzia serrata*] in its crude form can be extremely harmful and dangerous due to the existence of compounds other than Huperzine-A that are present in [crude form] *Huperzia serrata*." In addition:

- Chinese Medicinal Herbs of Hong Kong states that, "the [crude] herb is poisonous and has anesthetic effects".
- Herbal Drugs by Bisset states that "pharmacological testing has demonstrated considerable toxicity, with the occurrence of emetic and strong laxative properties".
- Martindale's Extra Pharmacopoeia (31st Edition) states that, "[it] is a traditional Chinese remedy used as a sedative and analgesic ... adverse effects include CNS depression and acute hepatoxicity".
- And, according to George A. Kraus, Professor of Organic Synthesis, Bioagricultural Chemistry & Toxicology, at Iowa State University, Department of Chemistry, "Lycopodine [another chemical constituent in crude *Huperzia serrata*] is a toxic alkaloid which causes illness in people and animals".

The bottom line is obvious. It is not just that cheap, low-grade crude form extracts are being promoted on the extensive favorable research— both efficacy and safety—of the purified compound, Hup A. These crude preparations carry with them the risk of significant toxicity. Don't use them.

In one of the first double-blind clinical studies, Huperzine A at a dose of 200 mcg twice daily produced measurable improvements in memory, cognitive function, and behavioral factors in 58% of AD patients. In contrast, in the placebo group only 36% showed improvement. However, more recent studies show that a higher dosage produces better results in AD. For example, in one double-blind study, 210 individuals with AD were randomized to receive placebo or Huperzine A (200 mcg or 400 mcg twice daily), for at least 16 weeks. Huperzine A 200 mcg twice daily did not produce any change in the Alzheimer's Disease Assessment Scale-cognitive subscale (ADAS-Cog), but Huperzine A at 400 mcg twice daily showed a 2.27-point improvement in ADAS-Cog at 11 weeks vs 0.29-point decline in the placebo group and a 1.92-point improvement vs 0.34-point improvement in the placebo arm at week 16. Hence, the recommended dosage for people with AD is now 400 mcg twice daily while the dosage of 200 mcg twice daily is used for MCI.

While Huperzine A is well-tolerated, side effects have been noted at the higher dosage level including hyperactivity, nasal obstruction, nausea, vomiting, diarrhea, insomnia, anxiety, dizziness, thirst, and constipation. One trial reported abnormalities in electrocardiogram (ECG) patterns (cardiac ischemia and arrhythmia). The bottom line is that at the high dosage level of 400 mcg twice daily, physician supervision is recommended.

The Gingipain Theory of Alzheimer's Disease

O.K. let me throw an interesting wrinkle in the Alzheimer's disease discussion. One of the most interesting and a real plausible theory on a key underlying cause of AD is the link between AD and gum disease. It looks like beta-amyloid seems to function as a sticky defense mechanism against bacterial infection in the brain. Researchers have found when they inject bacteria into the brains of mice the characteristic plaques of AD developed overnight. Human data show that 96% of patients with AD have in the key area of the brain in AD (the hippocampus) the presence of enzymes known as gingipains from the main bacteria involved in gum disease, *Porphyromonas gingivalis*. They have also found genetic material from *P. gingivalis* in the cerebral cortex—a region involved in conceptual thinking. Animal studies have shown conclusively that *P. gingivalis* gum disease leads to brain infection, amyloid production, tangles of tau protein and neural damage in the regions and nerves normally affected by AD. That is fairly conclusive evidence. How does *P. gingivalis* get in the brain? When dental plaque builds under the edge of your gums, it can form inflamed pockets in which *P. gingivalis* can thrive and release toxins and gingipains that can damage the lining of your gums and make it possible for *P. gingivalis* and other oral bacteria to enter the bloodstream and then the brain. Once in the brain, *P. gingivalis* will trigger the release of beta-amyloid. It is the brain's method of trying to contain the infection. In addition, it turns out the gingipains released by *P. gingivalis* break up the ApoE protein (see above) into fragments that can harm brain cells. The ApoE4 variant of this protein linked to AD contains more of the damaging fragments and explains why people with this variant are at a higher risk of developing AD.

Here is the bottom line from all of this research. Dental hygiene, proper immune function, and nutrition are all required to prevent gum and periodontal disease. Those same practices may also help prevent the development of AD.

Nature's Red Miracle

A vibrantly deep pigment known as astaxanthin may hold the key to living younger and longer as well as fighting off AD. Astaxanthin is available as a dietary supplement as well as being responsible for the color of sea animals having red or pink flesh, or outer shells. It is a member of the carotenoid family of pigments and has been crowned its "King" because of its unique benefits and actions in promoting health and protecting against cellular damage, especially in the brain, skin, and vascular system.

Although astaxanthin is found in some fish or krill oil supplements, the amounts in these sources are much lower than those provided from extracts of the microalgae *Haematococcus pluvialis*. For example, the level of astaxanthin naturally occurring in a capsule of fish or krill oil is in the range of 100 mcg (0.1 mg). That amount is not much compared to the 4 to 12 mg per capsule found in most astaxanthin supplements derived from *H. pluvialis*. This distinction is important based upon a growing body of scientific studies.

Among antioxidants that help prevents the cellular damage that contributes to not only AD, but also aging, cardiovascular disease, and cancer, astaxanthin is quite unique. First, astaxanthin is more than 65 times stronger than vitamin C and 50 times more powerful than beta-carotene. Second, one of the unique aspects of astaxanthin relates to its size and how it can span the entire thickness of the protective membrane that surrounds cells throughout the body. This size allows astaxanthin to protect both the outside and inside of the cell membrane against cellular damage.

One of the real special attributes of astaxanthin is its ability to cross the barrier that protects the brain from harmful compounds. This effect is quite unusual for carotenes. For example, popular carotenes like beta-carotene and lycopene do not cross either barrier. This ability of astaxanthin to cross the blood-brain barrier indicates that it may be particularly helpful in improving brain and eye health as well as protecting the brain against Alzheimer's disease, macular degeneration, and other degenerative disorders.

Astaxanthin also exerts some specific anti-inflammatory effects that make it quite useful in fighting many health conditions, but perhaps the most significant effect of astaxanthin may turn out to be its to protect the membrane system of mitochondria (the energy compartment of cells). By protecting the mitochondria from damage, astaxanthin can help boost cellular energy production. This effect has far reaching potential in improving many health conditions. After all, when a cell has more energy, it simply functions better. The energy boosting effects of astaxanthin has already been shown good use in improving muscle endurance as well as reducing eye fatigue.

There are now over 50 clinical and experimental studies that have shown astaxanthin to be helpful in the following conditions:

- *Brain Health.* Helps protect against aging and helps improve mental function.

- *Cardiovascular Health.* Protects vascular lining, promotes improved blood flow, and protects LDL cholesterol from becoming oxidized (damaged).
- *Eye Health.* Protects against eye fatigue, helps improve visual acuity and depth perception, and increases blood flow to eye tissues.
- *Sports Related Activities.* Promotes muscle endurance and protects against muscle damage.
- *Diabetes, insulin-resistance, and the metabolic syndrome.* Helps improve antioxidant status and protect against vascular damage.
- *Skin Health.* Reduces fine lines and wrinkles, improves skin elasticity, protects against sun damage, and prevents age spots and hyperpigmentation.
- *Immune health.* Protects against damage to immune cells.

The typical dosage recommendation for astaxanthin is 4 to 12 mg per day. Be sure to make sure the astaxanthin is produced from the *H. pluvialis* algae. It is the best source and significantly more beneficial than the synthetic form.

Case History: A New Passion for Living

My patients Mildred and George are a very interesting pair. When I first met them, they were bored with life. In their late seventies, they both felt they had nothing to live for. They were both in good health, especially for their age (I think the fact that they were on a very extensive nutritional and herbal supplement program was a big reason). They simply were consulting me to make sure that they were on the right track with their supplements. I made a few minor adjustments in their regimen. But my main "prescription" was for them to start off each day by discussing three memories from the past, three things they were grateful for, and three things they wanted to accomplish or learn more about in in the day.

The transformation was incredible. The laughter, joy, and passion for living was infectious the moment they entered into clinic—I could hear them and my receptionist laughing while I was still in my office down the hall. What happened, I asked? They told me that the little exercise that I prescribed reminded them of how thankful they are to still be here. It made them reconnect to all of the good things in life again. And, they felt "productive."

Key Considerations in Parkinson's Disease

Parkinson's disease results from damage to the nerves in the area of the brain that is responsible for controlling muscle tension and movement - the basal ganglia. The damaged cells are the ones needed to produce the neurotransmitter called dopamine. The disease usually begins as a slight tremor of one hand, arm, or leg. In the early stages the tremors are more apparent while the person is at rest, such as while sitting or standing, and are less noticeable when the hand or limb is being used. A typical early symptom of Parkinson's disease is "pill-rolling," in which the person appears to be rolling a pill back and forth between the fingers. As the disease progresses, symptoms often get worse. The tremors and weakness affect the limbs on both sides of the body. The hands and the head may shake continuously. The person may walk with stiff, shuffling steps. In many cases, the disease causes a permanent rigid stooped posture and an unblinking, fixed expression.

At this point in time, Parkinson's disease is best treated with drug therapy along with key dietary, nutritional, and herbal recommendations that can be used to address the underlying disease process and/or enhance the effectiveness of drug therapy.

The most popular drug used in PD is Sinemet® - a drug that contains two key ingredients: levodopa and carbidopa. Levodopa, or L-dopa, is the "middle step" in the conversion of the amino acid tyrosine into dopamine. L-dopa, but not dopamine (DA), crosses the blood-brain barrier. Carbidopa is a drug that works by ensuring that more L-dopa is converted to dopamine within the brain, where it is needed, and not within the other tissues of the body. Other drugs used include Eldepryl (selegiline or deprenyl), bromocriptine, and amantadine.

Unfortunately, although effective in the early stages of the disease in providing relief of symptoms, drug therapy does not stop the disease progression and it loses efficacy with time. Hence, the importance of the natural approach to try to make the drugs work longer as well as reduce common side effects. For example, simply eating a low protein diet can enhance the action of L-dopa therapy and is now a well-accepted supportive therapy. The usual recommendation is to eliminate good sources of dietary protein from breakfast and lunch while eating a typical dinner so that total daily protein intake is less than 50 g/day for men and 40 g/day for women. This simple dietary practice can offer an effective method for the reduction of tremors and other symptoms of Parkinson's disease during waking hours. Since L-dopa absorption is delayed or diminished by amino acids in protein meals, it is recommended that patients on L-dopa take their medication with a low protein meal.

Antioxidant Support in Parkinson's Disease

Given the abundance of data suggesting an excessive free radical burden contributes to PD, it is logical to consider that increasing antioxidant intake may offer some therapeutic benefit. Unfortunately, the research that exists on this line of therapy has focused on a rather limited number of antioxidant nutrients and the results have been rather disappointing. High dosages of vitamin E and C do not seem to impact PD.

Population-based studies have mostly indicated that high dietary intakes of antioxidant nutrients, especially vitamin E, may prevent Parkinson's disease.[1] The results from these preliminary studies led to a trial of high-dose vitamins C and E in early Parkinson's disease as well as a large study of high-dose vitamin E and the drug selegiline.

In the double-blind study in patients with early Parkinson's disease given 3,000 mg of vitamin C and 3,200 IU of vitamin E each day for a period of seven years, the supplement group fared better than the placebo group. Although all patients eventually required drug treatment, the patients receiving the vitamins were effectively able to delay the need for medication for up to 2 to 3 years longer. These results were quite promising, but a 10-year study with vitamin E only at a daily intake of 2,000 IU failed to show any real benefit in slowing or improving the disease. It is likely that a combination of nutrients and a very broad antioxidant supplement program may be required in order to see any significant benefit in preventing the progression of PD.

The combination of PQQ and CoQ10 discussed above is definitely indicated. PQQ especially has been shown to block some of the key triggers of PD in animal studies while CoQ10 has shown mixed effects in human clinical trials. For example, in one trial of CoQ10 supplementation, progression of PD was reduced by 44%, but in two other studies, a highly absorbable form of CoQ10 at a dosage of 100 mg three times daily produced no effect on PD symptoms. My thought is that CoQ10 may need adequate levels of PQQ to be effective. There have been no human studies with the PQQ+CoQ10 combination, but given the results in preclinical studies, safety, and *possible* benefit, I recommend it. I would also recommend the other supplements for MCI given above plus one other; a product called Enada.

Enada contains stabilized niacinamide adenine dinucleotide (NADH) - the activated form of vitamin B3 (niacin). NADH is required by the brain to make various neurotransmitters and to produce chemical energy. Human studies indicate that NADH is effective in raising the level of dopamine within the brain making it useful in Parkinson's disease. NADH supplementation with Enada™ has been shown to produce significant benefits in reducing symptoms as well as improving brain function in two clinical studies in PD patients. The dosage is 5 to 20 mg per day.

There is also an interesting botanical approach to PD: *Mucuna puriens* (velvet bean). The seed powder of the velvet bean has long been used in traditional Ayurvedic medicine for diseases including PD. It is a rich natural source of L-dopa, but other components also contribute to its medicinal actions. An extract of velvet bean was studied in sixty patients with Parkinson's disease (26 patients were taking Sinemet® before treatment with the extract and the remaining 34 were not taking any medication). Statistically significant reductions in symptom scores were seen from the beginning to the end of the 12-week study. The amount used in the study 7.5 grams of the extract dissolved in water three to six times daily. In another study, compared with Sinemet®, the 30 g velvet bean preparation led to a considerably faster onset of effect (34.6 v 68.5 minutes), reflected in shorter times to peak L-dopa concentrations in the blood, and fewer side effects. The researchers felt that the velvet bean might possess advantages over conventional L-dopa preparations.

Fava bean *(Vicia faba)* or broad bean is also a source of L-dopa. Anecdotal cases of symptomatic improvement after broad bean consumption have been described in patients with Parkinson's disease since 1913. In one clinical small study, 250 grams of cooked broad beans produced a substantial increase in L-dopa blood levels, which correlated with a substantial improvement in motor performance in PD patients. Individuals on medications like Sinemet* and L-dopa should be aware that broad bean consumption may increase L-dopa levels too high.

Key Recommendations for Eye Health

As we age, it's common to experience changes in vision. But while some changes are just a nuisance, others can cause serious impairment of vision. The good news is that nutrition plays an enormous role in the prevention and treatment of the leading causes of impaired vision in North America. And that means targeted supplements can help us maintain eye health, prevent eye diseases like cataracts and macular degeneration, and improve visual function when these conditions develop.

Packing your diet with richly colored fruits and vegetables is one of the best ways to lower your risk for cataracts and macular degeneration. Initially it was thought that this protection was the result of increased intake of antioxidant vitamins and minerals. However, we now know that various "non-essential" food components—lutein, zeaxanthin, lycopene, and flavonoids, among others—are even more important for eye health than traditional antioxidants like vitamins C and E or selenium.

In addition to a colorful diet, be sure to incorporate these six essential nutritional components that will keep your vision front and center.

Lutein and zeaxanthin

The carotenes lutein and zeaxanthin are critically important to the health of the macula. The macula is the part of the eye needed for sharp, central vision. It's what lets us see things that are straight ahead of us. Lutein and zeaxanthin help prevent oxidative damage, thereby protecting against macular degeneration.

Low levels of lutein and zeaxanthin within the macula represent a major risk factor for the disease. In fact, people with macular degeneration have 35 to 40 percent less lutein in their maculas than people without macular degeneration. In addition, new research shows that supplementing with lutein and zeaxanthin not only helps prevent macular degeneration, it can actually improve visual function in people who already have it. Specifically, in subjects with macular degeneration, 10 to 15 mg of lutein daily improves glare recovery, contrast sensitivity, and visual acuity.

Lutein is also important in preventing cataracts and improving visual function in people with existing cataracts. Like the macula, the human lens concentrates lutein and zeaxanthin. In fact, these are the only carotenes found in the human lens. Seven large studies have shown that the higher lutein intake is associated with decreased likelihood of needing cataract surgery. In addition, protecting against developing cataracts, lutein can also help improve visual function in people who have them.

Table 9.1 - Top 20 Plant Sources of Lutein, Zeaxanthin, and Lycopene

Corn
Kiwi fruit
Red grapes
Squash (zucchini, pumpkin, butternut, etc.)
Bell peppers (red>orange>green>yellow)
Greens (spinach, kale, chard, etc.)
Cucumber
Peas
Honeydew melon
Celery
Green grapes
Brussels sprouts

Scallions
Green beans
Orange
Broccoli
Apple
Mango
Peach
Tomato paste or juice

Flavonoid-rich extracts

Flavonoid-rich extracts of blueberry, bilberry, pine bark, or grape seed also offer valuable benefits in improving eye health, as well as protecting against cataracts and macular degeneration. Beyond their powerful antioxidant activity, these extracts have also been shown to exert positive effects on improving blood flow to the retina. They also improve visual processes—especially night vision. A daily dose of 150 to 300 mg of one of these flavonoid-rich extracts will support eye health.

Nutritional antioxidants

Nutritional antioxidants like beta-carotene, vitamins C and E, zinc, copper, and selenium are extremely important for eye health. While research has often focused on just one of these nutrients, studies conducted by the Age-Related Eye Disease Study Research Group (AREDS) confirm that these nutrients function better together than they do apart. Yet even something as simple as taking vitamin C or zinc can produce dramatic effects in preserving eye health. For example, several studies have demonstrated that vitamin C supplementation can prevent cataract formation, halt progression and, in some cases, significantly improve vision. One study conducted back in 1939 demonstrated that use of vitamin C supplements for 10 years or more was associated with a 77 percent lower rate of cataract formation. These results are astounding when you consider that cataracts are a source of a tremendous financial burden on our society. Cataract surgery is the most common major surgical procedure done in the United States each year for people on Medicare.

Zinc is perhaps the most important mineral for eye health. It plays an essential role in the retina's metabolism and the visual process. An early study in 1971 showed that in more than 90 percent of cataract cases, levels of zinc are very low. Zinc is also involved in protecting against macular degeneration. A two-year double-blind, placebo-controlled trial involving 151 subjects demonstrated that the group taking a zinc supplement had significantly less visual loss than the placebo group. Be sure to get 20 to 30 mg of zinc per day from your multiple vitamin and mineral formula.

Coenzyme Q10 (CoQ10) and Acetyl-L-carnitine

These two nutrients play a critical role in energy production. CoQ10 is to our cells what a spark plug is to a car engine. Acetyl-L-carnitine functions as the fuel injection system. Just as the car cannot function without that initial spark, cells in our body cannot function properly without CoQ10 and carnitine. CoQ10 and carnitine perform their functions primarily in the mitochondria—the cell's energy producing compartment.

Although the body makes some of its own CoQ10 and carnitine, research shows significant benefits with supplementation, particularly in patients with heart disease or those taking cholesterol-lowering drugs. In terms of eye health, the mitochondria within the retina are especially vulnerable to toxic byproducts of cell metabolism. That makes supplementation with acetyl-L-carnitine (a highly absorbable form of carnitine) and CoQ10 especially important. In one double-blind study, the combination of acetyl-L-carnitine (200 mg), omega-3 fatty acids (EPA 460 mg/DHA 320 mg), and CoQ10 (20 mg) was shown to improve visual function and macular alterations in the early stages of macular degeneration. In addition, it stopped the disease from progressing in 47 out of 48 cases.

Omega-3 Fatty Acids

Hardening of the arteries (atherosclerosis) is strongly associated with eye health. Just as in atherosclerosis, omega-3 fatty acids from fish oils play an important role in the prevention of eye conditions like macular degeneration. The recommended dosage of a fish oil supplement to support eye health is enough to provide approximately 1,000 mg of EPA+DHA—the two important omega-3 fatty acids.

NOTE: If you have any signs of visual impairment, you absolutely must be properly evaluated by a physician. I recommend is that you get a baseline eye exam and then follow the program for a minimum of six months before getting retested. Success is achieved if the condition has not worsened or if there are signs of improvement.

Fish Oils for Dry Eye Syndrome

Dry eye syndrome is a very common eye symptom as we age. Dry eyes happen either when you produce fewer tears, or when your tear film evaporates too quickly. As with many other vision problems, it becomes more common the older we get. In fact, approximately one in three people over 70 suffer from it.

Inflammation plays a central role in dry eye syndrome. Since fish oil supplementation have been shown to reduce inflammation, researchers began considering them as a treatment for dry eyes. And the research looks promising. For example, in a study published in the *International Journal of Ophthalmology*, 264 patients with dry eye were randomized to receive either 1,000 mg EPA+DHA (650 mg EPA and 350 mg DHA) daily or a placebo for three months. They were evaluated at several points throughout the study to look for improved tear production and signs of inflammation in the lining of the eyes.

The result? More than half–65 percent–of patients in the EPA+DHA group had significant improvement in their symptoms at 3 months. That's compared to only 33 percent of patients in placebo group. The improvement in symptoms was largely a result of reduced tear evaporation. It appears that EPA+DHA help retain the water content of the lining of the eye.

Typically, taking 1,000 mg EPA+DHA is an adequate dose, but that's just for general health promotion. When there is greater need or when used therapeutically, the recommended level is 2,000-3,000 mg per day. While the results from this study are excellent, my feeling is that they would have occurred faster and been even more impressive if a higher EPA+DHA dosage had been used.

Longevity Matrix Lifestyle Tune-Up #9–Focus on Dietary Variety and Spice/Herb it Up

People who eat a variety of different foods in their diets have a lower rate of obesity than people who consume pretty much the same foods day in and day out. This may be the result of the beneficial changes on the microbiome. Thinner people tend to have greater microbial diversity than those that are obese. The biggest determinate of microbiome diversity is dietary diversity.

Most Americans eat a very limited range of foods and consume a very monotonous diet as a result. It seems entirely possible that excessive calorie and food consumption in many people may be some sort of physiological craving gone awry. In other words, perhaps the brain is seeking to help improve nutritional intake by sending signals to eat, but somehow it is just causing excessive cravings for additional calories in general instead of giving the brain the specific nutrients it needs to feel satisfied.

Maybe the brain is requiring a greater variety of foods, but the message that gets relayed is to simply eat more of the same foods. So, the brain is constantly hungry. Despite this obvious possibility, there is not a lot of research in this area. There are numerous case histories in the medical literature of people having specific food cravings indicating some sort of physiological basis. For example, the eating of dirt or chewing ice cubes is often an indication of iron deficiency. Research done by the U.S. Army showed that when well-nourished men were placed on monotonous diets, it led to increased food craving for foods that were not provided in their monotonous diet. But there is little research into whether individuals who habitually consumed a monotonous diet are more likely to consume more calories than those consuming a more varied diet.

A study from researchers at the Harvard School of Public Health and NYU School of Medicine provides some evidence that dietary variety may help prevent obesity. To evaluate the role of food variety on body weight, researchers evaluated dietary data from the National Health and Nutrition Examination Survey (NHANES) 2003-2006 of over 7,000 men and non-pregnant, non-lactating women aged ≥20 years old. The subjects were dividing into groups 1 through 5 with the higher number reflecting greater dietary variety. Both men and women in the group with the greatest degree of dietary variety had a roughly 50% reduced risk for being obese. These results indicate that greater dietary variety is inversely associated with obesity in both sexes, indicating that greater healthful food variety may protect against excess body weight. This study explicitly recognizes the potential benefits of dietary variety in obesity management and provides the foundation to support its ongoing evaluation.

The bottom line is that I am a big proponent of eating a wide variety of health promoting foods. My reasons are that I appreciate the important role that eating a broad range of food components play in promoting human health. In particular, the importance of the long list of phytochemicals in fruits, vegetables, legumes, nuts, seeds, and other plant foods. We need variety in our diet to make sure we are getting the full spectrum of protection. Plus, I also think that a varied diet makes our food choices more interesting and less boring. Eating the same foods and menus over and over is a sure path to food boredom. Dietary variety wakes up the senses and makes eating more interesting and fun.

One of the great ways to add more variety to your diet and also pump up AMPk activity is the liberal use of herbs and spices. Some combinations of foods with herbs and spices are more appealing than others. Here are some pairings that can be used as a starting point. Again, my main goals here are to get you eating a greater variety of health promoting foods and also get in the habit of liberally adding herbs and spices to your foods.

Table 9.2–Matching Vegetables and Starches with Herbs and Spices

Asparagus

Chives	*Lemon Balm*
Pepper, black	*Sage*
Tarragon	*Thyme*

Beans, rice, and other grains

Cumin	*Garlic*
Mints	*Mustard seed*
Onions	*Oregano*
Horseradish	*Parsley*
Pepper, black	*Saffron*
Sage	*Thyme*
Turmeric	

Broccoli

Basil	*Dill*
Garlic	*Oregano*
Pepper, black	*Tarragon*
Thyme	*Turmeric*

Cabbage

Basil	*Cayenne (Red) pepper*
Cumin	*Dill*
Marjoram	*Mustard seed*
Pepper, black	*Sage*

Carrots

Anise	*Basil*
Chives	*Cinnamon*
Cloves	*Cumin*

Dill

Ginger

Marjoram

Mints

Mustard seed

Nutmeg

Parsley

Pepper, black

Sage

Tarragon

Thyme

Turmeric

Corn

Chives

Pepper, black

Saffron

Sage

Thyme

Eggplant

Basil

Cinnamon

Dill

Garlic

Marjoram

Mints

Mustard seed

Onions

Oregano

Parsley

Pepper, black

Sage

Thyme

Peas

Chives

Pepper, black

Rosemary

Tarragon

Thyme

Turmeric

Potatoes

Basil

Cayenne (Red) pepper

Chives

Coriander

Dill

Horseradish

Mustard seed

Oregano

Parsley

Pepper, black

Rosemary

Sage

Tarragon

Thyme

Turmeric

Pumpkin and Winter Squash

Basil	*Cardamom*
Cinnamon	*Cloves*
Ginger	*Marjoram*
Nutmeg	*Pepper, black*
Rosemary	*Sage*
Turmeric	

Spinach

Anise	*Basil*
Chives	*Cinnamon*
Dill	*Mustard seed*
Pepper, black	*Rosemary*
Thyme	*Turmeric*

Tomatoes

Basil	*Chives*
Coriander	*Dill*
Garlic	*Marjoram*
Oregano	*Parsley*
Pepper, black	*Rosemary*
Sage	*Tarragon*
Thyme	*Turmeric*

CHAPTER 10:

Strengthening Bones, Joints, and Muscles

We are designed to live an active, physical life thanks to our strong, sturdy, and flexible musculoskeletal system. However, the old adage, "use it or lose it," definitely applies in order to keep these structures young and functional. If we become inactive as we age, the bones weaken, and muscles lose strength. Making matters worse is that our joints are a common source of pain and inflammation. So, it becomes a bit of a vicious cycle as the more capacity they lose or pain we experience because of the inflammation, the more inactive we become. It doesn't have to be that way. There's a lot you can do to tune up and support your bones and muscles so that they'll serve you well no matter how long you live. Doing so takes commitment. But the payoffs are worth it: Greater strength, more stamina, increased flexibility, freedom from pain.

The Bones

Bones are not merely inert structures, like the beams or pillars of your house. They are dynamic living organs that require nurture and care. Your bones have several functions. They support the body and protect the soft organs inside. They permit movement, allowing us to walk, lift, and breathe. Bones also serve as a reservoir for minerals, especially calcium and phosphate, as well as magnesium and manganese. Like a kind of bank, bones allow us to deposit supplies of minerals and withdraw them later when the body needs them. Finally, and equally important, bone tissue is where most of our red and white blood cells are born.

Throughout your life, bones constantly remodeling. Each week you recycle up to seven percent of your bone mass. Normally, the rate of buildup and breakdown is the same. However, if the amount of bone lost exceeds the amount replaced, the bones become brittle and full of holes. This condition is called osteoporosis, or "porous bones." If we lack calcium or vitamin D, a condition called osteomalacia or "soft bones" can develop leading the bones to become weak and deformed.

Bone remodeling is controlled in part by chemical factors like hormones; vitamins like D, K, and B complex; minerals, not only calcium, but also magnesium, zinc, boron, etc.; stimulates the bones to absorb calcium. Other forces that trigger bone remodeling include stress and gravity. That's why weight-bearing exercise, such as running or weight training, promotes stronger bones.

The biggest threat to bone health is osteoporosis, a condition in which the bones lose both their supportive tissue (collagen matrix) and mineral content. Beginning in young adulthood, around age twenty-five, the bones become less efficient at absorbing and holding onto minerals. Normally, after the age of forty, there is a significant decrease in bone mass. The bones become less dense and less flexible, increasing the risk of fracture. Just about any bone in the skeleton can be affected, but bone loss is usually greatest in the hips, spine, and ribs. For women, menopause accelerates this process. By the age of seventy, women may lose up to fifty percent of their original bone mass and men can lose twenty-five percent. (Women have about thirty percent less bone mass to begin with.)

Osteoporosis leads to diminished bone strength, which then leads to an increased risk of fracture. Osteoporosis is now determined primarily by bone mineral density (BMD) testing and is defined by BMD scores less than or equal to -2.5 standard deviations below normal at the total hip, femoral neck, or lumbar spine.

Osteoporosis most commonly occurs in postmenopausal women, and the risk increases with age. Men are not immune to osteoporosis, though the risk is only about 25% compared to women. The prevalence of osteoporosis 4% in women between 50 and 59 years of age and rises to 52% in women age 80 and above. The big consequence of osteoporosis is fractures. It is estimated that osteoporosis causes approximately 1.5 million fractures every year. Of these, 250,000 are fractures of the hip. Even with considerable advances in medical care, up to 20% of women with hip fractures still die within a year of the fracture, and an additional 25% require long-term nursing care. Approximately half the women who suffer from a hip fracture are unable to walk without assistance.

The hip is not the only site where fractures result in serious consequences. Fractures of the spine bones (vertebral fractures) occur in a woman's mid-70s and cause significant pain as well as loss of height loss and an exaggerated kyphosis (hunchback) deformity. In addition to pain, restricted range of motion, changes in posture, restricted lung function, and digestive problems can all be caused by vertebral fractures of the thoracic or lumbar region or both. Once a vertebral fracture has occurred, there is at least a five- to sevenfold increase in the risk of additional vertebral fractures.

Nonetheless, hip fractures in men account for one third of all hip fractures and have a higher mortality than those in women. In addition, men break a hip suffer worse outcomes.

Osteoporosis affects more than twenty million people in the United States. Both men and women are at risk, but the risk for women is at least four times higher. That's partly due to the fact that during menopause their bodies no longer produce much estrogen and progesterone, hormones involved in maintaining bone mass.

Table 10.1 - Major Risk Factors for Osteoporosis in Women

- Family history of osteoporosis
- Gastric or small-bowel resection
- Heavy alcohol use
- Hyperparathyroidism
- Hyperthyroidism
- Inactivity
- Leanness
- Long-term corticosteroid therapy
- Long-term use of anticonvulsants
- Low calcium intake
- Nulliparity (never having been pregnant)
- Postmenopause
- Premature menopause (menopause before the age of 40)
- Short stature and small bones
- Smoking
- White or Asian race

Assessing Your Risk for Osteoporosis

Choose the item in each category that best describes you and fill in the point value for that item in the space to the right. In categories marked with an asterisk (*), you may choose more than one item.

Frame Size	Points
Small bones or petite	10
Medium frame, very lean	5
Medium frame, average or heavy build	0
Large frame, very lean	5
Large frame, heavy build	0
Score	_____

Ethnic Background

Caucasian	10
Asian	10
Other	0

Score_____

Activity Level

How often do you walk briskly, jog, engage in aerobics/sports, or perform hard physical labor, for at least 30 continuous minutes?

Seldom	30
1-2 times per week	20
3-4 times per week	5
5 or more times per week	0

Score_____

Smoking

Smoke 10 or more cigarettes a day	20
Smoke fewer than 10 cigarettes a day	10
Quit smoking	5
Never smoked	0

Score_____

Personal Health Factors*

Family history of osteoporosis	20
Longterm corticosteroid use	20
Longterm anticonvulsant use	20
Drink more than 3 glasses of alcohol each week	20
Drink more than 1 cup of coffee per day	10
Seldom get outside in the sunlight	10

Score_____

For women only:

Had ovaries removed	10
Premature menopause	10
Had no children	10

Score_____

Dietary Factors

Consume more than 4 oz. of meat on a daily basis	20
Drink soft drinks regularly	20
Consume the equivalent of 35 servings of vegetables each day	10
Consume at least 1 cup of green leafy vegetables each day	10
Take 1,000 mg of supplemental calcium	10
Consume a vegetarian diet	10

Score_____

Total Score_____

Interpretation

If your score is greater than 50, you are at significant risk for osteoporosis. However, you can reduce your score significantly by taking steps to reduce or eliminate risk factors. Start an exercise program; quit smoking; do not drink alcohol, coffee, or soft drinks (these leech calcium from the bones); take a good calcium supplement; and consume a diet low in protein and high in vegetables. These changes could take as many as 150 points off your total score.

If you are a woman, hormone replacement therapy may be appropriate for you, especially if you experienced an early menopause, had your ovaries surgically removed, or never had children. Both estrogen and progesterone have been shown to protect against bone loss. In women with established bone loss, these hormones may actually increase bone mass. I recommend bioidentical hormone replacement (discussed below).

In my opinion, for women who are at risk of osteoporosis or who have already experienced significant bone loss, the benefits of hormone therapy outweigh the risks. Those risks can be reduced by using bioidentical hormones (discussed below). The exception is in women at high risk for breast cancer or women with a disease aggravated by estrogen, such as active liver diseases or certain cardiovascular diseases. In these cases, a more natural approach is a better choice. This may involve using black cohosh extract, the most widely used herbal approach to menopausal symptoms.

Typically, black cohosh (*Cimicifuga racemosa*) extract is standardized for 27-deoxyacteine with a dosage based upon this compound of 2 mg twice daily. Clinical studies have shown that black cohosh relieves hot flashes as well as depression, night sweats, and vaginal atrophy. In fact, black cohosh has been shown to produce symptomatic relief comparable to that of hormone replacement therapy without the risk of serious side effects. Black cohosh offers a suitable natural alternative to HRT for menopause, especially where hormones are contraindicated, such as in women with a history of breast cancer, unexplained uterine bleeding, liver and gallbladder disease, pancreatitis, endometriosis, uterine fibroids or fibrocystic breast disease.

Magnesium supplementation is also very important during menopause as it can help improve blood vessel tone. Low magnesium levels are thought to contribute to the development of hot flashes by making blood vessels more sensitive to hormonal changes. By supplementing magnesium these blood vessels become more stable thereby eliminating the hot flash. Use the citrate form for best results and take 150 to 250 mg three times daily. Also, be sure to take grape seed or pine bark extract at 300 mg per day. It can help as well.

Monitoring Bone Loss

I recommend that all women have a baseline bone density study by the age of forty. Of course, there is nothing wrong with getting a bone density test in your twenties, especially if you are at high risk. I use the test in men only if there is some factor that may predispose them to osteoporosis such as long-term use of prednisone or other corticosteroid.

The bone density test assesses how much bone mass you currently have. The test will tell you whether you need to make an even more serious effort to maintain your bone. Information from the test can be used in later years to measure the rate at which bone loss occurs. Of course, a bone density determination may also tell you that you already have osteoporosis.

There are several techniques to measure BMD, but the gold standard is dual energy x-ray absorptiometry (DEXA). Other methods of assessing bone mass include computerized tomography (CT) scans, ultrasounds of the heel, and radiographs, none of which are as optimal for diagnosis and follow-up as the DEXA scan.

In addition to providing the most reliable measurement of bone density, the DEXA test requires less radiation exposure than a conventional radiograph or CT scan. Usually, the DEXA scan is used to measure both the hip and the lumbar spine densities. The hip is the preferred site for BMD testing, especially in women older than 60, because the spinal measurements can be unreliable. Although peripheral DEXA sites are accurate, they may be less useful because they may not correlate as well with fracture risk and BMD at the hip and spine. The guidelines for indications for BMD testing established by many reputable and independent organizations are as follows:

- Secondary causes of bone loss (e.g., steroid use, hyperparathyroidism)
- Radiological (X-ray) evidence of osteopenia (insufficient bone mineral density)
- All women 65 years and older (not only for a diagnosis, but also as a historical reference point to compare to in the future)
- Younger postmenopausal women with fractures due to fragile bones since menopause, low body weight, or family history of spine or hip fracture

Results of BMD tests are reported as standard deviations—either a Z-score or a T-score. A Z-score is based on the standard deviation from the mean BMD of women in the same age group. A T-score is based on the mean peak BMD of a normal, young woman. The World Health Organization's (WHO) criteria for the diagnosis of osteoporosis uses T-scores. A T-score below -2.5 is associated with osteoporosis. The classification of osteopenia signifies a BMD that is between normal and osteoporosis. Keep in mind that using the T-score versus a Z-score increases the likelihood for the classification of osteopenia. After all it is normal to lose some bone mass with aging.

Table 10.2 - Bone Mineral Density Score Interpretation

Status	T-score	Interpretation
Normal	Above -1	BMD within 1 SD of a young normal adult
Osteopenia	Between -1 and -2.5	BMD between 1 and 2.5 SD below a young normal adult
Osteoporosis	Below -2.5	BMD is 2.5 SD or more below a young normal adult

BMD = Bone mineral density; SD = standard deviation.

Once you know your current bone density, the next step is to monitor how fast your bones are breaking down. The easiest way to do this is to measure the products of bone loss in the urine. The tests I recommend is the Osteomark-NTX. The Osteomark-NTX (also known as urinary cross-linked N-telopeptides of type I collagen) is available through your doctor. This test provides quicker feedback on your direction of bone loss compared with DEXA, which can take up to 2 years to detect a therapeutic response. I want to stress something here. If you are a woman who cares about her health, it is absolutely essential that you monitor your bone density status and bone turnover.

Bioidentical Hormone Replacement Therapy

Approaching and during menopause, as estrogen levels decline, bone breakdown outpaces bone formation. Both estrogen replacement therapy (ERT) and hormone replacement therapy (HRT—the combination of estrogen and progesterone) reduce the rate of bone turnover and resorption leading to reduce fracture rates in postmenopausal women. In trials of 2 years in length, the average increase in BMD after estrogen or estrogen/progestogen was 6.8% at the lumbar spine and 4.1% at the femoral neck. However, there are significant risks with conventional, so I recommend bioidentical hormone therapy.

The bioidentical hormones most commonly used in menopause include estradiol, estrone, estriol, progesterone, and to a lesser extent, testosterone. Bioidentical hormones are made from either beta-sitosterol extracted from soybeans or from diosgenin extracted from Mexican Wild Yam (*Dioscorea villosa*). These compounds are then processed to create hormones that are biochemically identical to the hormones produced in your body. Bioidentical hormones require a prescription and are available from regular pharmacies or as non-patented forms prepared by compounding pharmacies. If you feel you are a strong candidate for hormonal therapy for osteoporosis, I recommend working with a licensed naturopathic doctor or other progressive health care practitioner familiar with bioidentical hormone therapy.

EstroSense for Women on Hormone Therapy

EstroSense is a dietary supplement that I strongly recommend for women on hormone replacement therapy (HRT) as it can help to properly detoxify and eliminate excess estrogen. I think it may reduce some of the risk for breast cancer in women taking HRT. and environmental toxins that can disrupt hormonal balance. The formula contains compounds found in cabbage-family vegetables such as indole-3-carbinole (I3C), diindolylmethane (DIM), sulforaphane, and calcium-d-glucarate (CDG). Studies have shown that increasing the intake of cabbage family vegetables or taking these compounds as dietary supplements significantly increased the conversion of estrogen from cancer-producing forms to non-toxic breakdown products.

Adding 500 grams per day of broccoli to your diet or taking IC3 (400 mg daily) or DIM (150 to 200 mg daily) shifts the ratio from bad to good estrogen breakdown products as determined by measuring these compounds in the urine. Specifically, the ratio when the body breaks down estrogen to 16-alpha-hydroxyestrone, this compound acts as a breast tumor promoter while the byproduct resulting from a better route of breakdown of estrogen, 2-hydroxyestrone, does not stimulate breast cancer cells. In women taking HRT or at high-risk for breast cancer, I recommend taking two capsules of EstroSense twice daily or by taking either 400 mg of IC3 or 200 mg daily) as well as making sure to have at least 3 servings of cabbage family foods per week.

Supplemental I3C, DIM, and sulforaphane reduces 16a-hydroxyestrone (16-OHE), a form of estrogen linked to increased risk for breast cancer, while increasing a healthier form of excreted estrogen called 2-hydroxyestrone (2-OHE).

Since I3C lowers 16-OHE estrogen levels, a double-blind study was done to see if it helps women with cervical dysplasia, a precancerous condition of the cervix. The women received either placebo, 200 mg, or 400 mg oral I3C daily for 12 weeks. In both groups receiving I3C, half of the women experienced a complete remission of CIN. None of the patients in the placebo group experienced complete remission. No adverse effects were noted in this or previous studies with I3C.

A Quick Look at Bisphosphonates

The most widely prescribed drugs for osteoporosis—prevention and treatment—are the bisphosphonates including such drugs as:

- Alendronate (Fosamax, Fosamax Plus D)
- Etidronate (Didronel)
- Ibandronate (Boniva)
- Pamidronate (Aredia)
- Risedronate (Actonel, Actonel W/Calcium)
- Tiludronate (Skelid)
- Zoledronic acid (Reclast, Zometa)

These drugs are a huge $8 billion business, yet they are of marginal benefit at best and carry with them significant risks. The first bisphosphonate was Fosamax. It's launch coincided with the publishing of a Merck-funded study called the Fracture Intervention Trial. At first glance the claims made in Merck's advertisements for Fosamax were quite impressive. Merck claimed that Fosamax reduced the rate of hip fracture compared to a placebo by 50%, but if you take a closer look the numbers do not seem so rosy. First of all, the women in the study were high risk women who had a history of a fracture due to osteoporosis. Next, when you look at the absolute number of hip fractures that occurred during the four-year trial it gives tremendous perspective. Only two out of a hundred women in the placebo group had a hip fracture during the trial compared to one out of a hundred in the Fosamax group. In other words, 98 women out of a hundred in the Fosamax group would have fared just as well on a placebo. Nonetheless, in severely high-risk individuals bisphosphonate therapy may offer some benefits, but we believe that in time non-drug measures will be shown to be even more effective. In fact, examination of the clinical studies with diet, lifestyle measures, and proper supplementation it appears the natural approach may be far superior.

An important consideration is that in the Fracture Intervention Trial and many others, the women studied were at extremely high risk for a fracture. Such women are a small group compared to the tens of millions of women identified by the expanded bone density determinations. In fact, bisphosphonates are just as often prescribed for women with osteopenia (bone mineral density that is lower than normal, but not low enough to be classified as osteoporosis) as they are for osteoporosis even though neither bisphosphonates nor other drugs have shown effectiveness or are indicated in the treatment of osteopenia despite considerable efforts of the drug companies to convince the doctors otherwise. Instead of relying on a drug to reduce the risk of osteoporosis and hip fracture, the more rational approach would be to focus on diet, lifestyle, and supplement strategies.

Case History: Saving Karen's Bones

Karen, then forty-nine years old, came to see me because of side effects related to hormone replacement therapy (Premphase: 0.625 estrogens and 5 mg medroxyprogesterone) she was taking for menopausal symptoms. She was also concerned that a CT bone density study had demonstrated significant bone loss, even though the Premphase was supposed to protect her bones. She complained of weight gain (twelve pounds in the six months since she had been taking Premphase), breast tenderness, and mood instability. I had Karen undergo a baseline Osteomark-NTX, which confirmed that she was losing bone at a rapid rate. I recommended the following program:

- Discontinue Premphase
- A high-potency multiple vitamin and mineral supplement
- Additional calcium and magnesium
- Flaxseed oil: One tablespoon daily.
- Black cohosh extract (Remifemin): Two tablets twice daily with each tablet supplying 1 mg 27-deoxyacteine.

Ten weeks after she began my program, Karen came back for a follow-up bone density test. Her results dropped from 44 to 26 units, a highly significant improvement. Karen comes back for bone monitoring every six months. Her results are always below

24, and at one check-up she scored a reassuringly low 21. I attribute this drop primarily to the black cohosh extract because she was already taking a multiple and extra calcium.

Preventing bone loss

Changes in diet and lifestyle can help you tune up your bones and reduce your risk of osteoporosis. My recommendations are:

- Consume a diet rich in whole, unprocessed foods (whole grains, legumes, vegetables, fruits, nuts, and seeds).
- While consuming enough protein is important, you do not want to overdo it. Protein is a concern in osteoporosis because diets high in protein can accelerate bone loss. Proteins are high in nitrogen and phosphorus. To buffer against these compounds, the body tends to pull calcium from bone. Keep protein intake below 100 g daily.
- Increase consumption of soy foods. Soy contains plant substances, known as phytoestrogens, that acts like estrogen in the body. These include genistein and daidzein. These substances enhance the positive effects of calcitonin on calcium metabolism and appear to protect against osteoporosis.
- Eliminate the intake of alcohol, caffeine, and sugar. Intake of these substances speeds up the rate of calcium loss from the body.
- Do not drink sodas or other soft drinks. In addition to their high sugar content, soft drinks are a hazard because they contain phosphates that tend to pull calcium from the bones (see below).
- Get regular exercise. Weight-bearing exercise puts healthy stress on the bones; to cope with the increased load, the bones work to boost their mass. Muscle activity pulls on bones, which increases their strength and vitality. Exercise picks up the pace at which the cardiovascular system delivers nutrients and oxygen to bones and carries away waste. It's never too late to begin exercising. The sooner you start, the better the impact will be on your bones.

The Great Milk Debate

The main source of calcium in the American diet is dairy products, but it is debatable how effective milk is in strengthening bones. While numerous clinical studies have demonstrated that calcium supplementation can slow down bone loss, it is less certain that high dietary calcium intake from milk prevents osteoporosis and bone fractures. People in countries with the highest dairy intake have the highest rate of hip fractures per capita. Hip fractures most often occur as a result of osteoporosis.

In analyzing data from the Nurses' Health Study, a study involving 77,761 women, researchers found no evidence that higher intakes of milk actually reduced fracture incidence. In fact, women who drank two or more glasses of milk per day had forty-five percent increased risk for hip fracture compared to women consuming one glass or less per week. In other words, the more milk consumed, the more likely a woman would experience a hip fracture. On the whole, despite what the dairy industry tells us, research simply does not support the idea that "every body needs milk." How then, should you get the calcium you need? Studies support the notion that sources of calcium from plant foods may be much more protective than milk. Plant foods rich in calcium include tofu, kale, spinach, turnip greens, and other green leafy vegetables. These foods also contain vitamin K1, which helps a protein in the bone, called osteocalcin, to "join hands" with calcium atoms, thus holding the calcium more securely within the bone. Studies have found that the higher the level of vitamin K (particularly K2, discussed below), the lower the risk of osteoporosis and hip fracture. The bottom line is that if you want to have healthy bones, do what cows do—eat greens.

Vitamin K, Osteoporosis and the Calcium Paradox

As people get older, they often experience the "calcium paradox." This refers to there being a lack of calcium in the bone and an increase of calcium in arteries and other soft tissue. Hence, the misplaced calcium leads to an increase in both osteoporosis and atherosclerosis. Everyone is familiar with osteoporosis, but an excess of calcium in arteries shows a greatly increased risk of cardiovascular death. It is the basis of the "Coronary Artery Scan" and the cardiac calcium score. This non-invasive CT scan (computed tomography) of the heart calculates the risk of developing coronary artery disease (CAD) by measuring the amount of calcified plaque in the coronary arteries. Plaque or calcium build-up in the coronary arteries causes heart disease or can lead to a heart attack. The coronary calcium scan is a better predictor of coronary events than cholesterol screening or other risk factor assessments.

There is substantial evidence that lack of vitamin K as well as vitamin D3 and magnesium in the body is the cause of the calcium paradox. These nutrients are critical in the normal metabolism of calcium. Deficiency of any of these nutrients can lead to loss of calcium from the bone and an increase in the calcification of the vascular and organ systems, but the role of vitamin K really stands out.

Vitamin K was first identified in 1936 to be a key factor in blood clotting. When chickens were fed a low-fat diet, they exhibited significantly lower coagulation capacity, resulting in severe bleeding. The lipid fraction of diet was analyzed, and a novel antihemorrhagic factor was discovered. This identified compound was given the first letter in the alphabet available, which coincided with the first letter of the German word "Koagulation" and deemed to be only essential for its requirement for preventing hemorrhaging. There are two main forms of vitamin K designated as K1 and K2. The first form, K1 or phylloquinone is derived from plant sources. K2 or menaquinone is produced by bacteria and found in some fermented foods. There are several different forms of K2 based upon the number of molecules in its chain. MK-7 is the most important supplemental form of vitamin K2. It is about 10 times more biologically active than MK-4, another form of K2.

Vitamin K is often neglected as a vitamin because the conventional wisdom is that deficiency is thought to be quite rare because there are good dietary sources of K1, and human needs are also because gut bacteria can produce K2. But it appears that the majority of K2 produced from K1 is the MK-4 form. Humans also convert some of the K1 (around 5-20%

into MK-4, but the conversion is ineffective in many). It is possible that if our gut bacterial flora, the microbiome, contains a good amount of *Bacillus subtillus*, we may manufacture more MK7, but we may benefit from dietary intake of K2 in the form of MK-7 for optimal health.

Since 1961 vitamin K1 injection has been given to all newborn babies to prevent hemorrhagic disease of the newborn. This condition occurs because of a lack of vitamin K. When a baby is born the intestinal tract is sterile. Since a major source of vitamin K (in the form of K2) is synthesized from gut bacteria and most women do not have high concentrations of vitamin K1 in their breast milk, the baby must rely on the amount of vitamin K delivered through the placenta before birth until the gut microflora gets established.

It turns out that while K1 is important in blood clotting and can actually be recycled. However, it also turns out that gut bacteria do not appear to provide optimal levels of vitamin K2, particularly MK-7, and that vitamin K2 is not recycled. That is why, as studies have shown, humans can develop a K2 deficiency in as little as seven days on a vitamin K2–deficient diet, which is one major factor in why inadequate vitamin K2 levels are so common.

Table 10.3 - Vitamin K2 Levels in Selected Foods (mcg/100 g)

Food	Amount	% MK-7 or MK-4
Natto	1103.4	100% MK-7
Goose Liver	369.0	100% MK-4
Gouda	76.3	94% MK-7
Brie	56.5	93.5% MK-7
Egg Yolk (Netherlands)	32.1	98% MK-4
Goose Leg	31.0	100% MK-4
Egg Yolk (US)	15.5	100% MK-4
Butter	15.0	100% MK-4
Chicken Liver	14.1	100% MK-4

Chicken Breast	8.9	100% MK-4
Chicken Leg	8.5	100% MK-4
Ground Beef	8.1	100% MK-4
Bacon	5.6	100% MK-4
Calf Liver	5.0	100% MK-4
Sauerkraut	4.8	92% MK-7
Whole Milk	1.0	100% MK-4
Salmon	0.5	100% MK-4
Egg White	0.4	100% MK-4

Vitamin K1 is abundant in the membrane of the chloroplast, the part of a plant cell that captures sunlight for photosynthesis. Rich sources of vitamin K1 are dark green leafy vegetables, broccoli, lettuce, cabbage, spinach, and green tea. Good sources are asparagus, oats, whole wheat, and fresh green peas.

When like cows, chickens or pigs consume green, chlorophyll-containing plants, the ingested K1 is converted to K2. Grain-fed animals have little K2 in their tissues, as animals, particularly herbivores, accumulate vitamin K2 in their tissues in direct proportion to the amount of K1 in their diet. Keep in mind the form of K2 in animal foods is MK-4, which is less active that MK-7. The best source of MK-7 is natto, a fermented soy food popular in Japan. A three-ounce serving of natto provides over 1,000 mcg of MK-7.

The recommended dietary intake (RDI) for vitamin K is a very low 90 mcg/day for adults. One cup of cooked kale or spinach has more than then times this amount, but all as vitamin K1. Most people are deficient in K2 because they do not eat enough vitamin K1 containing foods. Eating large quantities of foods very high in K1 may even give people all of the K2 they need, including MK-7, but since not many people are eating natto and given the importance of vitamin K2 as MK-7 in bone health (and preventing soft tissue calcification), I think it is smart to take a MK-7 supplement at a dosage of 50 mcg for general health and 180 mcg for osteoporosis or when there is calcification of soft tissues (e.g., when a person has a high coronary artery calcium score).

As mentioned above, vitamin K is responsible for converting the bone protein osteocalcin from its inactive form to its active form. MK-7 is much more effective than K1 or MK-4 in this regard. Osteocalcin is the major non-collagen protein found in our bones that anchors calcium into place within the bone. Most of the double-blind clinical studies with vitamin K1 in osteoporosis have shown only modest or mainly no effect on bone density and while studies with MK-4 have shown positive results in reducing bone loss and fracture rates, the dosage used (45 mg/day) was well beyond a nutritional effect and more likely the positive results are due to a drug-like effect at such high dosages. MK-7 has been found to be more potent and more bioavailable as well as to last longer in the body than MK-4.

In a landmark major clinical published in the March 23, 2013 issue of Osteoporosis International, MK-7 supplementation at relatively low dosage levels (180 mcg per day) produced tremendous effects on improving bone health. In the study, 244 healthy postmenopausal women took either the MK-7 or a placebo for 3 years. Bone mineral density of lumbar spine, total hip, and femoral neck was measured by DXA; bone strength measures of the femoral neck were also calculated. Vertebral fracture assessment was performed by DXA and used as measure for vertebral fractures. Measurements occurred at baseline and after 1, 2, and 3 years of treatment.

MK-7 intake significantly improved vitamin K status and active osteocalcin levels and decreased the age-related decline in bone mineral concentration (BMC) and BMD at the lumbar spine and femoral neck. It did not increase either measure at the total hip. Bone strength was also favorably affected by MK-7—a key determinant of fracture risk. Lastly, MK-7 significantly decreased the loss in vertebral height of the lower thoracic region at the mid-site of the vertebrae. These results highlight the importance of MK-7 supplementation in post-menopausal women.

Vitamin K2 is also critical in activating a calcium binding protein in blood vessels and other soft tissues of the body known as matrix Gla-protein (MGP). The protein is manufactured as needed in these tissues to block against tissue calcification. Vitamin K2 is required to activate MGP in order for it to become the strongest inhibitor of tissue calcification presently known. It is regarded as the only effective mechanism for preventing calcification in blood vessels. In other words, when vitamin K2 is deficient, MGP is not activated and calcium is deposited in vascular plaque leading to calcification of the blood vessel.

> NOTE: If you are taking anticoagulant drugs like Coumadin, consult your physician before taking any supplement with vitamin K.

Calcium Supplements in Osteoporosis

Supplementation of calcium has become the primary focus in both the prevention and treatment of osteoporosis. In a detailed meta-analysis, 15 double-blind trials, representing 1806 participants, demonstrated that calcium supplementation was more effective than placebo in reducing rates of bone loss after two or more years of treatment, but the actual degree of reduction in bone loss is not all that impressive, e.g., the difference in the amount of bone loss between calcium and placebo was 2.05% for the total body, 1.66% for the lumbar spine, and 1.64% for the hip. The risk of fractures of the vertebrae dropped 21 and non-vertebral fractures was reduced 14%. Again, these results with calcium alone are not that impressive, but they do show some benefit.

Closer examination of the largest study, the Women's Health Initiative, which enrolled more than 36,000 postmenopausal women, showed an important discovery. While overall data showed that supplementation with 1,000 mg/day of calcium and 400 IU/day of vitamin D decreased the risk of hip fractures by 12% when compared with placebo, when the analysis was restricted to women who actually took the tablets at least 80% of the time, calcium plus vitamin D significantly decreased hip fractures by 29% compared with placebo. That is a significant amount difference. This discovery leads to the question, "Did some of these other studies have the results clouded because they did not determine the results in woman who actually took the supplements 80% of the time?"

One question that has been asked often in the research on calcium supplementation and osteoporosis is if there is a difference in the absorption and efficacy of one calcium source versus another. Here is another surprise discovery, the reality is that clinical studies looking at the effect of different forms of calcium against osteoporosis and hip fracture have not shown an advantage of any one form especially when either form is given along with vitamin D. While it is true that ionized forms like calcium citrate are better absorbed than calcium carbonate by approximately 22% to 27%, either on an empty stomach or with meals, this difference represents an increase in net absorption of only a relatively small amount of calcium (e.g., with a 500 mg dose the difference is likely only 15-25 mg of calcium). The difference in absorption is probably not meaningful. Furthermore, there are studies using different measure of calcium absorption that indicate that when taken with food, calcium from the insoluble salt (e.g., carbonate) is fully as absorbable as from a soluble salt (e.g., citrate).

Also, higher dosages of calcium do not produce greater results. In a two-year study, 214 perimenopausal women received either 1,000 or 2,000 mg of calcium. While the control group actually lost 3.2% of the bone density of their spine, the calcium-treated groups increased their density by 1.6% (there was no difference between the two calcium groups). These results show a slight benefit with calcium supplementation prior to menopause in a prevention strategy, but taking 1,000 mg was just as good as 2,000 mg. So, more is not going to produce a greater effect.

Here are my practical recommendations on calcium supplementation. First, I do caution against using oyster shell, bone meal, or hydroxyapatite forms of calcium. Studies have indicated that these calcium supplements may contain substantial amounts of lead. While I prefer easily ionized forms of calcium like calcium citrate, the reality is that if taken with meals even calcium carbonate is effectively absorbed in most people. I also like tricalcium phosphate for the following reasons:

- Tricalcium phosphate provides 3 molecules of calcium for every molecule of phosphorus making it a highly efficient source of both calcium and phosphorus.
- Clinical studies indicate that consuming calcium with phosphorus in the form of tricalcium phosphate is more effective at building strong bones than consuming calcium alone.
- Calcium cannot be utilized in the absence of phosphorus.
- Approximately 50% of North American women are deficient in phosphorus.
- Phosphorus is an essential component of bone, with 85% of the phosphorus in your body found in your bones.
- Clinical research indicates that calcium supplements without phosphorus may actually decrease the phosphorus available to the body for bone health thus contributing to osteoporosis.

While too much phosphorus is not a good thing, especially when it is not accompanied by calcium (as in soft drinks and animal meats), so too is not enough phosphorus especially in regard to the absorption of calcium.

Vitamin D in Osteoporosis

In addition to studies that utilized calcium supplementation alone, there have been several studies that used calcium in combination with vitamin D (usually vitamin D3) as well as vitamin D alone. One study using vitamin D3 alone found that supplementation with 700 IU/day will reduce the annual rate of hip fracture from 1.3 to 0.5%—nearly a 60% reduction. Studies that combined vitamin D with calcium produced slightly better results. For example, in one study of 3,270 elderly women living in nursing homes, the hip fracture rate in those receiving 1,200 mg/day of calcium and 800 IU/day of vitamin D3 was reduced by 43% compared with the placebo group.

The result from studies imply that while vitamin D3 alone can be helpful, especially in elderly people living in nursing homes, people living further away from the equator, and those who do not regularly get outside, it should be combined with calcium for maximum benefits on bone health. Also, I recommend a dosage of 2,000 to 5,000 IU of vitamin D3 rather than the lower dosages used in a lot of these studies.

Silicon and BioSil in Osteoporosis

During bone growth and the early phases of bone calcification, silicon has an essential role in the formation of cross-links between collagen and proteoglycans. In animals, silicon-deficient diets have produced abnormal skull development and growth retardation, and supplemental silicon partially prevented bone loss in female rats that had ovaries removed.

A highly bioavailable form of silica (choline stabilized orthosilicic acid, tradename: BioSil) showed impressive clinical results in improving bone health in a double-blind study in postmenopausal women with low bone density. Compared to a control group receiving calcium and vitamin D alone, the addition of BioSil (6 mg per day) was able to increase the collagen content of the bone by 22% and increase BMD by 2% within the first year of use. The ability to improve the actual collagen matrix as well BMD indicates that BioSil produced greater bone tensile strength and flexibility, thereby greatly increasing the resistance to fractures. BioSil also helps improve collagen production in the skin leading to improvements in fine lines and wrinkles. Here is an important fact: changes in skin collagen with age correspond with changes in collagen in bone. Hence, evidence of decreased skin collagen (e.g., lots of wrinkles) is a clear indication of a lack of bone collagen and a risk for osteoporosis. The recommended dosage for BioSil is 6-10 mg per day.

Boron in Bone Health

In addition to vitamin K1, the high levels of many minerals like calcium and boron in green leafy vegetables may also be responsible for this protective effect. Supplementing the diet of postmenopausal women with 3mg/day of boron reduced urinary calcium excretion by 44% and dramatically increased the levels of 17-beta-estradiol, the most biologically active estrogen. It appears boron is required to activate certain hormones, including estrogen and vitamin D. Boron is also apparently required for the conversion of vitamin D to its most active form within the kidney. A boron deficiency may contribute greatly to osteoporosis as well as menopausal symptoms.

As fruits and vegetables are the main dietary sources of boron, diets low in these foods may be deficient in boron. Typically, the standard American diet is severely deficient in these foods. According to several large surveys, including the US Second National Health and Nutrition Examination, fewer than 10% of Americans met the minimum recommendation of two fruit servings and three vegetable servings per day, and only 51% ate one serving of vegetables per day.

In order to guarantee adequate boron levels in people with osteoporosis, I recommend supplementing the diet with a daily dose of 3–5 mg of boron.

Prunes for Bone Health

Prunes have been shown to help offset a woman's significantly increased risk for accelerated bone loss during the first three to five years after menopause. When 58 postmenopausal women ate about 12 prunes each day for 3 months, they were found to have higher blood levels of enzymes and growth factors that indicate bone formation than women who did not consume prunes. Plus, none of the women suffered any adverse gastrointestinal side effects. Prune's beneficial effects on bone formation may be due to their high concentration of phenolic compounds that act as antioxidants to curb bone loss. Prunes also provide a good supply of boron, a trace mineral integral to bone metabolism that is thought to play an important role in the prevention of osteoporosis. A single serving (100 g) of prunes provides 2 to 3 mg of boron.

Strontium in Osteoporosis

Strontium is a nonradioactive earth element physically and chemically similar to calcium. Strontium in large doses stimulates bone formation and reduces bone resorption. In one double-blind study, 680 mg per day of elemental strontium for 3 years was shown to reduce the risk of vertebral fractures and to increase BMD in 1649 postmenopausal women with osteoporosis. In the first year, there was a 49% reduction in the incidence of vertebral fractures in the strontium ranelate group and a 41% reduction at the end of 3 years. A 6.8% increase in BMD was seen at the lumbar spine after 3 years of strontium supplementation. There was also an 8.3% increase at the femoral neck.

In a two-year trial, 353 postmenopausal women with osteoporosis and a history of at least one vertebral fracture received a placebo or one of three different doses of strontium: 170 mg per day, 340 mg per day, or 680 mg per day. A small increase in lumbar BMD was seen with each dose of strontium, but the difference compared with placebo was statistically significant only for the highest dose. The incidence of new vertebral fractures was lowest (38.8%) with the lowest dose of strontium (170 mg), versus 54.7%, 56.7%, and 42.0% in the placebo, 340 mg/day, and 680 mg per day groups respectively. The fact that the highest dosage increased BMD the most, yet the lowest dosage had the greatest effect on preventing vertebral fractures indicates that the goal with strontium supplementation may not be trying to increase BMD to the highest possible degree. In addition, since there are potential adverse effects with strontium, including rickets, bone mineralization defects, and interference with vitamin D metabolism—it makes sense to use the lowest dosage as possible.

There are many questions to be answered about strontium including the question is strontium chloride (the most common form of strontium used in U.S. supplements) equal to the form used in the clinical trials (strontium ranelate)? Strontium chloride has not been the form used in the published research. Other questions relate to safety and long-term benefits. Until these questions are answered our advice is to consider supplementation with any strontium salt only as a last resort in elderly women who are at extremely high risk for fractures or who have a significant history of fractures.

Table 10.4 - Key Nutritional Supplements for Bone Health

- High-potency multiple-vitamin-and-mineral formula
- Key individual nutrients:
  - Calcium: 1,000 mg daily
  - Magnesium: 350 to 500 mg daily.
  - Vitamin D3: 2,000 to 5,000 IU daily (ideally measure blood levels and adjust dosage accordingly)
  - Vitamin B6: 25 to 50 mg daily
  - Folic acid: 800 mcg daily
  - Vitamin B12: 800 mcg daily
  - Vitamin K2 (MK-7): 180 mcg/day
- Fish oils: 1,000 mg EPA+DHA daily
- Choose one of the following:
  - Grape seed extract (>95% procyanidolic oligomers): 100 to 300 mg daily
  - Pine bark extract (>90% procyanidolic oligomers): 100 to 300 mg daily
  - Or, some other flavonoid-rich extract with a similar flavonoid content, "super greens formula" or other plant-based antioxidant that can provide an oxygen radical absorption capacity (ORAC) of 3,000 to 6,000 units or higher per day
- Specialty Supplements
  - Soy isoflavonoids: 90 mg per day

- ◦ Biosil: 6 mg per day
- ◦ Strontium: 170 to 680 mg per day (please read discussion)

Sarcopenia and Osteoporosis

Sarcopenia was discussed very early in this book in . As reminder, sarcopenia is the loss of skeletal muscle mass and strength as we age. Sarcopenia is to our muscle mass what osteoporosis is to our bones. The degree of sarcopenia as we age is predictor of mortality and disability. In addition to a significantly shorter life expectancy, sarcopenia is linked to decreased vitality, poor balance and gait speed, and increased falls and fractures. Just like in the prevention of osteoporosis where we want to build the bone while we are young to help us preserve it longer through the aging process the same is true for sarcopenia. And, just as it is important to engage in dietary, lifestyle, and exercise strategies to fight osteoporosis in our later years we must do the same to fight sarcopenia. As stressed very early in this book: You must build muscle to maintain your health. For more information on sarcopenia and what you can do about it, see Chapter 2, pages 24-27.

The Joints

The places where your bones meet are your joints. Joints help hold the skeleton together, and they also give it mobility. Because of these dual functions, the joints are under a lot of mechanical stress and prone to damage. Most joints contain a shock-absorbing, rubbery material called cartilage that prevents bone rubbing on bone and acts to prevent the ends of bone from damage. Osteoarthritis, the most common form of arthritis, results from loss or degeneration of cartilage. By age fifty, roughly eight of ten people have osteoarthritis to some extent. The joints most often affected are the hands and the weight-bearing joints, such as the knees, hips, and spine.

Osteoarthritis is generally a degenerative "wear and tear" process in our joints where after years of use, cartilage simply breaks down causing surrounding cells to release enzymes that destroy joint tissues. With age, the body loses its ability to repair the damage and produce normal cartilage.

Osteoarthritis usually sneaks up on you. You might first notice that your joints are a little stiff when you wake up in the morning. Later, you might feel pain when you move the joint; the pain goes away when you rest. Oddly, x-rays might show severe joint damage even though you don't feel much pain. Conversely, you might be in excruciating pain even though x-rays show little damage.

There are other forms of arthritis including gout and rheumatoid arthritis. These are briefly touched on below as well, but osteoarthritis is the major focus because it is by far the most common.

Assessing Your Joint Health

Circle the number that best describes the intensity of your symptoms on the following scale:

0 = I do not experience this symptom

1 = Mild

2 = Moderate

3 = Severe

> *NOTE: For any serious injury, consult a physician immediately. See a physician if you have severe pain, injuries to the joints, loss of function, or pain persisting for more than two weeks.*

		0	1	2	3
1.	Back pain	0	1	2	3
2.	Swollen knees/elbows	0	1	2	3
3.	Athletic injury	0	1	2	3

4.	Bursitis	0	1	2	3
5.	Tendonitis	0	1	2	3
6.	Joint pain/arthritis	0	1	2	3
7.	Morning stiffness	0	1	2	3
8.	Decreased range of motion or pain on movement	0	1	2	3
9.	Enlarged joints, especially on hands	0	1	2	3
10.	Joints crack and pop when in motion	0	1	2	3

TOTAL _____

Scoring
- 7 or more: High Priority
- 3-6: Moderate Priority
- 1-2: Low Priority

Interpreting Your Score

Chances are if you have problems with your joints, you are well aware of it. The results from your assessment will give you an idea of just how much attention to focus on tuning-up your joints. If you are over the age of 50, more than likely you are showing signs of osteoarthritis.

Dealing with Osteoarthritis

The best approach to preventing osteoarthritis, or slowing down its progression, is to enhance repair of the collagen matrix and regeneration by connective tissue cells. Dietary, lifestyle, and supplemental strategies all play a role.

- Your diet should be rich in plant foods. Such a diet will be rich in natural antioxidant compounds that can help fight inflammation.
- Reducing the intake of saturated fat and increasing the intake of omega-3 fatty acids from cold-water fish and flaxseed oil can also be helpful in fighting inflammation.

- Lose excess pounds. Losing weight is usually the most effective strategy for preventing stress on the joints.
- Vitamin C is crucial for maintaining healthy joints. One of the most important roles of vitamin C in the body is the manufacture of collagen. A large and important study, the Framingham Osteoarthritis Cohort Study, found that the group of people getting more vitamin C in their diet were only one third as likely to develop osteoarthritis as those with average vitamin C intake.
- Your body needs vitamins A and B$_6$, zinc, copper, and boron to make and maintain cartilage. Lack of any one of these may speed up the loss of cartilage, while adequate levels promote cartilage repair and synthesis. Copper, for example, is important in the function of an enzyme called lysyl oxidase, which helps collagen bind with another protein called elastin. There are several reports of people who enjoyed complete or near-complete improvement in osteoarthritis symptoms after taking boron in doses of 6 to 9 mg per day.
- Physical exercise is often very helpful in improving joint mobility and reducing pain in osteoarthritis. The best exercises are isometrics, walking, and swimming. Isometric exercise is a technique in which your effort is directed against a resistant object. (As an example, make a "hook" with all the fingers of both hands. Lock the "hooks" together and try to pull them apart.) These types of exercises increase circulation to the joint and strengthen surrounding muscles without placing excess strain on joints. Increasing muscle strength around joints affected with osteoarthritis has been shown to improve the clinical features and reduce pain.
- Physical therapy also helps. Among the various treatments available, short-wave diathermy, a method of administering deep heat, may offer benefit. Combining this with periodic ice massage, rest, and exercise appears to be the most effective approach. I have referred some of my osteoarthritis patients for acupuncture, which often provides a significant degree of relief.

Glucosamine sulfate

Glucosamine is a simple molecule, manufactured in the body from glucose and an amine. One of the primary physiologic roles of glucosamine is in the joints, where it stimulates the manufacture of molecules known as glycosaminoglycans (GAGs), key structural components of cartilage. Glucosamine also promotes the incorporation of sulfur into cartilage. Because of this effect, glucosamine sulfate (GS) is the best source of glucosamine.

As some people age, they apparently lose the ability to manufacture sufficient levels of glucosamine. The result is that synthesis of GAGs does not keep up with degradation. The inability to manufacture glucosamine at an adequate rate has been suggested to be the major factor leading to osteoarthritis.

There are no food sources of glucosamine. Commercially available sources of glucosamine are derived from chitin—the exoskeleton of shrimp, lobsters, and crabs. There is also now available a vegan form.

The use of GS in osteoarthritis has significant support in the medical literature. Numerous double-blind studies have shown GS to produce much better results compared with non-steroidal anti-inflammatory drugs (NSAIDs), placebo, or acetaminophen in relieving the pain and inflammation of osteoarthritis (OA). Although some of the studies comparing GS with NSAIDs or acetaminophen showed similar reduction in pain and symptom scores, only GS improved indexes of joint function or markers showing improvement of cartilage structure. Typically, the advantages of GS over these other treatments were seen after 2 to 4 weeks of use, but there is some evidence that the longer GS is used, the greater the therapeutic benefit.

Not all studies showed clear positive results, because a few exist that showed no greater benefit for GS over placebo in improving symptom scores. However, it must be kept in mind that the placebo response in OA is quite high and may confound the true benefit of GS and other approaches to OA. Fortunately, there were several studies that showed objective improvements.

The two longest placebo-controlled trials were 3 years in duration. The results from these studies showed, quite convincingly, that GS slowed down the progression of OA and in many cases produced regression of the disease, as noted by radiologic improvements, and significantly reduced the incidence of total joint replacement even after as much as 5 years after GS discontinuation.

In the first long-term study, 212 patients with knee OA were randomly assigned 1500 mg oral GS or placebo once daily for 3 years. Weight-bearing anteroposterior radiographs of each knee in full extension were taken at enrollment and after 1 and 3 years. Mean joint-space width of the medial compartment of the tibiofemoral joint was assessed by digital image analysis, whereas minimum joint-space width (i.e., at the narrowest point) was measured by visual inspection with a magnifying lens. The 106 patients on placebo had a progressive joint-space narrowing. In contrast, no significant joint-space loss occurred in the 106 patients on GS.

Other studies have shown that even if symptomatic improvement is not observed, GS may be exerting positive effects on joint structure. This effect was definitely shown in a study looking at cartilage metabolism in patients with OA of the knee, in response to muscle strength training in combination with treatment with either glucosamine, ibuprofen, or placebo. Glucosamine's reduction of cartilage breakdown products in the blood was statistically significant compared with both placebo and ibuprofen.

There have also been several head-to-head, double-blind studies also showed that GS produced much better results compared with anti-inflammatory drugs in relieving the pain and inflammation of OA, despite the fact that GS exhibited little direct anti-inflammatory effect and no direct analgesic or pain-relieving effects. Although anti-inflammatory drugs like aspirin and ibuprofen, and analgesics like acetaminophen offer purely symptomatic relief, GS appears to address the cause of OA. By promoting cartilage synthesis, thus treating the root of the problem, GS not only relieves the symptoms but also helps the body to repair damaged joints. The clinical effect is impressive, especially when glucosamine's safety and lack of side effects are considered.

The standard dosage for GS is 1,500 mg/day. It appears that administration as a single dosage may produce better results. Obese individuals may need higher dosages on the basis of body weight (e.g., 20 mg/kg body weight daily). Individuals taking diuretics may also need to take higher dosages. Athletes or individuals who are subjecting their joints to greater wear and tear may need to increase the dosage to 3,000 mg to maintain positive cartilage synthesis.

GS has an excellent safety record in animal and human studies. On the basis of these studies, many experts have recommended that GS be considered as a drug of choice for prolonged oral treatment of osteoarthritis.

Boosting Collagen Production

Collagen and supplements that impact collagen production are growing in popularity. Collagen is the abundant protein in the body and is not only important in the support of the skin but is also the main component of connective tissue such as tendons, ligaments, cartilage, bone, and blood vessels. As we age, it is critical that we strive to conserve the collagen content in our body.

The word collagen comes from the Greek word for glue. It is an appropriate root as collagen along with along with hyaluronic acid (a sticky mucopolysaccharide) from the ground substance or "intracellular cement" that literally holds us together. There are several different types of collagen but type II collagen is by far the most abundant in our body representing 30% of total body protein and up to 70% of the proteins in our connective tissues.

A lot happens in the collagen-rich support structure of the skin (i.e., the dermis) as we age. First and foremost, as we age the activity of the fibroblasts, the cells responsible for making collagen, elastin, and hyaluronic acid, slows down. As we age the dermis is also less able to protect itself from damage and is more prone to dehydration. All of these factors ultimately lead to a thinner dermis and structural changes that lead to skin looking old and weathered.

As we grow older, natural collagen production also slows in skin leading to increased tendency to form wrinkles. Loss of collagen in our joints may lead to osteoarthritis and the ligaments and tendons may also weaken. Bone is also rich in collagen. In fact, about 30 to 40% of bone is composed of collagen. It provides the structural matrix upon which mineralization of bone occurs. Collagen is to bone what 2X4s are to the frame of a house. Decreased collagen content of the bone is a key underlying factor in osteoporosis and low bone density. The amount of collagen determines the number of "bone mineral binding sites." If the collagen content is low, the bone becomes more brittle and fracture risk increases dramatically,

Obviously, the first thought that you may have to increase the collagen content of the body is simply to eat collagen or take a collagen supplement. However, it may not be that simple. Collagen supplements can provide the building blocks of collagen manufacture, but the key is to actually increase the activity of collagen-producing cells. Collagen supplements have shown mixed results in promoting joint health. In one recent study, a hydrolyzed collagen supplement at a dosage of 2 g per day was shown to produce considerable benefit in the treatment of osteoarthritis (OA) symptoms of the knee and hip. However, this collagen supplement also contains low molecular weight hyaluronic acid (HA). Studies with HA supplementation as well as natural eggshell membrane rich in HA in OA have also shown beneficial effects, so it's hard to know if the study results with collagen are due to the collagen or HA.

Natural Eggshell Membrane (NEM) is another source of collagen, HA, and other connective tissue components. Recent studies show that NEM brings fast relief to people suffering from the pain, stiffness, and impaired mobility of osteoarthritis and other joint health problems. In one clinical study, after 30 days of use NEM reduced pain by an average of 72% and improves flexibility by 44%, without side effects. Rather than simply supply collagen, it is thought that NEM boosts the production of critical joint molecules like type 2 collagen and glycosaminoglycans (GAGs), including chondroitin sulfate. GAGs are important component of cartilage, providing resistance to compression and contributing to the tensile strength of cartilage, tendons, and ligaments.

Palmitoylethanolamide (PEA) for Pain, Inflammation, and Osteoarthritis

While I believe everyone with osteoarthritis should use glucosamine sulfate or natural eggshell membrane, there are other natural approaches that can really help relieve the pain and inflammation. Of these, I am very excited about the research on PEA - a fatty substance produced in the body as well as found in god concentrations from food including organ meats, chicken egg yolk, olive oil, safflower and soy lecithin, peanuts, and several others.

PEA is technically referred to as a "pro-resolving lipid signaling molecule." What this means is that through impacting central control mechanisms within our cells, PEA has an ability to resolve inflammation and cellular stress. This extremely beneficial effect has been demonstrated in over 600 scientific investigations.

The potential clinical applications of PEA are quite broad, but research and popular use has focused on its use as an anti-inflammatory and pain-relieving agent in conditions like low back pain, sciatica, osteoarthritis, etc. Preclinical and human studies have also investigated its effects in depression, boosting mental function and memory, autism, multiple sclerosis, obesity, and the metabolic syndrome. While it shares many features comparable to cannabidiol (CBD), the advantage with PEA is that it has better science to support its use.

The health benefits of PEA involve a variety of effects including those on upon immune cells that control inflammation, particularly in the brain. PEA reduces the production of inflammatory compounds. But, the major effect of PEA is on receptors on cells that control all aspects of cellular function. These receptors are known as PPARs. PEA and other compounds that help activate PPARs reduce pain and also enhance metabolism by burning fat, reduce serum triglycerides, increase serum HDL cholesterol, improve blood sugar control, and promote weight loss.

PEA has extensive possible clinical applications due to its unique effects on factors that control cell function. The primary clinical research focus with PEA has been in the treatment of pain and inflammation. In that area of focus, there have been at least 21 clinical trials with PEA. These studies had a range of 20 to 636 patients and PEA was used for periods ranging from 14 days to 120 days. The dosage ranged from 300 mg to 1200 mg daily. The administration form of PEA was in most cases oral tablets and most common form of evaluation for pain was the visual analogue scale (VAS), where the patient makes a subjective assessment of her/his pain level on a scale of 0 to 10 where 0 is no pain and 10 is the worst imaginable pain. In all but one study, the clinical trials have largely reported significantly reduced pain intensity and an almost complete absence of side effects.

The largest of the double-blind studies, investigated the effects of PEA on lower back or sciatica pain. The results showed that PEA at a dosage of 600 mg per day and 300 mg per day were significantly more effective than a placebo with the higher dosage (600 mg) showing the greatest effect. The big finding of the study was the number needed to treat (NNT) to demonstrate a 50% reduction in pain. The NNT is considered a statistically reliable and readily interpretable measure to rank the efficacy of chronic pain treatments. The NNT is interpreted as the number of patients one would need to treat in order to get one more responder on the active treatment than one would have gotten had they been treated with a placebo. The lower the NNT, the higher the efficacy. In the study, PEA demonstrated a NNT of 1.5 meaning that out of 3 people two would be responders. For comparison, ibuprofen 400 mg has a NNT of 2.8; acetaminophen 600 mg has a NNT of 5; and codeine 60 mg has a NNT of 18.

This superiority to ibuprofen was also shown in a study that compared the effect of PEA versus ibuprofen for pain relief in temporomandibular joint (TMJ) osteoarthritis. The 24 patients (16 women and 8 men) aged 24 to 54 years were randomly divided into two groups: group A (12 subjects) received PEA 300 mg in the morning and 600 mg in the evening for 7 days and then 300 mg twice a day for 7 more days. Group B (12 subjects) received an extremely high dosage of ibuprofen at 600 mg three times a day for 2 weeks. Every patient recorded the intensity of spontaneous pain on a visual analog scale twice a day. Maximum mouth opening was recorded by a blind operator during the first visit and again after the 14th day of drug treatment. After two weeks of treatment the participants were evaluated. Results showed the pain decrease was significantly greater with PEA than with ibuprofen. Maximum mouth opening also improved more in group A than in group B. This study showed that PEA is effective in treating TMJ inflammatory pain and that it outperformed ibuprofen.

The most recent study with PEA was in the treatment of osteoarthritis of the knee. The 111 participants were randomized to receive 300 mg PEA, 600 mg PEA or placebo each day for 8 weeks. In the groups getting PEA, there was a significant reduction in the total symptom scores for knee osteoarthritis as well as the individual scores for pain, stiffness, and function as well as anxiety. There were no side effects with PEA in this study. While the 300 mg per day dosage was effective, the 600 mg per day dosage was even more so. Given its lack of side effects, the higher dosage is recommended.

Table 10.5 - PEA Shows Positive Clinical Benefits in Conditions Associated with Pain

- Low back pain
- Sciatic pain
- Osteoarthritis
- Fibromyalgia
- Carpal tunnel syndrome
- Peripheral neuropathies—diabetic neuropathy & chemotherapy-induced peripheral neuropathy
- Neuropathic pain—related to stroke & multiple sclerosis
- Dental pain

- Chronic pelvic and vaginal pain
- Postherpetic neuralgia

Several studies with PEA have used it in combination with standard drug therapy. For example, in the treatment of fibromyalgia, a syndrome characterized by persistent pain, depression, and poor sleep quality when PEA was combined with an antidepressant and pentagabin (Neurontin) compared to those on the drug approach alone, those receiving the PEA showed a greater than 50% lower score for fibromyalgia symptoms including pain. The researchers concluded "Our study confirms ... the added benefit and safety of PEA in the treatment of pain in patients affected by fibromyalgia."

In regard to PEA's antidepressant effects, this was proven in a randomized double-blind, and placebo-controlled study. PEA was used as an "add on" therapy to the drug citalopram (Celexa), a selective serotonin re-uptake inhibitor in patients with major depressive disorder . The 54 patients were randomized to receive either PEA (600 mg twice daily) or placebo in addition to citalopram for six weeks. Results showed a greater reduction in depression scores with PEA that were apparent after only 2 weeks of use. Thus, PEA exerts a rapid antidepressant effect. The advantage with PEA compared to the placebo group was evident throughout the trial period. At the end of the trial 100% of the patients in the PEA group experienced a ≥ 50% reduction in their depression score compared to 74% in the group takin only the antidepressant drug.

PEA also exerts a multitude of effects in models of degenerative brain diseases such as Alzheimer's disease, Parkinson's disease, and multiple sclerosis.

There are basically two forms of PEA available commercially. A synthetic form a powerful synthetic solvent and a natural derived form from safflower lecithin. Obviously, the natural form is preferred.

Most studies used a dosage of 300 mg twice daily or 600 mg daily. The exception is in depression where the dosage used is 600 mg twice daily. PEA is completely safe and nontoxic in No significant treatment related adverse effect with PEA has been noted in clinical trials in humans. There are no known drug interactions with PEA.

Curcumin for Osteoarthritis

Curcumin is the yellow pigment of turmeric (*Curcuma longa*)—the chief ingredient in curry—and one of the most intensely studied natural products available today. As of 2020, more than 8,000 scientific studies have been conducted focusing on curcumin. While curcumin has demonstrated significant activity in many experimental and clinical studies, its primary biological effects relate to its action as a broad-spectrum antioxidant and profound anti-inflammatory agent.

Curcumin has demonstrated significant anti-inflammatory activity in a variety of experimental models as well as clinical studies. In fact, in numerous studies, curcumin's anti-inflammatory effects have been shown to be comparable to the potent drugs hydrocortisone and phenylbutazone as well as over-the-counter anti-inflammatory agents such as ibuprofen. Some clinical studies have further substantiated curcumin's anti-inflammatory effects. While most anti-inflammatory drugs only impact one or maybe two of these mediators, curcumin exerts actions against all of them.

While there is a lot of excitement with curcumin, there is also some concern that clinical results will not be as impressive as preclinical studies in cell cultures and in animal models due to the fact that regular curcumin is poorly absorbed and rapidly metabolized and eliminated from the human body. Dosages as high as 12 grams of curcumin have failed to significantly raise blood levels. Fortunately, there are absorbable forms of curcumin such as Theracurmin® and Meriva® - the most clinically studied curcumin products on the market.

As it relates to osteoarthritis (OA), curcumin exerts a number of mechanisms that address much of the underlying disease process. Clinical studies also show some benefits in osteoarthritis. In the first double-blind study with curcumin in OA, 50 patients over 40 years old with knee osteoarthritis confirmed by X-ray took either 180 mg/day of curcumin (as Theracurmin) or a placebo daily for 8 weeks. Results showed that knee pain scores were significantly lower in the Theracurmin group than in the placebo group in those patients with moderate to severe symptoms. Theracurmin also lowered the use of celecoxib (Celebrex) much more significantly than placebo. While 60% of the placebo group still relied on Celebrex for adequate pain relief at the 8-week mark, only 32% of the Theracurmin group still needed the NSAID and there was a definite strong trend for eventual discontinuation. No major side effects were observed in the patients taking Theracurmin. This study is significant as it showed such a significant advantage over a placebo in such a short-term study. Generally, in osteoarthritis this requires a much larger study group and much longer periods of time. Therefore, for Theracurmin to show such clear benefit in this relatively small, short-term study bodes really well for people with osteoarthritis gaining immediate and noticeable benefits with curcumin.

Meriva has also been used with success in several studies. In the first study, 50 patients were given 1000 mg Meriva (providing 200 mg of curcumin) for 3 months, after which symptom scores decreased by 58%, walking distance in the treadmill test was prolonged from 76 to 332 meters, and the level of an inflammatory marker (C-reactive protein) in the blood decreased from 168 to 11.3 mg/L in the subpopulation with high C-reactive protein. In another study, 100 patients with osteoarthritis were given the same dosage of Meriva for 8 months. Just as in the previous study, symptom scores, walking distance, and blood measurements of inflammation were all significantly improved.

Gout

More than likely you are familiar with gout, an inflammatory arthritis triggered by crystallization of uric acid within the joints. It causes severe pain and swelling. Gout has now reached epidemic proportions in the Unites States as it now affects about 10 million people—or about 5% of the adult population. In addition, elevations in blood uric acid levels are found in over 43.3 million (21%) adults in the U.S.

Gout is strongly associated with metabolic syndrome, a group of health conditions characterized by central obesity, insulin resistance, high blood pressure and blood lipid issues that may lead to heart attack, diabetes and premature death.

Gout is the result of either increased synthesis of uric acid; reduced ability to excrete uric acid; or both over production and under excretion of uric acid. The first attack of gout is characterized by intense pain, usually involving only one joint, most often the first joint of the big toe. The first attacks usually occur at night and are usually preceded by a specific event, such as dietary excess, alcohol ingestion, trauma, certain drugs (mainly chemotherapy drugs, certain diuretics, and high dosages of niacin), or surgery.

Subsequent attacks are common, with the majority of gout patients having another attack within one year. That said, diet is often very effective in preventing subsequent gout attacks. The dietary treatment of gout involves the following guidelines:

- Elimination of alcohol intake. Alcohol increases uric acid production by accelerating purine breakdown. It also reduces uric acid excretion by increasing lactate production, which impairs kidney function. The net effect is a significant increase in serum uric acid levels. This explains why alcohol consumption is often a trigger in acute attacks of gout. Elimination of alcohol is all that is needed to reduce uric acid levels and prevent gouty arthritis in many individuals.

- Low-purine diet. Foods with high purine levels should be entirely omitted. These include organ meats, meats, shellfish, yeast (brewer's and baker's), herring, sardines, mackerel, and anchovies. Foods with moderate levels of purine should be eaten in moderation. These include dried legumes, spinach, asparagus, fish, and poultry.

- Achievement of ideal body weight. Weight reduction in obese individuals significantly reduces serum uric acid levels.

- Reduced consumption of sugar and refined carbohydrates. Simple sugars (refined sugar, honey, maple syrup, corn syrup, fructose, etc.) increase uric acid production.
- Low saturated fat intake. Saturated fats decrease uric acid excretion.
- Low protein intake. A high protein intake increases uric acid manufacture.
- Drink at least 48 ounces of water each day. Drinking lots of water keeps the urine diluted and promotes the excretion of uric acid.
- Consuming one-half pound of fresh cherries per day has been shown to be very effective in lowering uric acid levels, preventing attacks of gout, and reducing blood markers of inflammation. In the most recent study, researchers found that cherry intake (defined as one-half cup or 10 to 12 cherries or the equivalent in extract form) over a two-day period was associated with a 35-45% lower risk for gout attacks.

Rheumatoid Arthritis

Rheumatoid arthritis (RA) is a more severe form of arthritis. RA is an autoimmune reaction, in which antibodies formed by the immune system attack components of joint tissues. Yet what triggers this autoimmune reaction remains largely unknown. Speculation and investigation have centered around genetic factors, abnormal bowel permeability, lifestyle and nutritional factors, food allergies, and microorganisms. RA is a classic example of a multifactorial disease, wherein an assortment of genetic, dietary, and other factors contributes to the disease process.

The joints typically involved are the hands, feet, wrists, ankles, and knees. The onset of RA is usually gradual, but occasionally is quite abrupt. Fatigue, low-grade fever, weakness, joint stiffness, and vague joint pain may precede the appearance of painful, swollen joints by several weeks. Involved joints will characteristically be quite warm, tender, and swollen. The skin over the joint will take on a ruddy purplish hue.

Diet has been strongly implicated in RA for many years, in regard to both cause and cure. The major focus in dietary therapy is to eliminate food allergies, increase the intake of antioxidant nutrients, follow a vegetarian diet, and alter the intake of dietary fats and oils. A long-term study conducted in Norway at the Oslo Rheumatism Hospital showed that following these dietary principles can be "curative" in some individuals with RA, and significantly reduce symptoms in others.

The first step is a therapeutic fast or an elimination diet, followed by careful reintroduction of foods to detect allergens. Virtually any food can aggravate RA, but the most common offenders are wheat, corn, milk and other dairy products, beef, nightshade family foods (tomatoes, potatoes, eggplants, peppers, and tobacco) and coffee. After isolating and eliminating all allergens, a diet rich in whole foods, vegetables, and fiber, and low in sugar, meat, refined carbohydrates, and animal fats is recommended.

The importance of a predominantly vegetarian diet rich in fresh fruits and vegetables in the dietary treatment of RA cannot be overstated. Plant foods are the best sources of dietary antioxidants, including vitamin C, beta-carotene, vitamin E, selenium. Several studies have shown that the risk of RA is highest among people with the lowest levels of dietary antioxidants. An excellent source of antioxidants includes flavonoid-rich berries, such as cherries, cranberries, hawthorn berries, blueberries, blackberries, raspberries and strawberries. Carotenoids are beneficial antioxidants found in yellow and green vegetables, including squashes, yams, carrots and the cabbage family vegetables.

During flare-ups, fresh pineapple juice along with some fresh ginger root may help to relieve symptoms of RA due to their anti-inflammatory activity. Ginger possesses anti-inflammatory action by inhibiting the manufacture of inflammatory compounds and by the presence of an anti-inflammatory enzyme similar to bromelain, which is found in pineapple. In one clinical study, seven patients with RA in whom conventional drugs had provided only temporary or partial relief were treated with ginger. One patient took 50 g/day of lightly cooked ginger while the remaining six took either 5 g of fresh or 0.1-1 g of powdered ginger daily. All patients reported substantial improvement, including pain relief, joint mobility, and decrease in swelling and morning stiffness.

There are three key supplements for people with RA:

- *Fish oils* rich in eicosapentaenoic acid (EPA) and docosahexaenoic acid (DHA) have been shown to be extremely helpful in the relief of symptoms (morning stiffness and joint tenderness), fish oil supplementation has produced favorable changes in suppressing the production of inflammatory compounds secreted by white blood cells. improving psoriasis. The dosage used in the double-blind clinical studies has typically provided 3,000 mg of EPA+DHA.

- *Proteolytic enzymes* including fungal proteases, bromelain (pineapple enzyme), papain (papaya enzyme), and serratia peptidase (the "silkworm" enzyme) can be very helpful in RA and other inflammatory conditions. For anti-inflammatory effects, proteolytic enzyme products should be taken on an empty stomach. Take two capsules of Repair Gold from Enzymedica twice daily between meals.

- *Curcumin* (see above). Take either Theracurmin (180 mg daily) or Meriva (2,000 mg daily).

A Quick Look at Fibromyalgia

Fibromyalgia is characterized by generalized aches or stiffness of at least three anatomical sites for at least three months and six or more typical, reproducible tender points. It is also associated with fatigue; chronic headache; sleep disturbance; depression; numbing or tingling sensations in the extremities; the irritable bowel syndrome; and variation of symptoms in relation to activity, stress, and weather changes.

The cause of fibromyalgia is unknown. The primary treatment goals in fibromyalgia are to raise serotonin levels, improve sleep quality, and assure adequate magnesium levels. Here are key recommendations to improve fibromyalgia:

- *PEA* is a very important tool in patients with fibromyalgia who are experiencing a lot of pain. PEA works on central mechanisms to reduce pain. It also exerts some mood elevating effects helpful in these patients. Dosage if there is significant pain and/or depression: 600 mg twice daily.

- *5-Hydroxytryptophan* (5-HTP) is converted to the important neurotransmitter serotonin. 5-HTP is proving helpful since a deficiency of serotonin is linked to fibromyalgia. In one double-blind study, fifty patients with fibromyalgia were given either 5-HTP (100 mg) or a placebo three times per day. The group that received the 5-HTP experienced significant improvements in their symptoms. In contrast, the group that received the placebo did not improve much at all. Improvements were noted in all symptom categories: number of painful areas; morning stiffness; sleep patterns; anxiety; and fatigue. Although 5-HTP produces very good results within thirty days, even better results are obtained at ninety days of use. Dosage: 50 to 100 mg three times per day.
- *St. John's wort* (*Hypericum perforatum*) extract is often helpful in fibromyalgia because of its ability to improve mood and sleep quality. Dosage: (0.3% hypericin content) 900 to 1,800 mg daily. St. John's wort extract can be used in combination with 5-HTP and magnesium.
- *Magnesium* is critical to many cellular functions, including energy production, protein formation, and cellular replication. Low magnesium levels are a common finding in patients with fibromyalgia. The best food sources of magnesium are legumes, tofu, seeds, nuts, whole grains, and green leafy vegetables. Most Americans consume a low-magnesium diet because their diet is high in refined foods, meat, and dairy products. Magnesium supplementation has produced very good results in treating fibromyalgia. Dosage: magnesium (citrate, malate, fumarate, succinate, aspartate, or glycinate) 150–250 mg three times daily.
- *Bodywork* is a general term referring to therapies involving touch, including various massage techniques, chiropractic spinal adjustment and manipulation, Rolfing, reflexology, shiatsu, and many more. In fibromyalgia, gentle techniques such as Trager

massage, Feldenkrais, and Alexander technique seem to be most helpful.

Longevity Matrix Lifestyle Tune-Up Tip #10–Stretch to Stay Flexible (and Young)

One of the best habits you can develop to keep your musculoskeletal system healthy is regular physical stretching. What I mean by stretching is working to take your joints through their entire range of motion and actively taking the time to stretch the major muscle groups of the body.

My introduction to stretching came in 1980 when a friend of mine gave me the book *Stretching* by Bob Anderson and Jean Anderson. This husband and wife team has been a real driving force in helping people understand the importance of stretching. In 1968, at the age of 23, Bob began a personal physical fitness program, since he felt he was overweight and out of shape. He changed his diet, started eating less, and began running and cycling. He dropped 55 pounds over a period of time, and he soon was in much better physical condition. One day, while in a conditioning class in college, he discovered he could not reach much past his knees in a straight-legged sitting position. After discovering how tight he was, Bob started stretching. In several months he became much more limber; he found that stretching made running, cycling and other activities easier and more enjoyable and that it eliminated most of the muscular soreness that usually accompanies strenuous physical exertion.

After several years of exercising and stretching with Jean and a small group of friends, Bob gradually developed a method of stretching that could be taught to anyone. Soon, he was teaching his technique to others. He began working with professional teams, then college teams, other amateur athletes, and with a variety of people at sports medicine clinics, racquetball clubs, athletic clubs and running stores throughout the country.

Bob and Jean first published their book Stretching in 1975 and in four years sold over 35,000 copies by mail. The revised version was published in 1980 by Shelter Publications and has now sold over 2 million copies.

Although there are now other excellent books on the market on stretching, I encourage you to get Bob and Jean's book. It is still a great guide.

I must admit that even though I knew the value of stretching, I really didn't appreciate it until I turned forty a few years ago. When I started thinking about how I felt at forty compared to twenty or thirty, I realized that my body did not feel as flexible as it did earlier. I knew that I had to really make stretching more of a priority. I am happy to tell you that it has really paid off.

Another stimulus for paying more attention to stretching was watching just how flexible my two young children are and comparing that to how stiff and inflexible most elderly people are. The older people that I have had as patients and have known personally who are much younger than their years all had excellent flexibility.

When done properly, stretching can do more than just increase flexibility and make you feel younger. The confirmed benefits of stretching include:

- contributing to enhanced physical fitness.
- enhancing the ability to learn and perform skilled movements.
- increasing mental and physical relaxation.
- enhancing the development of body awareness.
- reducing risk of injury to joints, muscles, and tendons.
- reducing muscular soreness and tension.
- Reducing joint pain due to stimulation of the production of chemicals which lubricate the joints.

To gain the benefits of stretching it is important to follow these simple guidelines.

- Warm-up to stretch. Perform some exercises such as push-ups, jumping jacks, or go for a brisk walk to warm up the muscles before you stretch. It is not a good idea to attempt to stretch before your muscles are warm as it could lead to pulls and tears in the muscle.

- Stretch after your warm-up and during the cool down period after exercise for maximum results.
- Isolate the particular muscle you are stretching. For example, you are better off trying to stretch one hamstring at a time than both hamstrings at once. By isolating the muscle you are stretching, you experience resistance from fewer muscle groups, which gives you greater control over the stretch and allows you to more easily change its intensity.
- The stretch must be slow and controlled. Do not bob or jerk when stretching, slow and steady is the approach. Hold the stretch for a minimum of 15 seconds. As you become more flexible, you will be able to hold the stretch longer. But, in the beginning 10 seconds may feel like an eternity.
- Breathe during a stretch. The proper way to breathe during a stretch is to inhale slowly through the nose, expanding the abdomen (not the chest); hold the breath a moment; then exhale slowly through the mouth.
- Stretch in the proper sequence. As a general rule, you should stretch in the following sequence:
  - stretch your back (upper and lower) first
  - stretch your neck after stretching your back
  - stretch your sides before stretching your legs
  - stretch your buttocks before stretching your groin or your hamstrings
  - stretch your calves before stretching your hamstrings
  - stretch your shins before stretching your quadriceps (if you do shin stretches)
  - stretch your arms before stretching your chest
- Do not overstretch. Stretch only to the point of discomfort. You should feel tension in your muscle, but not pain. Do not feel you have to regain or gain flexibility all at once. The tortoise approach definitely wins this race. If you stretch properly, you should not be sore the day after you have stretched. If you are, then it may be

an indication that you are overstretching and that you need to go easier on your muscles by reducing the intensity of some (or all) of the stretches you perform. Overstretching can actually reduce flexibility because it can damage the muscles.

Here is a sample stretching routine to get you started:
- Low back stretch. Lie on your back. Hug knees to chest.
- Neck stretch. Tilt your ear to your shoulder and hold. Repeat other side.
- Lateral side stretch. Extend arm overhead, place opposite hand on hip. Bend sideways at hip. Repeat with other side.
- Calf stretch. Keep your back leg straight and heel on the ground. Move your front foot as far forward as you can but keep your back heel on the ground. Place both hands above bent knee. Move hips forward. Repeat with other side.
- Hamstrings stretches. Start with one leg straight supporting your weight. Now place the other leg straight in front of you about six inches. Point the toe of your forward foot up and with your opposite hand touch your pointed toe. Repeat with other side.
- Quadriceps stretch. Standing next to something for balance such as a wall or heavy chair and raise one leg behind you and grab hold of your foot. The upper part of the leg should remain in a vertical position as you pull your foot upwards. Repeat with other side.
- Tricep stretch. Place hand behind your head to the middle of your back. Your elbow points up. Push your elbow down with your other hand. Repeat with other side.
- Full body stretch. Raise your arms over head, stand on your toes and reach for the sky. Flex and extend fingers.

CHAPTER 11:

Keys to Healthier Hair, Skin, and Nails

There is a reason why radiant, vibrant, and lustrous looking hair, skin, and nails have long been associated with good health. What you see on the outside reflects what is going on in the inside. While most people try and improve the appearance of these tissues from the outside alone, the real key to healthy skin, beautiful hair, and strong nails is building them from the inside out through good nutrition and key dietary supplements. Skin, hair, and nails are derived from dynamic, living tissue. And, like all living tissue they need proper nourishment. Since hair and nails are derived from skin cells, the nutrients required for healthy skin are the same nutrients required for healthy hair and nails.

Collectively, the skin and its associated tissues—oil and sweat glands, hair, and nails—are known as the integumentary system. *Integumentary* means "covering." Imagine going into a clothing store and seeing a mannequin wearing a special coat. A sign near the mannequin boasts that the coat is waterproof and washable. It's sturdy, but it's also astoundingly flexible—no matter what size you are, it will always fit you like. . . well, like a glove. This remarkable coat automatically adjusts to the outside temperature—when things heat up, it will cool you down; when things get chilly, it will keep you warm. What's more, it automatically darkens to protect you against sunlight. Amazingly, if it suffers small tears or minor burns, it will mend itself in just a few days. Best of all, the manufacturer guarantees that, if you give it proper care, the coat will last you a lifetime. It is a pretty amazing coat we have isn't it.

Skin

The skin is the largest organ of the body and accounts for about seven percent of your weight, about nine pounds for most people. If you were to peel it off and lay it on the ground, it would cover about twenty-one square feet—about the size of the top of a twin mattress. It varies in thickness from one to four millimeters, or about one sixteenth of an inch at most.

Thin as it is, the skin is composed of several layers. The outermost portion is the epidermis (*derm-* means skin), and it serves as the body's main protective shield. Below that is the dermis, a thicker layer where most of the business of living goes on. Below the dermis is the subcutaneous tissue, which contains larger blood vessels and fat cells.

The epidermis skin cells are born in the from the deepest of its 4 layers and migrate upward. By the time they reach the surface they are no longer living. Each day you shed millions of these dead cells through washing or abrasion. Much of the "dust" in your house is actually dead skin cells. As you slough them off, new cells rise to take their place. You grow a completely new epidermis every five to seven weeks.

The dermis miles of nerve fibers, blood vessels, and lymphatic vessels, as well as millions of oil glands and sweat glands. Most of the dermis consists of flexible connective tissue that forms a matrix that holds everything together and also allow skin to stretch and return to its original shape. Structural proteins, especially collagen (discussed below), as well as elastic fibers called elastin, and sulfur are all critical to the health and function of this matrix. Collagen and related structures comprise roughly 75% of skin's dry weight.

Tune-Up Tip: Avoid Excessive Sun Exposure and Use Sun Block

You need a little bit of sunlight so your body can make its own supply of vitamin D. The cells in your outer skin layer (the epidermis) store the raw materials for making the vitamin. When sunlight penetrates the layer, it starts the conversion process. But you don't need a lot of light for this to happen—fifteen minutes a day should do it.

Too much sunlight is not good for the skin. Ultraviolet light can rip through cells and destroy their membranes, causing them to leak their contents. This leakage is what causes the redness, itching, and irritation of sunburn. If the cells die in massive numbers, the skin peels off in chunks. Such damage—whether it occurs in a few intense episodes or more gradually, over a period of time—puts you at risk of skin cancer, especially the deadly form known as melanoma.

If you plan to spend more than twenty minutes or so outdoors, wear protective clothing, sunglasses, and a hat. And, please use sunscreen. The strength of sun-blocking creams and lotions are based on the SPF (sun protection factor). The higher the number, the stronger the protection of your sunscreen. So which rating should you use? 10 SPF? 15 SPF? 30 SPF? These ratings indicate how much longer the sunscreen's use will allow you to be in the sun without getting a sunburn. Example: If you usually start to burn after about 20 minutes, proper use of SPF 2 protects you for about 40 minutes and proper use of SPF 15 protects you for about five hours ($15 \times 20 = 300$ minutes). However, because these figures are derived from a laboratory setting and several important factors—including reflections, altitude, wind, the angle of the sun, the presence on your skin of water or sweat, etc.—reduce the effectiveness of sunscreens as a practical matter, most doctors and the American Academy of Dermatology say the safest approach is for everyone to wear at least 15 SPF, even on a cloudy day.

This recommendation makes particularly good sense with children. Here is a sobering thought, 90% of the sun-related damage that can lead to skin cancer occurs prior to age 18. Due to the thinning of the atmosphere's ozone layer, a person born today is twice as likely to develop skin cancer as someone born only a decade ago—and 12 times as likely as someone born 50 years ago!

Keep an Eye on Your Moles

One of the deadliest skin cancers is melanoma. This cancer arises from moles on the body and is often referred to as black mole cancer. Fortunately, melanoma almost always occurs on the skin surface. You don't see other cancers that may grow undetected inside the body. But you can often spot melanoma – and get treatment before it poses a serious health problem.

To find melanoma, however, you must check yourself routinely – once every few months. Report any suspicious moles to your physician or a dermatologist. Look for moles characteristic of these ABCDs:

A –Asymmetrical shape

B – Border is irregular

C – Color varies from one area to another

D – Diameter larger than a pencil eraser

If you notice a mole that is different from others, or that changes, itches or bleeds, you should make an appointment to see a dermatologist.

Tuning Up Your Skin

The best strategy for supporting the skin is to provide it with highest-quality nutrition possible. Overall, I think the best diet for healthy skin, hair, and nails is the modified "Mediterranean Diet." That is probably not surprising to you by this time, I have recommended it throughout this book for good reason. There are also some specific overarching strategies for achieving "beauty from within." Getting the right types of oils in the diet, especially the essential fatty acids, along with boosting collagen, and protecting against oxidative damage are key steps for healthy looking and more youthful skin.

A Wrinkle in Time

Why does skin wrinkle? The main reason skin wrinkles are the cumulative effects of free radical damage. This damage may be the result of exposure to the elements–sun, wind, and pollution all take their toll–but exposure to internal free radicals is also a major cause. So too is normal aging. Over time, the amount of fat stored in layer just below the dermis tends to diminish. Thus, there is less "bulk" material to support the skin layer, causing it to sag. As we age, the collagen in our skin loses its ability to hold its shape. The molecules that must "link arms" and form a cohesive structure lose their grip. The fibers become literally fewer and farther between. As the network of collagen shrinks, the skin becomes thinner and less elastic. The glands that secret natural skin oils wither away, causing skin to become dry and itchy. To prevent wrinkles from forming, eat a diet rich in antioxidants and avoid smoking cigarettes and environmental exposure to free radicals.

Boosting Collagen Production

As discussed in the last chapter, collagen and supplements that impact collagen production is growing in popularity for supporting skin and joint health. A lot happens in the collagen-rich support structure of the skin (i.e., the dermis) as we age. First and foremost, as we age the activity of the fibroblasts, the cells responsible for making collagen, elastin, and hyaluronic acid, slows down. As we age the dermis is also less able to protect itself from damage and is more prone to dehydration. All of these factors ultimately lead to a thinner dermis and structural changes that lead to skin looking old, wrinkled, and weathered.

Collagen dietary supplements are a big business worldwide with an enormous greater than $4 billion market. They are derived from a variety of sources, including the skin, bones and connective tissues of cows, chicken, pigs and fish. When denatured by heat, collagen forms gelatin, which has been used for centuries as a food source and traditional medicine. So, in other words, gelatin is a source of collagen peptides. In fact, there is evidence that gelatin provides identical benefits to collagen peptides. Collagen sources are broken down a little more than gelatin to manufacture hydrolyzed collagen or collagen peptides. The benefit is that collagen peptides have a higher water-solubility and no gelation properties, allowing them to be conveniently formulated into not only powdered mixes, but also hot and cold liquid drinks.

Gelatin and collagen peptides can provide valuable amino acids to the skin, hair, joints, and connective tissue. Collagen is an excellent source of proline and hydroxyproline amino acids. However, these amino acids are deemed non-essential because our body can make them in most circumstances. That said, perhaps the preformed proline-rich small peptides and hydroxyproline are utilized pre-formed and that helps the fibroblasts out in collagen synthesis. Gelatin and collagen supplements have been shown to help maintain skin elasticity and hydration, which may help minimize the appearance of skin aging. Supplementing with collagen may also boost nail growth. One study showed it increased nail growth 12% and reduced breakage.

Here is my take on gelatin and collagen supplements. I don't think they provide that much special nutrition over a diet sufficient in protein. Let's say you owned a ladder manufacturing plant. You would need the vertical and horizontal pieces, right? But you can have all of the ladder pieces in the world and it would do you no good in making ladders if your factory did not have the workers or machinery to actually assemble the pieces to make a ladder. In the body, the collagen factory in skin is the fibroblast. My feeling is that yes, we need the building blocks, but most of us have plenty of collagen building blocks. More important is that we need to have all of the machinery in the fibroblast working and turned on to make collagen.

One of the most interesting and well-documented approaches to actually increasing the manufacture of collagen is the use of a highly bioavailable from of silica (choline stabilized orthosilicic acid or BioSil®). Initially research focused on the ability of Biosil to increase the levels of hydroxyproline, the key amino acid required for the production of collagen and elastin. Clinical studies with Biosil showed impressive results in women (ages 40 to 65 years) with signs of sun-damage and premature aging of the skin. Those receiving 10 mg of Biosil daily experienced 30% improvements in shallow, fine lines and 55% increased skin elasticity, and a significant reduction in brittle nail and hair. As described in the last chapter, there is a link between low levels of collagen causing wrinkles in the skin and loss of the collagen matrix in bone leading to osteoporosis. So, not only does BioSil benefit the health of the skin, it helps support nail and bone health too.

Plant flavonoids are critical in supporting healthy collagen. In general, flavonoids produce an antioxidant activity that is more potent and effective against a broader range of oxidants than the traditional antioxidant nutrients like vitamins C and E, beta-carotene, selenium, and zinc. This effect goes a long way in protecting collagen structures from damage. Especially beneficial to collagen structures are the blue or purple pigments—the anthocyanidins and PCOs (short for proanthocyanidin oligomers) - that are found in grapes, blueberries, red kidney beans, and many other foods. These flavonoids can also be found in pine bark and grape seed extracts. Anthocyanidins, PCOs and other flavonoids affect collagen metabolism in many ways:

- They have the unique ability to actually crosslink collagen fibers resulting in reinforcement of the natural crosslinking of collagen that forms the so-called collagen matrix of connective tissue (ground substance, cartilage, tendon, etc.).

- They prevent free radical damage with their potent antioxidant action.
- They inhibit destruction to collagen structures by enzymes secreted by our own white blood cells during inflammation.
- They prevent the release and synthesis of compounds that promote inflammation.

To ensure sufficient levels of these beneficial flavonoids increase your intake of richly colored berries and other fruit, drink green tea, and red kidney beans. It is also a good idea to supplement your diet with a PCO extract like grape seed or pine bark at a dosage of 150 to 300 mg daily.

A high potency multiple vitamin and mineral formula is also a key to healthy skin and boosting collagen production. They are part of the machinery in the fibroblast that are needed to make collagen. Each day you shed millions of skin cells and as you slough them off, new cells rise to take their place. You need all of your essential nutrients for skin cells to form properly. In particular, zinc is extremely important in skin cell manufacture and wound healing. A key sign of low zinc is the presence of white lines on the fingernails, indicating poor wound healing of the nail bed even after the least trauma.

Sulfur is also especially important nutrient for the skin, hair, and nails because it acts to stabilize the support structures of these tissues like collagen and other components of the connective tissue matrix. MSM (methyl-sulfonyl-methane) is a major form of sulfur in the human body and the sulfur-containing amino acids methionine and cysteine also play valuable roles. For example, about a quarter of your collagen is made of cysteine (cysteine contains atoms of sulfur) which forms especially sticky bonds with other neighboring proteins. The strength and water-binding potential of collagen is important in supporting the epidermis and dermis in ways that helps keep your skin remain supple and smooth. Cysteine, methionine, and MSM are also important in preventing brittle or weak nails. To ensure optimal sulfur levels, I recommend taking at least 1,000 mg of MSM daily.

The Importance of Essential Fatty Acids

Vitamin F is a term that is not used much anymore. It was used initially to highlight the importance of the only two official essential fatty acids: linoleic (an omega-6 fat) and alpha-linolenic acid (an omega-3 fat). These fats are considered essential nutrients because the body cannot manufacture them, they must be ingested. In general, a deficiency of essential fatty acids (EFAs) can be so vague and broad that symptoms typically are written off as one of a myriad of other causes. Suffice to say surveys suggest that Americans are up to 80% deficient in the essential fatty acids and the long chain omega-3 fatty acids EPA and DHA. One of the hallmark features of EFA deficiency is dry skin, cracked nails, dry lifeless hair, and dry mucous membranes.

Table 11.1 - Signs and symptoms typical, but not exclusive to essential fatty acid deficiency.

- Dry skin
- Cracked nails
- Dry lifeless hair
- Dry mucous membranes, tear ducts, mouth, vagina
- Fatigue, malaise, lack luster energy
- Lack of endurance
- Maldigestion, gas, bloating
- Constipation
- Immune weakness
- frequent colds, and sickness
- Aching sore joints
- Angina, chest pain
- Depression
- Lack of motivation
- Forgetfulness
- Forgetfulness, uh oh!!
- High blood pressure
- History of cardiovascular disease

- Arthritis

In addition to frequently eating raw nuts and seeds, and avocados in your diet and supplementing with fish oils, I recommend incorporating one tablespoon of flaxseed oil daily. Flaxseed oil is one of the best sources of both EFAs. Do not cook with flaxseed oil, it is far too fragile and is easily damaged by heat and light. You can add it to foods after they have been cooked or use it as a salad dressing. Taking flaxseed oil by swigging it down or by the tablespoon is not very palatable. Use it as a salad dressing, dip your bread into it, add it to your hot or cold cereal, or spray it over your popcorn. Here is a simple salad dressing featuring flaxseed oil that is easy to make:

Flaxseed Oil Basic Salad Dressing
Place all ingredients into a salad bowl and whisk together until smooth and creamy. This recipe is quick and delicious!
- 4 tablespoon organic flaxseed oil
- 1 1/2 tablespoon lemon juice
- 1 medium garlic clove, crushed
- Pinch of sea salt or salt-free seasoning
- Fresh ground pepper to taste

Jazz up this basic recipe to your own personal taste by using your favorite herbs and spices.

Cooking Oils

The best oils to cook with in baking recipes, stir fries, and sautés, are the monounsaturated oils and coconut oil. Olive oil and avocado oil are by far the most popular monounsaturated fats in use. Coconut oil is also a very good choice. In cooking, the smoke point of an oil or fat is the temperature at which it begins to break down to glycerol and free fatty acids and produce bluish smoke. The glycerol is then further broken down to acrolein—a rather toxic substance that is also extremely irritating to the eyes and throat.

Table 11.2 - The Smoke Points of Various Cooking Oils:

Oil	Quality	Smoke Point
Avocado oil	Refined	500°F
Butter		250-300°F
Canola oil	Refined or Expeller Press	375-450°F
Canola oil	High Oleic	475°F
Coconut oil	Extra Virgin (Unrefined)	350°F
Coconut oil	Refined	450°F
Corn oil	Unrefined	352°F
Corn oil	Refined	450°F
Cottonseed oil		420°F
Flaxseed oil	Unrefined	225°F
Ghee (Indian Clarified Butter)		485°F
Grapeseed oil		420°F
Hemp oil		330°F
Lard		370°F
Macadamia nut oil		413°F
Olive oil	Extra virgin	375-405°F
Olive oil	Virgin	391°F
Olive oil	Extra light	468°F
Peanut oil	Unrefined	320°F
Peanut oil	Refined	450°F
Rice bran oil		490°F
Safflower oil	Unrefined	225°F
Safflower oil	Semi-refined	320°F

Safflower oil	Refined	510°F
Sesame oil	Unrefined	350°F
Soybean oil	Unrefined	320°F
Soybean oil	Refined	460°F
Sunflower oil	Unrefined	437°F
Sunflower oil, high oleic	Unrefined	320°F
Sunflower oil	Refined	440°F
Walnut oil	Unrefined	320°F

Antioxidant Protection for the Skin

Boosting dietary antioxidant intake by eating plenty of richly colored fruit and vegetables is a key goal in supporting skin health. It is not only important for making the skin look healthier and have fewer wrinkles, it is important in fighting skin cancer. Carotenoids like beta-carotene, lutein, and lycopene are important to focus on through dietary intake (see Table 9.1 - Top 20 Plant Sources of Lutein, Zeaxanthin, and Lycopene) and I would also recommend supplementing with astaxanthin, the "King of Carotenoids." Astaxanthin supplementation positively affects skin health and appearance and has an ability to accumulate in the skin when taken internally enables it to improve all four layers of the skin. In one study of 49 middle aged women who were divided into two groups and took either 4 mg of astaxanthin per day or a placebo for six weeks. Positive results were found across the various test methods:

- In the self-assessment (questionnaire), over 50% of the subjects taking astaxanthin rated improvements in all areas.
- Dermatologist assessment found improvements in all areas tested: Fine lines and wrinkles, elasticity and dryness.
- Clinical instruments used in measuring skin moisture and elasticity recorded improvements.
- Before and after photos showed visible improvements in fine lines, wrinkles and elasticity.

Tune-Up Tip: Ironing Out Wrinkles

The most popular antiwrinkle and antiaging products contain natural compounds known as fruit acids or alpha-hydroxy acids (AHAs for short). Examples are glycolic, lactic, tartaric, malic, and citric acids. Of these glycolic acid (from sugar cane) is by far the most common.

First used in 1974, AHAs were quickly adopted as renaissance materials by the cosmetic and dermatology world. Besides ironing out wrinkles, AHA-containing preparations are used as moisturizers in the treatment of dry skin, acne, and age spots. They also help your skin look younger. Dermatologists use AHAs to perform chemical peels of the skin—a procedure where the AHAs literally dissolve or peel away layers of skin. The amount of free acid in the product determines whether it will moisturize, eliminate wrinkles, or act as a chemical peel. The higher the percentage of AHA, the greater the peeling effect. While dermatologists use products with seventy percent free acids, most over-the-counter AHA products contain only four percent—the minimum amount needed to produce skin cell renewal.

Use AHA-containing products according to label recommendations. If you use AHAs, be aware that your skin is now even more vulnerable to the negative effects of the sun. Use an effective sun block before exposing your skin to the sun.

Dealing with Some Specific Age-related Skin Issues

The recommendations above regarding tuning up the skin go a long way in making your skin look younger, but I wanted to also address age spots and cellulite.

Age Spots

As we get older, large, freckle-like discolorations appear on the skin. These blemishes—commonly called age spots—result from the build-up of a dark substance produced by your cells, known as lipofuscin. This material is mostly debris from molecules that have been partially destroyed by free radical damage. Actually, lipofuscin collects in many tissues throughout your body, including your brain, where it may play a major role in causing age-related memory loss. But the spots are only visible on the skin. The number and severity of age spots is a good indication of the level of oxidative damage that has occurred throughout the body.

It is easier to prevent lipofuscin deposits than to reverse them. The smartest strategy is to avoid excessive sun exposure and to use sunblock. Also make sure your intake of antioxidants, especially beta-carotene, is high. If you are prone to age spots, eat dark green leafy vegetables, carrots, yams, and other foods high in carotenes. You can also take 4 to 12 mg of astaxanthin.

Now, if you are really bothered by age spots or sun damage, I recommend Intense Pulsed Light (IPL) Photofacial. IPL is a laser light treatment that targets pigment issues, such as brown spots, sun damage and red spots, and acne rosacea. The bright light passes through the epidermis, drawing out the pigment producing cells and dispersing the uneven pigment. IPL Photofacial can be used on the face, neck, chest, shoulders, back arms, legs and just about anywhere else.

I had an IPL Photofacial and the results were incredible. I think it made me look 20 years younger. It was amazing. IPL Photofacial is not for everyone; it works best for light-skinned people who have had a lot of sun damage. It does not work on darker skin tones and can actually lead to darkening of patches. It is relatively painless and takes about 45 minutes. My results after one treatment were dramatic, but some people may need 3-5 treatments about four weeks apart for maximum benefit. And, you may need to repeat treatment on an annual basis for optimal results.

Cellulite

As stressed above, with age, the collagen matrix in the dermis becomes weaker. When that happens, the fat cells below can start to migrate, pushing up into the layer above. The connective tissue between cells also weakens, allowing the fat cells to become swollen. As a result, the skin over these regions can develop pits and ridges—the so-called "mattress phenomenon"—and the fatty areas can feel like granules or buckshot. The common name for this condition is *cellulite*.

Cellulite is a cosmetic problem, not a medical one, but because it is unsightly it can cause great distress in those who have it. Due to sex differences in skin tissue, women are more than nine times as likely to develop cellulite as men. Women who are overweight are far more likely to have cellulite than slender women or athletes. In men, the development of cellulite is likely the result of a deficiency in male hormones, especially testosterone. The regions most likely affected are the thighs and buttocks; less frequently cellulite develops in the lower abdomen, the nape of the neck, and upper arms.

Generally, the number of fat cells in your body is determined by heredity. While you can't control the number of cells you have, to a significant extent you can control how big those cells get. The goal is to maintain a slim subcutaneous fat layer, and the first choice of methods for achieving should be no surprise: exercise, maintain a healthy weight, and eat a healthy, low-fat diet. Lose excess weight, but do so gradually, especially if you are a woman over age forty. If weight loss occurs too quickly, the mattress phenomenon can be more apparent, especially in people whose skin and connective tissues are undergoing the normal changes associated with aging.

You can also take steps to improve circulation to the affected area and to increase the integrity of connective tissue. Massage is helpful, because it stimulates better flow of both blood and lymph. You can administer massage yourself, using your hand or a brush. The idea is to gently push against the affected tissue, with strokes moving in the direction toward the heart.

Many cosmetic formulas and herbal preparations claim that they can "cure" cellulite. I am dubious of such claims, because they are usually made without scientific data to back them up. However, research has shown that certain botanical compounds can provide good results for many patients. I recommend using a combination of oral and topical products that strengthen connective tissues.

An extract of centella (*Centella asiatica*, or Gotu kola) supports connective tissue metabolism by stimulating the body to produce structural components known as glycosaminoglycans (GAGs). GAGs are the major components of the so-called ground substance in which collagen fibers are embedded. Use of centella extract helps perhaps six to eight out of ten women who try it for improving the appearance of their cellulite. The dose is 30 mg of a product containing seventy percent triterpenic acids, taken three times per day.

Hair

For many people, a good head of hair is important for self-esteem and a sense of well-being. Unfortunately, for most people hair loss is a predictable, if distressing, tradeoff for living a long life. Part of the problem comes from genetics, but dietary factors as well as years of using shampoos, conditioners, coloring agents, and other harsh chemicals can take their toll on our hair. Exposure to sun and wind, coupled with constant combing, brushing, and blow-drying, doesn't help either.

In most cases, hair loss is a normal part of aging. By the age of forty or so, the rate of hair growth slows down. The hair follicles just run out of steam. New coarse hairs are not replaced as quickly as old ones are lost. Instead, fine hairs grow in their place. Both men and women suffer from age-related hair loss, but the problem is more apparent in men.

Hair growth is controlled by hormones, especially male hormones (androgens such as testosterone), but thyroid and adrenal hormones also play a part. The typical pattern of baldness seen in men—loss of hair beginning at the temples, followed by further loss along the top of the head—is the result of genetics. For decades, the hair grows normally, responding to stimulation from androgens in the hair follicle. But then a gene that has been inactive all this time suddenly switches on, causing changes in the way follicles respond to testosterone. The growth cycle shortens. Hairs don't grow long enough to emerge from the skin before they fall out. The higher a man's testosterone level, the greater the risk of baldness. This link may be the basis for the fact that many women think that bald men are sexier!

While there is not a lot success with male-patterned baldness, there is a lot that can be done for hair loss in women. It is one of the most common complaints from female patients in clinical practice. Often it is just the perception that hair is falling out at an increasing rate, but it still needs to be investigated. I have heard many women complain that other doctors dismiss hair loss as "nothing to worry about"—after all, minor hair loss is certainly not a life-threatening disorder. But these women feel frustrated—because the hair loss is a big deal to them, and I certainly understand why.

So, we have to do a little work. First, here is a simple test called the "hair pull test" that can help determine the relative formation of new hair. It involves taking a few strands between their thumb and forefinger and pulling on them gently. Hairs that are in an active growth phase should remain rooted in place while hairs in a resting state should come out more easily. By knowing approximately how many hairs were pulled and the number that came out, the percentage of hair follicles in a resting or growth state can be determined. So, if 20 hairs were pulled and 2 come out, then the frequency of resting hair follicles is 10%. As a rough guide, a 10% telogen frequency is excellent, up to 25% is typical, over 35% is problematic. It means that there is less hairs that are in the growth phase. I just did the test myself, grabbed about twenty strands, and am thrilled that none of my hairs pulled out. If you were not so lucky or if it is clear to you that your hair loss is real there are five common causes of hair loss in women that you need to explore: (1) female pattern hair loss; (2) drugs; (3) nutritional deficiencies; (4) hypothyroidism; and (5) the presence of antigliadin antibodies.

Female Pattern Hair Loss

Women can suffer from hormone-related hair loss just like men. The female pattern hair loss, however, is more diffuse than the characteristic male pattern baldness. It is a relatively common condition affecting approximately 30% of women before the age of 50. Although genetic factors are clearly significant, testosterone excess, insulin resistance, the polycystic ovarian syndrome, and low antioxidant status are also associated with female pattern hair loss. Four possible recommendations to help slow down this genetically predisposed process are: (1) improve blood sugar regulation through dietary, lifestyle, and supplementary measures; (2) increase antioxidant intake; (3) use saw palmetto extract; and (4) consider bioidentical hormone replacement therapy:

- **Improving blood sugar control** may help improve hormonal factors linked to female pattern hair loss. Follow those guidelines given in Chapter 5.

- **Increase antioxidant intake**. Free radicals have been shown to play a central role (along with testosterone) in male pattern baldness. Higher levels of these damaging compounds are found in the hair follicles in men (and presumably women) with male pattern baldness. The reason? Lowers levels of the protective antioxidant glutathione. Free radical damage has been shown to play a central role (along with testosterone) in male pattern baldness. Higher levels of these damaging compounds are found in the hair follicles in men (and presumably women) with male pattern baldness. This appears due to lower levels of glutathione. The use of glutathione sparing antioxidants like vitamin C, N-acetylcysteine, alpha lipoic acid and flavonoids may help slow down the process.

- **Use saw palmetto extract**. This herbal medicine is a popular therapy for benign prostatic hyperplasia (BPH) in men. It works by slowing down the enzyme that converts testosterone to a more potent form, dihydrotestosterone (DHT). In women, saw palmetto extract may relieve androgen-related alopecia by reducing the formation of DHT. The dosage for the extract standardized to contain 85-95% fatty acids and sterols is 320 mg per day.

- **Consider bioidentical hormone replacement therapy**. The female hormones estrogen and progesterone will counteract the effects of testosterone on hair loss in women, especially in those experiencing hair loss during or after menopause. This therapy was discussed in Chapter 10.

Drug-Induced Hair Loss

A long list of drugs can cause hair loss, but it should not be interpreted that simply because a woman is complaining of hair loss and is taking one of these drugs that the drug is the single cause of her hair loss. Of course, for some drugs, most notably chemotherapy agents like fluorouracil; they are obviously the cause because they are such powerful inhibitors of hair growth. When medically appropriate, natural alternatives to suspected culprits of hair loss should be employed (see Table 11.3).

Table 11.3 - Classes of Drugs that Can Cause Hair Loss

Class	Examples
Antibiotics	Gentamycin, chloramphenicol
Anticoagulants	Coumadin, heparin
Antidepressants	Prozac, desipramine, lithium
Antiepileptics	Valproic acid, Dilantin
Cardiovascular drugs	Angiotensin-converting enzyme inhibitors, beta-blockers
Chemotherapy drugs	Adriamycin, vincristine, etoposide
Endocrine drugs	Bromocriptine, Clomid, danazol
Gout medications	Colchicine, allopurinol
Lipid-lowering drugs	Gemfibrozil, fenofibrate
Nonsteroidal anti-inflammatory drugs	Ibuprofen, indomethacin, naproxen
Ulcer medications	Tagamet, Zantac

Nutritional Deficiency

A deficiency of any number of nutrients can lead to significant hair loss. Zinc, vitamin A, essential fatty acids, and iron are the most important. If a person's finger nails have horizontal white lines it may indicate poor wound healing of the nail bed even with the most minor of trauma, which may be a sign of low zinc levels (although white lines in the finger nails are popularly considered a sign of zinc deficiency—look at the finger nails of a carpenter or anyone else whose work causes regular trauma to the fingers). If the back of the arms bumpy and rough, it may represent hyperkeratosis, a common sign of vitamin A deficiency. If the elbows are very dry and cracked it may be due to essential fatty acid deficiency. For evaluating iron status, a blood test called serum ferritin evaluation is recommended. If the serum ferritin is less than 30 mg/L, iron intake must be increased via diet and supplementation. When serum ferritin levels fall below this level, hair growth and regeneration is impaired, as the body seeks to conserve the iron. There is a very strong association between low body iron stores and diffuse hair loss in women when serum ferritin levels are below 30 serum ferritin levels below or equal to mg/L. After 2 months, reassess serum ferritin levels. Improvements in serum ferritin often correlate with improved health of the hair and the halting of excessive hair loss.

Typically, women with noticeable generalized hair loss suffer from apparent deficiencies of all of these nutrients. The treatment of hair loss secondary to nutritional deficiency is straightforward—increase dietary intake of these nutrients and supplement appropriately. One caveat is that many of these women may not be secreting enough stomach acid. In these cases, hydrochloric acid supplementation at meals may be all that is necessary. A general recommendation for women with hair loss related to nutritional status is to take a high-potency multivitamin and mineral formula that contains iron, along with 1 tablespoon of flaxseed oil per day. As stated above, if serum ferritin levels are below 30 mg/L, women can consume iron-rich foods and supplement with additional iron.

One general recommendation for hair loss is to take BioSil, the stabilized and highly absorbable form on silica. Studies show that BioSil increases levels of hydroxyproline, the key amino acid required for the production of collagen and elastin—compounds that are essential to the strength, thickness, and elasticity of hair. In one double-blind study, 48 women with fine hair were given 10 mg BioSil daily for 9 months. Results showed quite clearly that BioSil had a positive effect on tensile strength including elasticity as well as produced thicker hair.

Hypothyroidism

Up to 20 percent of the adult female population has mild to severe hypothyroidism. Hair loss is one of the cardinal signs of hypothyroidism. Given the importance of adequate thyroid hormone to human health, I tend to be aggressive in recommending thyroid hormone replacement when lab tests show even mild hypothyroidism. For more information see Chapter 5, pages 123-130.

Table 11.4 - Signs and Symptoms of Hypothyroidism

Hair loss
Dry, rough skin
Course, dry, and brittle hair
Thin and brittle nails
Depression
Weight gain
Sensitivity to cold weather
Cold hands or feet
Elevated cholesterol and triglyceride levels
Menstrual abnormalities in women.
Muscle weakness and joint stiffness
Shortness of breath
Constipation

Intolerance to Gluten

The protein gluten and its derivative gliadin are found primarily in wheat, barley, and rye grains. Some people make antibodies to gliadin.

Their presence also triggers production of cross-reacting antibodies that can attack the hair follicles. This situation can cause hair loss including alopecia areata, an autoimmune disease characterized by patches of virtually complete hair loss.

Most often the presence of antibodies to gliadin in the blood indicates celiac disease, an intestinal disease characterized by structural abnormalities in the small intestine leading to malabsorption. In many cases, removing gluten from the diet allows the intestine to revert to its normal structure and function. Many people with gluten intolerance do not exhibit overt gastrointestinal symptoms. Instead, they may have indirect signs, such as hair loss. I consider ordering a test to detect gluten sensitivity in patients with general hair loss, especially if they also have gastrointestinal symptoms. I also recommend taking a gluten-digesting enzyme for anyone with gluten sensitivity or intolerance.

Nails

Your fingernails and toenails are part of your epidermis. Like hair, they contain hard keratin. Nails look pink, but they are actually relatively clear. The pink color comes from the blood vessels underneath. Nails grow from a root beneath the skin. As they push outward, they grow away from the skin to which they are attached, producing the white part (or free edge) that we trim away. The cuticle is a fold of skin that overlaps and protects the corner of the nail. On average, a nail grows about two hundredths of an inch in a week. The nail on the middle finger grows fastest, the pinkie slower, and the toenails slowest of all. With age, toenail growth tends to slow down considerably, and the nails become thick and ridged.

Biotin for Strong Nails and Healthy Hair

Biotin is a popular recommendation to increase the strength of nails and promote health hair. Early research on biotin in this application came from the veterinary literature. Biotin was shown to increase the strength and hardness of hooves in pigs and horses. Human studies have shown that biotin supplementation (2,500 mcg per day) can produce a 25%

increase in the thickness of the nail plate in patients diagnosed with brittle nails of unknown cause and up to 91% of patients taking this dosage will experience definite improvement. However, despite its impressive results in people with brittle nails, biotin supplementation has not been shown to produce much impact on nail strength in people with normal nail strength.

In regard to the beneficial effects of biotin on the health of hair, it possibly reflects an ability to improve the metabolism of scalp oils similar to biotin's effects in seborrheic dermatitis, a common condition that is associated with excessive oiliness (seborrhea) and dandruff. The dandruff of seborrhea may be yellowish and either dry or greasy. In addition, scaly bumps may coalesce to form large plaques or patches. Seborrheic dermatitis usually occurs either in infancy (usually between two and twelve weeks of age) or in the middle-aged or elderly and has a prognosis of lifelong recurrence.

MSM for Strong Nails and Healthy Hair

Methylsulfonylmethane (MSM) was discussed above. It is a physiological form of sulfur that is available as a dietary supplement. It has shown benefits for joint health, sports nutrition, immune function, and is gaining popularity as a nutritional supplement for supporting the health of hair, skin and nails. In a double-blind clinical stud, 63 subjects ingested either 1g or 3g per day of MSM. Results showed that MSM supplementation showed statistically significant improvements in the condition of hair and nails as determined by expert grading and subject self-assessment. MSM appears to benefit hair and nail health possibly by its action on keratin which is a major building block for hair and nails. The higher concentration (3g/day) of MSM appeared to deliver quicker and stronger benefits, as compared to the lower concentration of 1g/day. For general support of healthy hair and nails, I recommend 1,000 mg per day. If there is an issue of poor nail health, especially weak, peeling, and brittle nails, I recommend 3,000 mg per day.

Longevity Matrix Lifestyle Tune-Up Tip #11—Connect with Nature

Most Americans spend 90% of their lives indoors separated from fresh air, natural sunlight, and nature. I do not think that this is healthy. There is something extremely refreshing (and calming) that happens when we can get in touch with nature, whether it is simply a walk through a park, tending to our lawns, gardening, going on a picnic, or getting out in the wilderness for a weekend of camping. For your lifestyle tune-up try to engage in at least one outdoor activity a week. Make it a high priority. I try to get outdoors every day. But, since I can't always get out and enjoy nature as much as I would like, I try to find other ways to commune with nature. Here are some simple tips:

- **Adopt a plant.** Plants are not only a way to get in touch with nature they are phenomenal air filters, especially if you work in an office building. Much of the pollution that is generated in a large office building is the outgassing of the material used in buildings or in maintaining the structure. Machines or cleaners used within the structure can also create this out-gassing. There are many sources, including foam insulation, plywood, particulate fibers, plastics, inks, oils, as well as out-gassing from business machines such as fax machines and copiers. In 1973, NASA found that the tightly contained air inside Skylab was contaminated with more than 100 toxic chemicals. Without effective purification, space travel would be impossible. Fortunately, NASA was tipped off by the CIA that the Russians were experimenting with plants as air purifiers. The NASA scientists learned that virtually all indoor plants clean the air of almost all known contaminants. The contaminants are sucked into the leaves and migrate into the soil where microorganisms associated with the roots break them down and turn them into plant food. Using sealed growth chambers, NASA scientists demonstrated that common house plants were the most effective purifiers of our most common pollutants. The more plants you have in the office building or house, the purer the air becomes.

- **Listen to sounds of nature.** In my office, car, and home, I usually have a recording of sounds of nature playing in the background. The recordings are of beautifully relaxing music intertwined with sounds of nature like the sounds at an isolated beach, waterfall, or forest. I find myself being more productive and relaxed when these gentle sounds are playing. I highly recommend it.

- **If you use a computer, use nature scenes as your desktop wallpaper and screensaver.** I know that this may seem like a real stretch, but I cannot tell you how much pleasure I get from watching the nature scenes on my computer screen during the course of my day while I am on the phone or not using my computer.

CHAPTER 12.

Advanced Superfood and Supplement Recommendations

I n this final chapter I want to provide some of the key superfoods and supplements that I utilize on a daily basis. Basically, I am answering the question "what do you take, Dr. Murray?" Now, keep in mind that I am a true "health nut" and can also afford to invest in foods and supplements to support and build my health. What I have laid out in all the preceding chapters can be affordable to most. And, it is important to keep in mind that the foundation of the Longevity Matrix is a lifestyle, attitude, and diet that everyone can afford. The foundation supplements are the next level of support and those are affordable to most. Just a reminder, the foundation supplements are a multiple vitamin-mineral formula, extra vitamin C and D3, a plant-based antioxidant, and a high-quality fish oil. Most of what I am laying out here in this chapter is an ideal plan for those who are both committed and can afford it, but there is also valuable information that is also affordable to almost everyone. I also have included some information on andropause and low testosterone at the end of this chapter.

Superfoods for Living Better, Stronger, and Longer

What is a superfood? In order to provide some framework for discussion, my definition of a superfood is one that provides exceptional health benefits. Obviously, virtually any food, herb, or spice has the potential to be a superfood. But, most often a superfoods list focuses on berries; exotic superfruits like acai, goji, noni, and others; kale and other dark green vegetables; fatty fish such as salmon, mackerel and sardines; many legumes (peanuts, lentils, beans) and whole grains. While I agree with these sorts of foods being worthy on any superfood list, my list is different because my general diet recommendations already focus on so many superfoods.

Obviously, if you have come to this point of the book you have seen several dietary themes over and over again. One of the keys to eating a diet that promotes health and longevity is focusing on flavonoids, a type of plant pigment and a member of the larger polyphenol family. As a class of compounds, flavonoids are often referred sometimes called "nature's biological response modifiers" because of their anti-inflammatory, antiallergic, antiviral, and anticancer properties. Many of the superfoods owe their benefits to their flavonoid content. While different flavonoids have different effects in the body, the key factor may not be a high intake of any one particular flavonoid, but rather a high total flavonoid intake that also provides a high variety of flavonoids rather than any one particular flavonoid class. Remember, there are over 8,000 different types of flavonoids out there in nature.

What the research also shows is that it does not seem to matter where the flavonoids come from dietary sources or through supplements containing flavonoid-rich extracts. The caveat is that the dosage must be sufficient, and the total intake must come from a variety of sources. So, with this caveat on the importance of proanthocyanidins in mind, what is an effective dosage of flavonoids? Based upon my interpretation of all of this data, I believe that the total flavonoid intake for general health should be at least 500 mg from a wide variety of sources. My flavonoid intake is exceptionally high because of my dietary and supplementation strategy.

For many years I have consciously sought to achieve a minimum of 2,000 mg per day and usually go well beyond this total on most days. Here is a list of the high flavonoid foods and supplements that I consume on a daily basis to reach this goal:

Dietary sources:	Daily dosage	Flavonoid content
Berries	1 cup	205 mg
Raw cacao powder	3 tablespoons	85 mg
Tea (green or herbal)	12 ounces	400 mg
Decaffeinated coffee	12 ounces	400 mg
Nuts	1/2 cup	85 mg
General diet not included above	-	150 mg
Supplement sources:		
Micronized diosmin*	600 mg	600 mg
Resveratrol	500 mg	500 mg
Cacao flavanols	375 mg	375 mg
Green Tea Phytosome®	300 mg	100 mg
Grape seed extract	300 mg	300 mg

*from VeinSense (Natural Factors)

To help you calculate the flavonoid content I am providing a table of the approximate flavonoid content of selected foods. The values are derived from multiple sources, but primarily the USDA Database for the Flavonoid Content of Selected Foods, Release 3.1 (December 2013). Results vary considerably based upon numerous factors including the water content of the selected source, analytical method, exact species or type of the selected food, and other factors. In general, smaller more dense fruit will provide a higher content of flavonoids than larger, more woody fruit. For example, a smaller, denser blueberry or apple will have a higher content of flavonoids than a larger, higher water content blueberry or apple. The key is to try to hit that 500 mg per day target and remember these foods have numerous other beneficial compounds in them besides flavonoids.

Table 12.1–Approximate Flavonoid Content of Selected Foods in Milligrams (mg) per 3½ oz (100 g) Serving*

Foods	Flavanols	Anthocyanins	4Oxoflavonoids	Total
Fruits				
Apples	30	15	15	60
Apricots	25	-	15	40
Black berries	15	350	2	367
Blueberries	15	190	5	205
Cherries, sweet	40	75	5	120
Cranberries	20	150	50	275
Currants, black	15	200	150	415
Grapefruit	-	-	50	50
Grapes, black	4	125	20	149
Grapes, green	10	-	4	14
Grapes, red	4	80	3	87
Lemons, without peel	-	-	83	83
Oranges, all commercial types	-	-	101	101
Peaches	21	7	2	30
Pears	27	4	4	20
Plums, black	140	54	40	234
Raspberries	20	135	10	165
Strawberries	12	75	9	96

Vegetables				
Cabbage, red (raw)	-	210	3	213
Kale, raw	-	-	135	135
Onions, red (raw)	-	53	235	288
Parsley	-	-	330	330
Radishes, raw	-	100	2	102
Nuts and Seeds				
Almonds	7	4	10	21
Chia seeds	-	-	34	34
Hazelnuts	12	11	-	23
Pecans	25	25	-	50
Miscellaneous				
Cacao powder	8,500	-	-	8,500
Cocoa powder, unsweetened	378	-	-	378
Chocolate, dark semisweet	65	-	-	65
Tea, black brewed	119	-	4	123
Tea, green brewed	128	-	5	133
Wine, red	125	80	3	208

*Flavanols include catechins and proanthocyanins; 4Oxoflavonoids include flavanones, flavones, and flavonols (including quercetin).

My Top Seven Superfoods

Before getting to my superfoods list, I like to say that when it comes to superfoods, Americans suffer from xenophilia. Let's examine the meaning of this term. "Xeno" means foreign and "philia" means love. So, what I am referring to is my feeling that we tend to think of exotic, foreign sounding fruits and vegetables as being much more of a superfood that the wondrous common fruits and vegetables that are very accessible to us. For example, in the past decade or so various "superfruits" have dominated new product introductions in health food stores. However, I am not sure that the health benefits provided by "exotic" superfruits are significantly greater than those provided by familiar fruits.

Table 12.2 - Superfruits: Familiar vs. Exotic

Familiar	Exotic
Apples	Acai
Black currant	Baobab
Blueberry	Camu Camu
Cranberry	Goji
Grape	Mangosteen
Strawberry	Maqui
Pomegranate	Noni

There is also little doubt that many common fruits, vegetables, legumes, nuts, seeds, spices, herbs, and other foods are worthy of superfood status. That said, there are seven superfoods that I try to ingest on a daily basis because of their exceptional health properties:

- Berries
- Raw Cacao Powder and Dark Chocolate
- Green tea
- Bee pollen
- Ground flaxseeds
- Whey protein
- PGX

I am passionate about these seven superfoods and definitely make them a big focus in my daily routine. But they are not the only "superfoods" that I consume. In fact, I think my whole diet is focused on health promoting foods. You can do the same and enjoy better health, higher energy levels, and greater clarity of thought as a result.

Berries

I know that I started off by saying that my list was different and here I go and start it off with a superfood that makes everybody's list—berries. But, making a commitment to consume one cup of some sort of berry every day is a vital step to maintain or improve your health. While some lists just focus on one type of berry, my message again is to eat a variety. Whether it is blackberries, blueberries, raspberries, strawberries, cranberry, currants, acai, goji, or any other berry you are getting a magical superfood. Berries are rich in vital nutrients and phytochemicals like flavonoids, yet low in calories making them an excellent food choice for those who have a sweet tooth and are attempting to improve their quality of nutrition without increasing the caloric content of their diet. In other words, berries are perfect diet foods.

Most of the research on the beneficial effects of berries has focused on blueberries, cranberries, black currants and strawberries, but there is so much overlap that it is a bit like splitting hairs. Other fruit sources are in the same mix, especially pomegranate, amla (gooseberry), grapes (with seeds), and cherries. While I have stressed the importance of flavonoids, berries contain many other beneficial phytochemicals. For example, while blueberries are higher in anthocyanidin flavonoids, strawberries are a much better source of the anticancer compound ellagic acid. In one study, strawberries topped a list of eight foods most linked to lower rates of cancer deaths among a group of 1,271 elderly people in New Jersey. Those eating the most strawberries were three times less likely to develop cancer than those eating few or no strawberries. Again, the key is eating a variety of different type of berries on a regular basis to make sure you are getting an array of flavonoids and other beneficial compounds that act in a synergetic fashion. Another key is to choose organic berries because conventional sources are often laced with pesticide and herbicide residues.

Raw Cacao Powder and Dark Chocolate

Cacao is not a misspelling of cocoa. Both come from the beans of the cacao tree, but raw cacao beans are minimally processed to produce raw cacao powder by crushing the beans to remove the fat to produce a powder. It looks a lot like cocoa powder, but the latter is roasted and in process loses many of the key compounds and living enzymes.

Of all the foods available on planet Earth, perhaps the most magical and loved are those from cacao, especially chocolate. The old saying is that nine out of 10 people say they like chocolate, and the tenth is lying. The world consumes more than 7 million tons of chocolate each year, and sales in the United States alone are predicted to reach $22.4 billion in 2017.

This delectably seemingly addictive food is produced from the beans of the cacao tree whose official name *Theobroma cacao* reflects the longstanding love for chocolate (*theobroma* being the Greek word for "food of the gods"). In the United States, the average person consumes about 12 pounds of chocolate per year. That pales in comparison to the Swiss, where the average person consumes about 22 pounds of chocolate yearly. Based upon a lot of evidence, Americans might be healthier if they tried to match the Swiss intake.

Chocolate has been referred to as nature's best medicine. I am not going to go that far as I believe raw cacao is much better, but I will say that including chocolate in your diet has many health benefits. At the center of these health benefits are the flavonoids of chocolate. While these plant pigments are responsible for many of the health benefits of many fruits and medicinal plants, with chocolate they are in a much more sensually pleasing vehicle. Also, there is evidence that not only is chocolate rich in flavonoids, but that factors in chocolate somehow dramatically increase the absorption of these compounds. The key flavonoids are flavanols similar to those found in green tea as well as proanthocyanidins (also called procyanidins) similar to those found in grape seed extracts, berries, and pine bark extract. Chocolate is very well endowed with both of these compounds. In fact, flavonoids constitute as much as 48% of the dry weight of the cocoa bean.

There are several ways that I get my chocolate fix including the special brew that I have almost every day that I create with organic raw cacao powder. For that and practical recommendations on selecting dark chocolate, see page 350.

Green Tea

Drinking herbal teas provides many health benefits, but without question the most popular tea is derived from *Camellia sinensis*, the source of both green tea and black tea. Black tea is by far the most popular of the two as green tea represents only 20 percent of the nearly 2.5 million tons of dried tea produced each year. In other words, four times as much black tea is produced and consumed as green tea. Though black tea is more popular, green tea provides greater health benefits.

The difference between green and black teas results from the manufacturing process. To produce black tea, the leaves are allowed to oxidize. What this means is that a series of chemical reactions are allowed to take place that result in the browning of the tea leaves and the production of flavor and aroma compounds. Unfortunately, during oxidation enzymes present in the tea convert the polyphenols into substances with much less biological activity. In contrast, green tea is produced by lightly steaming the fresh-cut leaf. Steaming prevents the enzymes from converting polyphenols, so oxidation does not take place. Oolong tea is partially oxidized.

Although green tea contains vitamins and minerals, the polyphenols are the primary keys to the magic it produces. The usual concentration of total polyphenols, a larger category of plant compounds that includes flavonoids, in dried green tea leaf is around 8% to 12%.

In order to gain the health benefits from green tea, a sufficient dosage of the polyphenols must be achieved. For example, one study sought to determine the dose effect of green tea on antioxidant protection. In the study, 15 healthy volunteers consumed 500 ml of green tea with different contents of solids (1.4, 1.6, 1.8, and 2.0 g per liter). Ingestion of the lowest dosage produced no change in plasma antioxidant capacity. At the highest dosage, the effects increased the plasma antioxidant capacity the greatest at 1 and 4 hours after ingestion. This study is extremely significant as it indicates that some of the studies failing to show health benefits with green tea ingestion may have been due to insufficient dosage.

Here is an example of the magical effect of green tea. In addition to exerting direct antioxidant activity on its own, green tea increases the activity of antioxidant enzymes within the body. The human antioxidant system involves not only the use of dietary compounds like green tea polyphenols, but also a number of enzymes produced by cells to deactivate damaging compounds. This magical effect is important because often nutritionists only look at the direct action of the food component as an antioxidant instead of looking at the total effect on the body's antioxidant system. The antioxidant effects of green tea far exceed its direct antioxidant effects.

The same is true for green tea's anticancer effects. Yes, green tea polyphenols exert many direct anticancer actions, but they also have the ability to impact many of the body's own anticancer mechanisms. Population-based studies clearly attest to the anticancer effects of green tea consumption. The forms of cancer that appear to be best prevented by green tea are those of the gastrointestinal tract, including cancers of the stomach, small intestine, pancreas, and colon; the lung; and estrogen-related cancers, including most breast cancers; skin cancer; and prostate cancer.

Its effects against breast cancer are quite interesting. In addition to inhibition of the interaction of estrogen with its receptors in breast tissue, the polyphenol compounds in green tea also block genetic factors that promote the interaction of tumor promoters, hormones, and growth factors with their receptors—a kind of sealing-off effect—in breast tissue. Experimental and epidemiologic studies demonstrated a protective effect against breast cancer, and clinical results confirmed that green tea might be helpful as a treatment for early-stage breast cancer.

Similar to studies on antioxidant activity, however, results in fighting cancer seem to be dependent upon a sufficient dosage. The takeaway message is that in order to see a statistically significant effect, higher dosages of green tea or green tea extract have to be consumed, i.e., a minimum of 600 mg total polyphenols per day. In terms of getting that dosage of polyphenols from drinking green tea it requires an intake of 4 to 6 cups of green tea. That is a lot of tea, but not an unrealistic goal.

There are more than 150 varieties of the green tea plant used in the commercial marketplace. Not surprisingly, there are many different quality grades of tea. Here is my suggestion, sample a variety of brands and types of green tea to find the one that you really enjoy the most. While brewing and drinking of tea is an art, and all over the world there are tea ceremonies celebrated with reverence, in the United States, most consumers simply steep their tea bags in hot water for an unspecified time. The longer it is steeped, the higher the content of polyphenols.

Bee Pollen

Bees are amazing and absolutely critical to life on earth given their essential role in pollinating plants. Albert Einstein is often quoted as saying "If the bee disappears from the surface of the earth, man would have no more than four years to live." Recently, there has been an alarming decline in bee numbers in North America due to a phenomenon known as Colony Collapse Disorder (CCD). There are a lot of factors suggested as a cause of CCD with pesticides, pathogens, and bee keeping practices, but no single factor has been found with enough consistency to suggest that it is the sole cause.

In addition to its role in pollination, bees also provide us with some wondrous nutritional products. Not only the sweetness of honey, but also the tremendous health benefits offered by bee pollen, propolis, and royal jelly. Here is a brief description of these products:

- *Bee pollen* comes from the male germ cell of flowering plants. As the honeybee travels from flower to flower, it fertilizes the female germ cell. Honeybees enable the reproduction of more than 80% of the world's grains, fruits, vegetables, and legumes. The pollen is collected and brought to the hive, where the bees add enzymes and nectar to the pollen. It is important to recognize that one teaspoon of bee pollen would take a single bee working eight hours a day for one month to gather.

- *Propolis* is the resinous substance collected by bees from the leaf buds and barks of trees, especially poplar and conifer trees. The bees use the propolis, along with beeswax, to construct the hive. Propolis has antimicrobial activities that help the hive block out viruses, bacteria, and other organisms.

- *Royal jelly* is a thick, milky substance produced by worker bees to feed the queen bee. The worker bees mix honey and bee pollen with enzymes in the glands of their throats to produce royal jelly. Royal jelly is believed to be a useful nutritional supplement because of the queen bee's superior size, strength, stamina, and longevity compared with other bees.

Pure and simple, I take 2 tablespoons of bee pollen every day because I notice that it gives me higher energy levels. Bee pollen is often referred to as "nature's most perfect food." It is especially rich in protein (typically containing 35-40% total protein) and it is a complete protein meaning it contains all eight essential amino acids. In fact, bee pollen is higher in protein content than any animal source and about half of its protein is in the form of free amino acids that are ready to be used directly by the body. Bee pollen also provides significant levels of B vitamins, vitamin C, carotenes, minerals, DNA, RNA, numerous flavonoid molecules, and plant hormones.

Propolis and royal jelly have similar nutritional qualities to pollen but considerably higher levels of different biologically active compounds.

Royal jelly contains approximately 12% protein, 5% to 6% lipids, and 12% to 15% carbohydrates.

The health benefits of bee products are much heralded but insufficiently researched. Some overlap exists in the uses of pollen, propolis, and royal jelly to promote health. Here are my dosage recommendations.

- Bee pollen: usually 1 to 2 tablespoons daily
- Propolis: 100 to 500 mg three times daily
- Royal jelly: 50 to 250 mg of royal jelly one to two times daily

---

WARNING: If you have never used bee pollen, it is recommended to start with just a few granules a day and gradually build up to the full dosage of one to two tablespoons daily. Although rare, allergic reactions have been reported and are the most common side effects with bee pollen and other products. Allergic reactions to a food, including bee pollen, can range from mild to severe. The reaction is generally related to the amount of the allergen ingested, hence the reason for starting with just a few granules a day. If allergy symptoms such as hay fever-like symptoms (itchy eyes, runny nose, scratchy throat), shortness of breath, itchy skin or hives, or gastrointestinal pain occurs at any time while building up to the full dosage, discontinue use of bee pollen or other bee product. If symptoms are significant, seek appropriate medical care.

Ground Flaxseeds

The major health benefits of flaxseeds centers around their rich content of essential fatty acids and fiber components known as lignans. In fact, ground flaxseeds are the most abundant sources of lignans. Population studies, as well as experimental studies in humans and animals, have demonstrated that lignans exert significant anticancer effects, especially breast and prostate cancer. Lignins can bind to sex hormone receptors and interfere with the cancer-promoting effects of estrogen on breast tissue and testosterone in prostate tissue. Lignans also increase the production of a compound known as sex hormone binding globulin (SHBG). This protein regulates sex hormone levels.

Dr. Paul Gross, director of the breast cancer prevention program at the Princess Margaret Hospital and the Toronto Hospital, conducted a study that showed flaxseed in the diet may shrink breast cancers. His study involved 50 women who had recently been diagnosed with breast cancer. While waiting for their surgery, the women were divided into 2 groups. One group received a daily muffin containing 25 grams (a little less than 2 tablespoons) of ground flaxseed. The others were prescribed ordinary muffins. After surgery, the investigators found that women who had received the flaxseed muffins had much slower-growing tumors than the others.

As detailed in Chapter 8, ground flaxseeds have also been shown to be helpful in lowering blood pressure and improving blood lipid profiles.

When buying ground flaxseeds it is highly recommended to purchase them in a vacuum-sealed package as once flaxseeds are ground, they are prone to oxidation and spoilage. FortiFlax from Barlean's and the various offerings from Spectrum Essentials are the leading brands of ground flaxseeds in the marketplace and are properly packaged to insure freshness.

My goal with ground flaxseeds is to try to get 2 to 4 tablespoons daily. That provides a daily dosage of 15 to 30 g of ground flaxseeds. Most often, I just spoon ground flax into my mouth, but here are some quick serving ideas:

- Add ground flaxseeds to smoothies.
- Sprinkle ground flaxseeds onto hot or cold cereal.
- Mix in ground flaxseeds with yogurt.
- To give cooked vegetables a nuttier flavor, sprinkle some ground flaxseeds on top of them.

Whey Protein

Whey is a natural by-product of the cheese making process. Cow's milk has about 6.25% protein. Of that protein, 80% is casein (another type of protein) and the remaining 20% is whey. When cheese is made, it uses the casein molecules leaving whey. Whey protein is made via filtering off the other components of whey such as lactose, fats, and minerals.

Whey protein has the highest biological value of all proteins. In order to assess the quality of a protein, scientists measure the proportion of the amino acids that are absorbed, retained, and used in the body to determine the protein's *biological value* (BV). Whey protein is a complete protein in that it contains all essential and non-essential amino acids. One of the key reasons why the BV of whey protein is so high is that it has the highest concentrations of glutamine and branched chain amino acids (BCAAs) found in nature. Glutamine and branched chain amino acids are critical to cellular health, muscle growth, and protein synthesis.

Glutamine, the most abundant amino acid in the body, is involved in more metabolic processes than any other amino acid. Glutamine is especially important as a source of fuel for white blood cells, and for cells that divide rapidly, such as those that line the intestine. It has become an important component of intravenous feeding mixes in hospitals, since double-blind studies have shown that it dramatically increases survival in critically ill subjects. Supplementation with glutamine has been shown to heal peptic ulcers, enhance energy levels, boost immune function, and fight infections.

Although the most popular use of whey protein is by body builders and athletes looking to increase their protein intake, nearly everyone can gain benefit by adding whey protein to their diet. Whey protein is especially important to help fight off sarcopenia and age-related muscle loss. It is also a useful aid for weight loss, nutritional support for recovery from surgery, and to offset some of the negative effects of radiation therapy and chemotherapy.

Table 12.3–Benefits of Whey Protein

- Whey protein has the highest biological value of any protein.
- Whey protein is a rich source of glutamine, the most abundant amino acid in the body.
- Whey protein is a rich source of branched chain amino acids (BCAAs) that are metabolized directly into muscle tissue and are the first ones used during periods of exercise.
- Whey protein is an excellent source of leucine. Individuals who exercise benefit from diets high in the essential amino acid leucine and have more lean muscle tissue and less body fat compared to individuals whose diet contains lower levels of leucine.
- Whey protein is a soluble, easy to digest protein and is efficiently absorbed into the body.
- Whey protein intake prior to a meal improves blood sugar control.
- Whey protein contains bioactive components that help stimulate the release of three appetite-suppressing hormones from the gut: cholecystokinin (CCK), peptide tyrosine-tyrosine (PYY), and glucagon-like peptide-1 (GLP-1).

My dosage recommendation for whey protein is based upon your level of activity. Specifically, how much exercise are you regularly engaged in. If you are very active and regularly workout then my recommendation is 50 grams per day. If you get little exercise, then it is 25 grams per day.

You can find whey protein powder in a variety of flavors including vanilla, chocolate, and strawberry available in pre-measured individual serving packets and bulk canisters. Usually these sorts of protein powders are found in the "body building" section of a health food store. The highest quality is often referred to as micro-filtered or ultra-filtered whey protein concentrates. One of the easiest ways to use whey protein is as a component in smoothies. I also have several whey protein-based nutrition bars available on the market available exclusive through iHerb.com.

PolyGlycoPlex (PGX)

I have mentioned PGX in several places. As a reminder, it is produced in a patented process that allows three natural fibers (konjac root, alginate, xanthan gum) to coalesce and form a matrix that has a higher level of viscosity, gel-forming properties, and has more expansion with water, than any other fiber. In essence, it is a "super" fiber with all of the beneficial effects of fiber but are magnified and more easily attained with PGX. It is available in granules, capsules, nutritional bars, drink mixes, and weight loss meal replacement formulas.

Clinical studies published in major medical journals and presented at the world's major medical conferences have shown PGX to exert the following benefits:

- Increases the level of compounds that block the appetite and promote satiety.
- Decreases the level of compounds that stimulate overeating.
- When taken prior to a meal can increase the feeling in fullness, very hungry to very full.
- It reduces the glycemic index of any food, beverage, or meal by as much as 70%.
- Increases insulin sensitivity and promotes improved blood sugar control.
- Helps stabilize blood sugar levels to reduce food cravings.

PGX has the ability to address some of the core underlying reasons why weight loss and blood sugar control are often so difficult to achieve. I played a role in the development of PGX, so some may say that I am severely biased. My response is that I am biased, but it is not because of any financial benefit (there is none). My bias is a reflection of the powerful effect that I have seen this safe and effective natural product have on changing people's lives including my own! I want everyone who has struggled with weight loss to give PGX a try. Here are my practical recommendations on how to use PGX:

- In most cases, I recommend starting with 2 ½ grams of PGX® before meals.
- After 1 to 2 weeks, increase the dosage to 5 grams of PGX® before meals at least 3 times per day.
- If you consider yourself to be heavy, you may find that 5 grams of PGX® with each meal will reduce your appetite substantially.
- To get 2 ½ grams of PGX you can choose:
    - 3 to 4 capsules of PGX Daily Ultra Matrix Softgels
    - 1 stick pack of granules from PGX® Daily Singles
    - 1 scoop of Satisfast Vegan Protein powder
    - 1 scoop of Satisfast Whey Protein Energy Drink
    - 1 scoop of SlimStyles Weight Loss Drink Mix
- These products can be found in health food stores throughout North America and through a number of Internet retailers including iHerb.com.
- Take medications 1 hour before or after taking PGX. Be sure to consult your physician.
- PGX can be taken in combination with other supplements.
- For more practical information on how to use PGX, go to www. PGX.com.

Advanced Supplementation Program

One of the most frequent questions that I get is "What supplements do you take?" Well, I have promised myself for years that I would write an article or outline in a book exactly what I take and why. That is what I am going to do here. I am also going to add some recommendations for men dealing with andropause and low testosterone.

You will notice that I refer to my genetics and increased risk factors for certain diseases in my reasons for taking certain supplements. There is little doubt that the future of medicine, including diet and supplement recommendations, will all be personalized in the future based upon our genetics, risk factors, lifestyle, and environmental exposures.

While our genes are important, it turns out that they need specific instructions to follow on what to do, how to do it, and when. It is amazing to consider that a human liver cell contains the same DNA as a brain cell, yet somehow it knows to express only the code needed to make itself a liver cell. So, if these instructions are not found in the DNA where do they come from? Scientists discovered an array of chemical markers and switches that lie along the length of the double helix of DNA. Collectively these factors are referred to as the "epigenome." An analogy would be that DNA is like a computer (hardware) while the epigenome is like complex software. The hardware is important, for sure, but it is the software that actually tells the DNA what to do.

It is commonly held that our DNA determines who we are, but through the study of epigenetics that view is changing. Originally it was thought that an individual's epigenome was firmly established during early fetal development, but we now know that the epigenome can change in response to diet, environmental factors, lifestyle choices, and even our habitual thoughts. Damage to the epigenome can produce what are referred to as epigenetic marks or epimutations. Unlike damage to DNA that produces genetic mutations or genetic defects, it turns out that epimutations are reversible by various compounds in food.

All of this discussion on genetics is important because of the big point that is being made—food affects how genes are expressed throughout an individual's lifetime. Various other factors such as environmental toxins, stress, and even our habitual thoughts and attitude remodel our epigenomes lifelong in a beneficial or detrimental way. The future will be about understanding how to avoid the detrimental factors while utilizing those that are beneficial.

Although genetic factors are obviously important to our health and can certainly determine our risk for disease, in most cases, the entire set of genetic factors linked to many inherited predisposition are termed "susceptibility genes" as they modify the risk of the disease but are neither necessary nor sufficient for the disease to necessary develop. In other words, rather than acting as the primary cause the genetic predisposition simply sets the stage for the environmental or dietary factor to initiate the destructive process. The very term predisposition clearly indicates that something else needs to occur. Just like a parched forest may be predisposed to a forest fire, if there is a big rain, or no match or spark is lit, then there is no fire. But if there is something that ignites the fire, it may burn out of control. For many inherited diseases less than 10% of those with increased genetic susceptibility actually develop the disease. Again, nutrition is one of the key variables. I am using the results from my genetic profile and family history to reduce the risks not only with my diet, lifestyle, and attitude, but also through proper scientifically based supplementation. *Nutrigenomics* refers to the emerging science studying the effects and mechanisms of nutrients and other food compounds have in altering the expression of our genes to improve our health.

One of the key tools in nutrigenomics is looking how a difference in just one single building block of our DNA (genes) interacts with dietary compounds to influence health and disease. with diet, disease, and other health conditions. A building block of DNA is a nucleotide, so the term used to describe this difference is a single nucleotide polymorphism or SNP.

SNPs are being shown to be factors in the risk for just about every chronic health condition. Grouping several different SNPs together is also showing great promise. For example, certain SNPs are associated with a reduced resting metabolic rate, whether an individual will lose weight on a low- to moderate-fat diet or a diet that is higher in fat (especially more monounsaturated fats), the odds of weight gain on a high-dairy diet or a diet low in vitamin D, or enhanced weight loss on a high-fiber diet.

There is much to be discovered in the process of developing complete personalized diet and supplement programs, but we don't need to wait to start making rational choices to reduce our risk for aging, inflammaging, and chronic disease until that time. We can move forward with reasonable certainty based upon the current tools available including genetic assessment as well as examining the microbiome.

Dr. Murray's Personalized Supplementation Plan

You will see that I take a lot of supplements. The way that I organize them is by creating a little mini factory. I use 60 small 3-ounce Dixie cups and small plastic pill bags that I get from Amazon (Plymor 3" x 3" Plastic Reclosable Zipper Bags). I line up six rows of ten cups and place the daily amount of each supplement that I take (noted after the name of the supplement below). I take only one packet daily just before a meal. I also take a few supplements on an empty stomach twice per day. I do not put these in the packets.

Foundation Supplements:

- Men's 50+ Multistart (Natural Factors)—4 tablets
    - I developed this multiple vitamin and mineral when I was working with Natural Factors. I have been taking it for 20 years now and still like it very much.
- BioCoenzymated Active B Complex (Natural Factors)—3 capsules
    - This formula offers balanced ratios and clinically supported doses of the active form of B vitamins. Based upon some of my SNPs, I do not effectively activate B vitamins. This genetic variation or "polymorphism" makes me susceptible to many health conditions, especially heart disease and Alzheimer's disease. In order for B vitamins to be utilized effectively by the body they must be converted into an active coenzyme form. For example, the coenzyme form of folate is 5-methyltetrahydrofolate (5-MTHF). It is formed in the body from regular folate with the aid of an enzyme known as 5-MTHF reductase. But some people, including me, have a genetic type (SNP) with deficient activity of this enzyme to form the active coenzyme. Without the active coenzyme, certain biochemical reactions cannot take place that are critical to the functioning of the cell and our overall health. Taking B vitamins already in their active coenzymated forms

allows the body to bypass the deficient enzymatic conversion for immediate utilization.

- Aqua Biome Fish Oil with Meriva—4 capsules
  ○ This product combine's the world's cleanest and most optimal fish oil with Meriva, the most well-researched enhanced form of curcumin. Aqua Biome exceeds quality control standards and eco-friendly certifications to become the first Fish Oil to receive Clean Label Project Certification—it tests the lowest of any commercially available fish oil for pollutants, contaminants, and heavy metals, such as lead, cadmium, arsenic, and mercury. Aqua Biome fish oil formulas provide the optimal ratio of Omega-3 fatty acids DHA, EPA, and DPA. I take 4 capsules, which provides over 1,500 mg of omega-3 fatty acids and 2,000 mg of Meriva.
- Vitamin D3 & K2 (Natural Factors)—1 capsule
  ○ Contains the bioactive and highly bioavailable forms of vitamin D (D3) and vitamin K2 (MK-7).

Polyphenol and Flavonoid-rich Extracts:
- Grape Seed Extract 100 mg—3 capsules
  ○ The benefits of the procyanidolic oligomers of grape seed were highlighted throughout the Longevity Matrix.
- Green Tea Phytosome 50 mg—3
  ○ The Phytosome form of flavonoid-rich extracts produce better absorption and clinical results. The technology involves binding the components of the extract to phosphatidylcholine. This fatty substance is produced from sunflower oil and is also key component of our cellular membranes throughout the body. Phosphatidylcholine is not merely an emulsifier or carrier of the flavonoid; it has also been shown to help to repair cell membranes. Hence, these two components of work in a synergistic way to protect and repair cells. Scientific research indicates that the Phytosome form produces better results

than regular extracts because the active components are better absorbed and has the added benefit of the phosphatidylcholine.

- Resveratrol 500 mg—2
  - Resveratrol is a plant compound similar to flavonoids found in low levels in the skin of red grapes, red wine, cocoa powder, baking chocolate, dark chocolate, peanuts, and mulberry skin. Most resveratrol supplements use Japanese knotweed (*Polygonum cuspidatum*) as the source. Resveratrol activates an enzyme known as sirtuin 1 that plays an important role in the regulation of cellular life spans; it also promotes improved insulin sensitivity.
- Green Coffee Bean Extract—2
  - Green coffee bean extract is rich in chlorogenic acid, a compound that has been shown to improve glucose metabolism, inhibit the accumulation of fat, and decrease the absorption of glucose in the intestines. Roasting coffee beans destroys most of the chlorogenic acid, so drinking coffee will not yield these benefits. Only raw green coffee beans contain a significant amount of this health-promoting compound.
- Vein Sense (Natural Factors)—2 capsules
  - I have varicose veins, so I love this product that I developed when I was at Natural Factors. It contains diosmin, a citrus flavonoid, in a micronized form for better absorption and utilization, along with standardized extracts of Butcher's broom and horse chestnut seeds. It provides excellent support for healthy vein structure and function throughout the body.

Carotenoids:
- Astaxanthin 4 mg - 2
- Lutein 40 mg - 1
- Lycopene 30 mg - 1

Detoxification, Metabolism, and Mitochondrial Support:
- Berberine 500 mg (Enzymedica)—3
  - The benefits of berberine include beneficial changes to the microbiome; activation of AMPk; positive effects on the immune system (particularly macrophages); lowering blood pressure, cholesterol, and blood sugar levels; and enhancement of mitochondrial function.
- Liver Detox (Enzymedica)—2
  - This formula was mentioned in Chapter 5. It contains premium ingredients for supporting detoxification reactions including N-acetylcysteine, milk thistle Phytosome (Siliphos), and SelenoExcell.
- Alpha Lipoic Acid 400 mg—1
  - Unlike vitamin E which is primarily fat soluble and vitamin C which is water soluble, ALA can quench either water- or fat-soluble free radicals both inside the cell and outside in the intracellular spaces. It is often described as "nature's perfect antioxidant." It has been shown to improve blood sugar control, activate AMPk and metabolism to promote weight loss, and exert very positive effects in protecting and enhancing liver function.
- SAMe 100 mg—2
  - S-Adenosylmethionine (SAMe) is involved in over 40 biochemical reactions in the body. It is critical in the manufacture of many body components especially brain chemicals as well as in detoxification reactions. SAMe is also required in the manufacture of all sulfur-containing compounds in the human body including glutathione and various sulfur-containing cartilage components including chondroitin sulfate. The beneficial effects of SAMe supplementation are far-reaching due to its central role in so many metabolic processes. Currently, there are five main

uses of SAMe: depression, osteoarthritis, fibromyalgia, liver disorders, and migraine headaches.

- Ubiquinol 200 mg—1
  - Ubiquinol is the best absorbed form of coenzyme Q10 (CoQ10), an essential component of the mitochondria - the energy producing unit of the cells of our body. CoQ10 is involved in the manufacture of ATP, the energy currency of all body processes. Generally, CoQ10 levels decline with aging. Low levels are also seen in many health conditions, especially in people taking statins or dealing with a cardiovascular disease such as angina, high blood pressure, mitral valve prolapse, and congestive heart failure. I take CoQ10 (and PQQ) primarily as an insurance policy that my mitochondria, especially in the brain, are functioning optimally.
- Bio PQQ 20 mg—1
  - Like CoQ10, PQQ is critical to mitochondrial function. It protects mitochondria from oxidative and also stimulates the generation of new mitochondria, supporting efficient energy production, especially in energy-hungry tissues like the brain and the heart. PQQ also displays anti-inflammatory activity; and may further benefit neurological health by influencing gene expression and preventing the development of Parkinson's disease and Alzheimer's disease. PQQ has also been shown to activate AMPk and lower LDL cholesterol. The combination of PQQ and CoQ10 has been shown to enhance memory and mental function in older adults better than either agent given alone.

Skin and Connective Tissue Support:

- Biosil 5 mg—2 capsules
  - BioSil is a highly bioavailable from of silica (choline stabilized orthosilicic acid). BioSil acts on cells known as fibroblast in the skin to increase the production of collagen and elastin to

produce impressive results in improving shallow, fine lines; skin elasticity; and the health of nails and hair.

- MSM as OptiMSM 1,000 mg—1 tablet
  - MSM (methyl-sulfonyl-methane) is the major form of sulfur in the human body and maybe one of the most important supplements that I take. Sulfur is a critical element for all cells and body tissues, especially the skin and joints. As far back as the 1930s, researchers demonstrated that individuals with arthritis are commonly deficient in sulfur. Sulfur is also necessary for proper liver detoxification.

Hormonal and Prostate Support:
- Saw Palmetto Extract (85-95% fatty acids and sterols) 320 mg—2
  - Numerous double-blind studies have shown saw palmetto extract to significantly improve the signs and symptoms of benign prostatic hyperplasia (BPH)—a condition that affects approximately 5 to 10% at age 30 and increases in incidence to eventually affect over 90% in men over 85 years of age. Roughly 90% of men with mild to moderate BPH experience some improvement in symptoms during the first 4 to 6 weeks of therapy. All major symptoms of BPH are improved, especially increased nighttime urination (nocturia). The mechanism of action is related to improving the hormonal metabolism within the prostate gland.
- AndroSense T-Correct (Natural Factors)—4
  - Androsense T-Correct is an identical formula to EstroSense, which was discussed for women on hormone replacement therapy or who are at higher risk for breast cancer. Androsense T-Correct (or EstroSense) is recommended for men for proper testosterone metabolism. The formula features diindolylmethane (DIM), indole-3-carbinole (I3C), sulforaphane, and calcium-d-glucarate (CDG), concentrated nutrients found in cabbage-family vegetables that support proper estrogen metabolism. The also contain a wide range of

additional supportive agents that enhance detoxification of sex hormones and also offers protection against prostate cancer.

o Both men and women convert testosterone into estrogen. In men, however only about a tenth of the testosterone they produce is usually converted into estrogen. In women it is just the opposite, most of their testosterone is converted into estrogen. What controls the conversion of testosterone to estrogen in both men and women is an enzyme called aromatase. If this enzyme is too active in men, it will mean lower testosterone and higher estrogen levels. If they are prescribed testosterone and the activity of aromatase is too high, it could increase the risk for some of the conditions linked to excess estrogen in men, especially prostate cancer.

o There are a number of dietary factors that influence aromatase activity. Most notable is a high carbohydrate diet because it can lead to insulin resistance and obesity. Insulin resistance is probably the main reason why many men are experiencing too low of testosterone and higher levels of estrogen as they age (often referred to as andropause, which is discussed below).

o One of the problems in hormonal metabolism in men as they age is that too much testosterone is converting into estrogen. This can produce such things as loss of energy, weight gain, fatigue, depression, and difficulty maintaining lean muscle mass. A man getting "man boobs" is an obvious sign of what is referred to as estrogen dominance, but sometimes the effects of too little testosterone and too much estrogen is less obvious. Many men on prescription testosterone also run the risk of increased conversion to estrogen as well as disruption of normal hormonal metabolism. Androsense T-Correct is designed specifically to support normal metabolism of both testosterone and estrogen.

- MacaRich (Natural Factors)—2
  - ○ Maca is becoming increasingly popular in the United States. Maca is the common name for *Lepidium meyenii*, a plant in the broccoli family that is grown exclusively in Peru. It looks a lot like a turnip. One of maca's most renowned benefits is the enhancement of sexual desire and function for both men and women. Clinical trials confirm these properties, including maca's benefits in erectile function. Maca does not appear to directly affect the level of testosterone, but rather acts on the entire endocrine system to reduce the harmful effects of stress while improving mood, energy, and endurance. There are many forms and types of maca. For general health, I like raw maca powder, especially from black roots at a dosage When stronger effects are desired, more concentrated extracts like MacaRich made from the whole tubers that have been gelatinized (removal of the starch) are preferred at a dosage of 1,000 to 1,5000 mg per day. Otherwise the daily dosage for maca is 3 to 6 grams.

Between Meal or Empty Stomach Supplements:
- Natto-K (Enzymedica)—2
  - ○ Natto-K contains nattokinase and other enzymes useful in promoting vascular health.
- (PEA)+ (Enzyme Science)—4
  - ○ Palmitoylethanolamide (PEA) was discussed on page 421. In addition to its anti-inflammatory, pain relieving, and antidepressant effects, it also plays a key role in our endocannabinoid system (ECS). The ECS is responsible for helping cells maintain homeostasis. Many of the benefits people are currently looking to receive from CBD are more likely achieved by using PEA instead. Four capsules of (PEA)+ provides 600 mg of PEA and 1,000 mg of Meriva.

Nighttime Supplements:
- Endo Sleep (Emerald Health Bioceuticals)—2
    - Endo Sleep provide full-spectrum endocannabinoid support through its proprietary mixture of non-hemp-/cannabis-based ingredients known as Phytocann. This powerful herbal mix is then synergized with melatonin, passionflower and PharmaGABA to promote deep, restful and rejuvenating sleep. I love this formula. It is amazing in how well-rested and energized I feel after a good night's sleep.
- Magnesium citrate or bisglycinate drink mix 250-300 mg
    - I am a big fan of a nighttime dosage of magnesium to promote relaxation and recovery. There are a number of companies marketing these magnesium drink mixes. I prefer the Natural Factors version as I like its taste and mouthfeel.

Andropause and Low T

Men experience their own hormonal changes as they get older. Often referred to as "andropause, "male menopause," or "man-opause," this event has some superficial similarities to menopause. But, while all women go through menopause, not all men go through andropause.

Andropause reflects the appearance of signs and symptoms related to the slow, but steady reduction in the hormones testosterone and dehydroepiandrosterone in middle-aged men. Decreased testosterone naturally occurs as men age, but in andropause or its more technically correct term of "hypogonadism" levels drop below the normal range for a given age.

In case you have not seen the ads for "Low T" on TV or in press, there is a big push by suppliers of prescription testosterone preparations to get men hooked on the quick fix of testosterone therapy. Suffice it to say, that this whole area of andropause and Low T is fraught with controversy.

Do low levels of testosterone produce symptoms in middle-aged men? Absolutely. In fact, the classic symptoms have been recognized for over 70 years ago when two American physicians, Carl Heller, M.D., and

Gordon Myers, M.D., showed the effectiveness of testosterone treatment for symptoms of fatigue, depression, irritability, reduced libido, erectile dysfunction, night sweats, and hot flashes.

Subsequent studies over the years have definitely found that some, but not all men, with low age-adjusted testosterone levels show these sorts of symptoms as well as improvement with testosterone therapy. If you are curious if you have low T, get a blood test to measure your testosterone levels (I recommend testing for both total and free testosterone). Normally, depending upon the lab, the bottom of a man's normal total testosterone range is about 300 nanograms per deciliter (ng/dl) and the upper limit is about 800ng/dl. A free testosterone level below 5 ng/dl is also indicative of low T.

What Causes Low T?

Testosterone levels naturally decline 10% every decade after age 30 or roughly 1% per year. That is normal, what is not normal is when testosterone levels drop faster than this rate. There are a number of factors that can lead to low testosterone including:

- Obesity, diabetes, and insulin resistance are the main causes of low testosterone today. The level of total and free testosterone is reduced in obese men in proportion to the level of obesity. Making matters worse is that estrogen is increased.

- Chronic inflammation is another risk factor for low testosterone. Insulin resistance is the key factor in causing silent inflammation and high levels of high-sensitivity C-reactive protein (CRP).

- Increased exposure to "xenoestrogens"—compounds in food and the environment that exert estrogenic effects including pesticides; phthalates (plastics); tobacco smoke byproducts; heavy metals (lead, mercury, etc.), and various solvents. Xenoestrogens enhance the effects of estrogen in men leading to lower production of testosterone.

- Lack of physical activity. On the flip side, one of the quickest ways to boost testosterone production is regular bouts of short intense exercise, especially weightlifting.
- Stress has a negative effect on testosterone levels by increasing the release of the adrenal hormone cortisol.

Boosting Testosterone

If your testosterone level is too low, your doctor may suggest testosterone replacement therapy (TRT). Testosterone is available as an injection, patch, gel applied to the skin, or pellets implanted under your skin. In my opinion a topical gel is the least invasive.

Before opting for TRT to boost testosterone levels in men with low T, the best approach to boosting testosterone levels is addressing underlying issues by improving the action of insulin, achieving ideal body weight, and improving blood sugar control. Weight loss alone has been shown to increase testosterone levels by 50%. Beyond these basic measures there are a number of natural products that may be helpful. Again, I would try all of these measures for at least 3 months before opting for TRT:

- Zinc is perhaps the most critical trace mineral for male sexual function and is found in high concentrations within the prostate, testes and particularly high amounts are also found in the semen (approximately 2.5 mg of zinc is lost per ejaculate). It is involved in virtually every aspect of male reproduction, including testosterone metabolism. Several studies support the use of zinc supplementation in the treatment of low sperm counts, especially in the presence of low testosterone levels. In these studies, zinc has shown an ability to raise both sperm counts and testosterone levels. Many men may be suffering from low T simply because they are lacking sufficient zinc. Daily supplementation of 30 to 45 mg per day is recommended to insure adequate zinc levels.

- Fenugreek contains a number of active plant steroids, most notably fenuside and protodioscin. Fenugreek extracts have shown promising results in improving libido and testosterone levels in several human clinical studies. In one double-blind study, the group taking 600 mg of special fenugreek extract daily reported improved libido (81.5%), recovery time (66.7%), and quality of sexual performance (63%) as well as a mild effect in boosting testosterone levels. In another study, 50 male subjects between the age of 35 to 65 years took 500 mg per day of a 20% protodioscin content fenugreek extract. Free testosterone levels were improved in 90% of the study population as much as 46%.

- *Eurycoma longifolia* (tongkat ali or longjack) is a flowering plant native to Indonesia, Malaysia that is heavily promoted as a testosterone booster and sexual performance enhancer. There is some evidence to support these claims along with concerns over fake products on the market. In one study in men with Low T, a daily dosage of 200 mg of a standardized water-soluble extract of longjack produced a 46% increase in total testosterone levels with 90% of the subjects achieving testosterone levels within the reference range for their age. In another study, thirteen physically active males (ages 57–72 years) given 400 mg of longjack extract daily for 5 weeks demonstrated a 15% increase in serum testosterone and a 61% increase in free testosterone levels. Positive results have also been noted for improving sperm counts and sexual well-being.

- *Tribulus terrestris* (Tribulus) has been used traditionally in Ayurvedic medicine as a tonic and aphrodisiac and in European folk medicine to increase sexual potency. While studies in healthy males with normal testosterone levels have not shown Tribulus to raise testosterone levels, there is some clinical evidence that it may be effective in raising testosterone levels in men with low T. A 2012 study showed that consuming six grams of tribulus root for 60 days raised testosterone levels by 16% and improved erections and frequency of sex in men with low sperm counts. Typical dosage for tribulus extracts is 100 to 250 mg per day.

- Chrysin is a flavonoid that has been shown to be an inhibitor of the aromatase enzyme that converts testosterone to estrogen. Chrysin is available as a dietary supplement, but it has a low bioavailability. Natural sources like royal jelly and propolis may contain other factors that improve absorption. I really like royal jelly for low T even though there are no clinical investigations in this application. Royal jelly is produced by nurse bees that mix honey and bee pollen with enzymes in the glands of their throats to produce a thick, milky substance that they then feed to the queen bee. Royal jelly is a concentrated food as evident by the queen bee's superior size, astounding ovulation, stamina, and longevity. The scientific investigation into the health promoting properties of royal jelly has focused on its ability to lower blood cholesterol levels, but I think it exerts far greater benefits. The typical dosage is 50 mg to 100 mg per day.

There are a lot of options in natural medicine for men to improve their declining testosterone, libido, and sexual performance. However, realistic expectations are required along with some common sense. If a man is overweight, does not exercise, and causes significant stress on his system because of other dietary and lifestyle factors, none of these natural products are likely to produce the real magic that he is looking for.

If after 3 months, testosterone do not rise above 300 ng/dl, I would recommend TRT with a gel (e.g., Androgel or Testim) and use the lowest dosage possible to get testosterone levels to the low end of normal (i.e., 300-500 ng/dl). Though more and more data are coming out all the time on TRT safety, I do NOT recommend trying to boost testosterone levels above these levels. I think it is better to error on the side of safety with any hormone therapy.

Longevity Matrix Lifestyle Tune-Up #12–Develop a Strategy to be "Awe Inspired"

The field of positive psychology is providing valuable insights on exactly how our emotions influence the way our body works (our physiology). One area of body function that is very closely tied to our emotional experiences is the functioning of our immune system. Our emotional state not only influences how well we are protected from infection, but also the degree of inflammation that we may suffer from. Two studies have found that the most powerful emotion in fighting inflammation is the feeling of awe.

While there have been a lot of studies on the impact of emotions on physical health, in general, these emotions are most often all lumped together. Negative emotions like grief, sadness, shame, fear, and anger are all viewed as having pretty much the same effects. The same is true for all positive emotions grouped into the general category of optimism or positive mood. What needs to be answered is if all positive emotions are created equal or is there a way to boost certain body functions by focusing on experiencing more of a particular positive emotion.

In an effort to better understand the different effects of various positive emotions, researchers conducted two studies at the University of California-Berkeley. The first study featured 94 freshman undergraduates who completed a questionnaire and provided a sample of the fluid from their inner cheek (oral mucosal transudate [OMT]). In the second study, 119 freshmen completed a questionnaire on their home computers using a secure website and then went to the lab for a follow up session where the sample of fluid from their inner cheek, the OMT, was collected and another questionnaire was given.

In both studies, interleukin-6 (IL-6) was measured from OMT samples. IL-6 is an important marker for inflammation that is influenced by the immune system. Higher IL-6 levels are associated with greater inflammation. In the first study, a questionnaire known as the Positive and Negative Affect Schedule (PANAS) was used to determine emotional status. In the second study, two additional questionnaires were used, the

Dispositional Positive Emotion Scale (DPES) and The Big Five Personality Inventory were added as outcomes measures in addition to PANAS.

In both studies, positive emotions were associated with lower IL-6. These means that emotions like awe, amusement, compassion, contentment, joy, love, and pride were linked to lower levels of inflammation. In the second study, researchers were able to dig deeper into the type of positive emotion that had the most significant impact on IL-6 levels because the DPES does a better job of subclassifying the positive emotions. Surprisingly, they found that awe had the strongest correlation to lower levels of IL-6 compared to any of the other emotions. In fact, only the degree of awe was able to significantly predict levels of IL-6. On the day the OMT was taken in the second study, the participants who reported feeling the most awe, wonder and amazement, that day had the lowest levels of IL-6. Joy, contentment, pride and awe were all strongly correlated with lower levels of IL-6; however, awe was the strongest predictor of low IL-6 levels.

The takeaway message from these studies is that it stresses the importance of fostering feelings of awe in our lives to positively influence the immune system and reduce inflammation.

So, how do we get more feelings of awe in our life? Let me share what positive psychology has learned about awe. It is not what I would have expected. It turns out that awe is most often linked to feelings of social connectedness and social exploration. So from a practical perspective, the first step in feeling more awe in your life is to become more socially engaged. This goal is especially important if you are older of dealing with depression, because these situations often lead to social isolation. Here are some recommendations to become more socially engaged:

- Get connected online. Using email, the Internet, and Web-based social networks such as Facebook or Twitter can make a big difference in helping people feel more connected.
- Encourage positive relationships. A person is never too old to learn how to be a better friend, parent, mentor, or better listener. Personal development is a never-ending process.

- Join a club or church. In today's world, there are always opportunities to find places to socialize that are positive and healthful.
- Volunteer. There is perhaps no greater opportunity to feel connected than by finding a way to volunteer time and energy towards a greater good. It is perhaps the most powerful way of connecting to people outside of our deepest personal relationships.

The health benefits of increased socialization are significant. Many of these benefits may be related to fighting inflammation and studies indicate that people who feel connected and have strong social relationships have lower levels of inflammatory markers in their blood.

What research has also shown is what inspires most people to feel awe is usually pretty simple. What is interesting is that activities such as seeing a sunset, listening to music, walking in nature, or being creative, have been shown to exert a positive impact on the immune system. These effects may be related to feelings of awe.

For me, the things that really make me say "wow" are research studies like these that I am sharing with you here in this Tune-Up Tip. I am constantly reading studies that create an awe-inspired appreciation of the wonder of nature or the way in which our body and mind function. Of course, just looking around at nature or the stars is pretty awe inspiring to me as well. My final message to you is to find a something that you can enjoy on a daily basis that makes you feel awe. It is important!

RESOURCES

www.TheLongevityMatrix.com

If you are looking for chapter references, meal plans, recipes, and other useful information to live better, stronger, and longer then please visit the dedicated website for *The Longevity Matrix*.

www.DoctorMurray.com

Please visit my professional website for free content and answers to over 100 health conditions as well as nutrition, dietary supplements, and other natural approaches to improving your health. Be sure to sign up for my free weekly email newsletter.

www.DoctorMurraySuperfoods.com

I have developed a line of functional foods and ingredients to improve your health that are exclusively available online through iHerb.com but you can check out all of the offerings here including really innovative nutrition bars, protein powders, PerfeKt Sea Salt, AllSweet Plus, and much more.

www.Enzymedica.com

I am the Chief Science Officer for Enzymedica, a leading digestive care and whole-body wellness company that provides a wide range of dietary supplements to improve your health. Enymedica's lead product is Digest Gold, which is by far the best selling digestive enzyme supplement in North America.

ABOUT THE AUTHOR

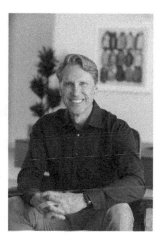

Michael T. Murray, N.D. is widely regarded as one of the world's leading authorities on natural medicine. Dr. Murray is a graduate, faculty member, and serves on the Board of Regents of Bastyr University. With Dr. Joseph Pizzorno, he is co-author of *A Textbook of Natural Medicine*, the definitive textbook on naturopathic medicine for physicians. They have also written the *Encyclopedia of Natural Medicine* and *The Encyclopedia of Healing Foods*. Dr. Murray has also written over 30 other books including *The Magic of Food*; *Dr. Murray's Total Body Tune-Up*; *The Pill Book Guide to Natural Medicines*; and *What the Drug Companies Won't Tell You and Your Doctor Doesn't Know*.

Since 1985, as a consultant within the natural product industry, Dr. Murray has played a major role in bringing many safe and effective dietary supplements to North America, including glucosamine sulfate; curcumin; standardized herbal extracts from ginkgo, saw palmetto, St. John's wort, etc.; enteric-coated peppermint oil; PharmaGABA; and PGX.

Dr. Murray bases much of his work on a massive database of original scientific studies from the medical literature that he has been compiling for over 40 years. This research provides strong evidence on the effectiveness of diet, vitamins, minerals, herbs, and other natural measures in the maintenance of health and the treatment of disease. According to Dr. Murray:

502 | THE **LONGEVITY** MATRIX

"One of the great myths about natural medicine is it is not scientific. The fact of the matter is that for most common illnesses there is tremendous support in the medical literature for a more natural approach."

Dr. Murray has dedicated his life to educating physicians, patients, and the general public on the tremendous healing power of nature. In addition to his books, which have cumulative sales of over six million copies, Dr. Murray has written numerous articles for major publications, appeared on thousands of radio and TV programs, and lectured to hundreds of thousand people worldwide.

In recognition of his work, Dr. Murray has been the recipient of numerous awards and honors over the years including several denoting lifetime achievement such as the Benedict Lust Award in 2015 from the American Association of Naturopathic Physicians and also in 2015 the Mission Award from Bastyr University. In 2016, he was recognized as "The Voice of Natural Medicine" by the Nutrition Business Journal for his commitment to the advancement of evidence-based approaches to health and healing with natural products.

For more information, free educational resources, and to sign up for a free bi-weekly email newsletter from Dr. Murray, go to DoctorMurray.com.